Workbook and Lab Manual for Mosby's Pharmacy Technician: Principles and Practice

Fourth Edition

Workbook Material Provided by:

Marcy May, MEd, CPhT, PhTR
Adjunct, Associate Professor
Austin Community College
Austin, Texas

ELSEVIER

ELSEVIER

3251 Riverport Lane
St. Louis, Missouri 63043

WORKBOOK AND LAB MANUAL FOR MOSBY'S
PHARMACY TECHNICIAN: PRINCIPLES AND PRACTICE,
FOURTH EDITION

ISBN: 978-1-4557-5180-8

Notices

Knowledge and best practice in this field are constantly changing. As new research and experience broaden our understanding, changes in research methods, professional practices, or medical treatment may become necessary.

Practitioners and researchers must always rely on their own experience and knowledge in evaluating and using any information, methods, compounds, or experiments described herein. In using such information or methods they should be mindful of their own safety and the safety of others, including parties for whom they have a professional responsibility.

With respect to any drug or pharmaceutical products identified, readers are advised to check the most current information provided (i) on procedures featured or (ii) by the manufacturer of each product to be administered, to verify the recommended dose or formula, the method and duration of administration, and contraindications. It is the responsibility of practitioners, relying on their own experience and knowledge of their patients, to make diagnoses, to determine dosages and the best treatment for each individual patient, and to take all appropriate safety precautions.

To the fullest extent of the law, neither the Publisher nor the authors, contributors, or editors, assume any liability for any injury and/or damage to persons or property as a matter of products liability, negligence or otherwise, or from any use or operation of any methods, products, instructions, or ideas contained in the material herein.

Executive Content Strategist: Jennifer Janson
Content Development Manager: Luke Held
Senior Content Development Specialist: Jennifer Bertucci
Publishing Services Manager: Hemamalini Rajendrababu
Project Manager: Nisha Selvaraj
Cover Designer: Gopalakrishnan Venkatraman

Working together
to grow libraries in
developing countries

www.elsevier.com • www.bookaid.org

Printed in United States of America

Last digit is the print number: 9   8   7   6   5   4   3   2   1

Preface

This student workbook and lab manual is designed to help you master the information and skills presented in your textbook, *Mosby's Pharmacy Technician: Principles and Practice*, 4th edition. The various types of exercises will challenge your knowledge, help further reinforce key content, allow you to gauge your understanding of the subject matter, and demonstrate important concepts in the lab setting. This combination workbook and lab manual is divided into three separate areas for each chapter in the textbook: Reinforce Key Concepts, Reflect Critically, and Relate to Practice. Each of these three sections focuses on activities for students that will maximize their understanding of the content taught in the book.

The types of activities available in this workbook and lab manual are listed and described below.

REINFORCE KEY CONCEPTS

- *Terms and Definitions:* Terms and definitions are listed, preceded by a letter. You are to read each statement following the list, and write in the letter that represents the correct response. This exercise helps you recall the many terms that are introduced to you in each chapter. Your textbook conveniently lists this information at the beginning of each chapter. If you find you are not sure of any of your responses, you can easily turn to the appropriate chapter to refresh your memory.
- *Fill in the Blanks:* Complete each statement by filling in the blanks. This exercise gives you the opportunity to specifically apply the vocabulary you have learned within the context of pharmacy.
- *True or False:* Test your knowledge of the validity of the statements. If you think a statement is true, write a "T" in the blank preceding the statement; if you believe it is a false statement, write in an "F." Completing these exercises helps you immediately to recognize content of which you are unsure. You can then review and strengthen your understanding of the material by re-reading that particular section in your textbook.
- *Multiple Choice:* You are to select the one best answer to complete the numbered questions by circling the letter preceding the answer you have selected. This is the type of question in which your first response is usually

the correct reply. If you are not sure, then you can easily review the subject in question.
- *System Identifier:* Each chapter devoted to a body system features an illustration of the system with its organs numbered. You are asked to identify the organs contained in the body system. This visual exercise helps further reinforce your knowledge of anatomy. Questions in these chapters test you on the anatomy and physiology of the system, diseases and conditions that may occur within this system, and the medications prescribed to treat such illnesses.
- *Matching:* These exercises provide you with essential practice in matching controlled substance drug schedules with given drug names. Ease of recognition is essential in your chosen profession. If you are not sure of some of your responses, you can then refer back to your textbook for further study.
- *Conversion and Calculation:* These questions require you to convert measurements, thereby applying what you have learned.
- *Research Activities:* You are asked to use the Internet as a research tool to assist you in locating essential information. Featured websites address such topics as the scope of practice for pharmacy technicians and where to find information on controlled substances and recalls.

REFLECT CRITICALLY

- *Critical Thinking:* This exercise tests your accumulated knowledge of each chapter by giving you scenarios to solve. You are asked to draw upon your knowledge of pharmacy and direct it to specific situations. This is a good test of your understanding of key concepts. If any of these questions stump you, refer back to your textbook for further study, or ask your instructor for clarification.

RELATE TO PRACTICE

- *Lab Activities:* Labs for each chapter will help you master such skills as gram staining, inventory management, compounding, and aseptic technique. These labs offer you many opportunities for hands-on reinforcements of what you have learned in your textbook.

Contents

1 History of Medicine and Pharmacy

TERMS AND DEFINITIONS

Select the correct term from the following list and write the corresponding letter in the blank next to the statement.

A. Apothecary
B. Bloodletting
C. Caduceus
D. Dogma
E. Herbals
F. Hippocratic oath
G. Inpatient pharmacy
H. Laudanum
I. Leeches
J. Maggots
K. Medicine
L. Opioid
M. Opium
N. Outpatient pharmacy
O. Pharmacist
P. Pharmacy
Q. Pharmacy clerk
R. Pharmacy technician
S. PTCB
T. Shaman
U. Staff of Asclepius
V. Trephining

_____ 1. The practice of draining blood, which was thought to release illness

_____ 2. The science and art of dealing with the maintenance of health and the prevention, alleviation, or cure of disease

_____ 3. Segmented worms that attach to the skin of a host and engorge themselves on the host's blood

_____ 4. A wingless staff with one snake wrapped around it

_____ 5. Latin term for pharmacist

_____ 6. A pharmacy in a hospital or institutional setting

_____ 7. A person who holds a high place of honor in a tribe as a healer and spiritual mediator

_____ 8. A staff with two entwined snakes and two wings at the top

_____ 9. A principle or set of principles laid down by an authority as incontrovertibly true

_____10. A mixture of opium and alcohol used through the 1800s to treat dozens of illnesses

_____11. Pharmacies that serve patients in their communities; pharmacies that are not in inpatient facilities

_____12. Fly larvae that feed on dead tissue; used in medicine to clean wounds not responding to routine antibiotics

_____13. Person who assists a pharmacist by filling prescriptions and performing other nondiscretionary tasks

_____14. A practice of making an opening in the head to allow disease to leave the body

_____15. Person who dispenses drugs and counsels patients on medication use and any interactions it may have with food or other drugs

_____16. A substance made from or using herbs

_____17. Person who assists the pharmacist at the front counter of the pharmacy; the person who accepts payment for medications

_____18. Any agent that binds to opioid receptors

_____19. Place where drugs are sold

_____20. Issues a national exam for pharmacy technicians

_____21. An oath taken by physicians concerning the ethics and practice of medicine

_____22. An analgesic that is made from the poppy plant

1

TRUE OR FALSE

Write T or F next to each statement.

_____ 1. Currently there are no nationally standardized requirements for pharmacy technicians.

_____ 2. Technicians have been perceived as posing a threat to pharmacy.

_____ 3. All pharmacists believe that technicians may take jobs away from pharmacists or increase the liability to the pharmacist if someone who is not properly trained makes a mistake.

_____ 4. As the roles of pharmacist and pharmacy technician become more clearly defined, new concerns arise.

_____ 5. All states require technicians to be certified as pharmacy technicians before they are employed.

_____ 6. Doctors are eager to have pharmacists write orders, especially when the medications are simple.

_____ 7. Pharmacies requiring a certain level of education from their technicians allows for expansion of job duties and higher pay for pharmacy technicians.

_____ 8. The pharmacy clerk regularly enters new prescription orders into the computer.

_____ 9. The pharmacy technician has become what the traditional pharmacist once was.

_____10. Education in understanding trade/generic drug names and instruction in billing procedures are some of the curricula provided specifically for future pharmacy technicians.

MULTIPLE CHOICE

Complete each question by circling the best answer.

1. In early America, physicians were:
   A. Responsible for diagnosing conditions
   B. Responsible for preparing the necessary remedy
   C. The first druggists
   D. All of the above

2. The division between physicians and pharmacists began after the:
   A. Korean War
   B. Civil War
   C. Vietnam War
   D. Cold War

3. Early remedies in American history included:
   A. Cinchona bark (quinine) to treat malaria
   B. Mercury to treat syphilis
   C. Opium and alcohol to treat pain
   D. All of the above

4. The first pharmacy technicians were:
   A. Military personnel
   B. High school graduates
   C. Family members of the pharmacist
   D. Certified pharmacy technicians (CPhTs)

5. In some states, today's typical pharmacy technician:
   A. Is required to do an array of tasks
   B. Is required to be educated and receive on-the-job training
   C. Is a family member of the pharmacist
   D. Both A and B

6. How can technicians gain the trust of the patients they serve?
   A. Education
   B. Training
   C. Good communication skills
   D. All of the above

7. The concept that doctors act only for the good of the patient and keep confidential what they learn about their patients reflects the:
   A. Galenic oath
   B. Corpus Hippocratum
   C. Hippocratic oath
   D. De Materia Medica

8. The effectiveness of the opium and alcohol mixture known as laudanum was surpassed only by its:
   A. Addictiveness
   B. Availability
   C. Adverse effects
   D. All of the above

9. Some of the instruments used earliest for bloodletting were:
   A. Thorns
   B. Sharp bones
   C. Shark teeth
   D. All of the above

10. The first synthetic drug, a(n) _____, was derived from a chemical dye found to inhibit bacterial growth.
    A. Opioid
    B. Penicillin
    C. Sulfonamide
    D. Cephalosporin

FILL IN THE BLANKS

Answer each question by completing the statement in the space provided.

1. _____ have been used for centuries for minor ailments such as intestinal problems, arthritis, and gout.

2. Many ancient treatments for illness were based on the _____ or _____ of the believers.

3. The most common form of treatment, _____, still has remained in many cultures as the only way to cure illness.

4. The origin of the term _____ _____ stems from the belief that too much of the black bile humor resulted in a person showing signs of melancholy.

5. Digestion of the type of _____ that resembled the organ affected by disease also was believed to cure illnesses.

6. As new scientists emerge and new methods are devised to test hypotheses, the results can lead to _____ _____.

7. Remedies used in early American history included cinchona bark (quinine) for the treatment of _____.

8. _____ vaccination was stopped in 1971 because of its total eradication worldwide.

9. _____ _____ was marketed as a tonic and contained extracts of cocaine and caffeine until 1905.

10. New job positions are constantly being created for those technicians who have the necessary _____ and _____ to fulfill them.

MATCHING

Match the following people who have influenced the history of medicine with their correct description.

A. Aristotle
B. Asclepius
C. Roger Bacon
D. Francis Crick and James Watson
E. Gerhard Domagk
F. Alexander Fleming
G. Galen
H. Hippocrates
I. Gregor Mendel
J. Florence Nightingale
K. Paracelsus
L. Louis Pasteur

_____ 1. Scientist and monk, known as the father of genetics

_____ 2. A great physician, hero of his time in ancient Greece, and associated with healing

_____ 3. Greek scientist and philosopher who described much of human anatomy from observations he made from dissections of other animals, which included in-depth descriptions of the brain, heart, lungs, and blood vessels

_____ 4. Greek philosopher and physician, considered the father of medicine

_____ 5. English scientist responsible for scientific methods

_____ 6. Greek physician who proved that blood flowed through arteries

_____ 7. Swiss physician, philosopher, and scientist; introduced laudanum

_____ 8. Developed sulfonamides and synthetic antibiotics

_____ 9. Discovered the molecular structure of DNA—the double helix

_____ 10. Nurse responsible for improving the unsanitary conditions at a British base hospital, reducing the death count

_____ 11. Discovered penicillin, first antibiotic

_____ 12. French scientist, discovered several vaccines and invented pasteurization

SHORT ANSWER

Write a short response to each question in the space provided.

1. Name four duties of pharmacy technicians in a hospital (inpatient) setting:

   A. _____

   B. _____

   C. _____

   D. _____

2. Name two areas of pharmacy in which a pharmacist can specialize:

   A. _____

   B. _____

3. Name two areas of pharmacy in which a pharmacy technician can specialize:

   A. _____

   B. _____

4. What is the difference between an opioid and opium?

   _____

   _____

   _____

5. What must a technician do to gain the trust of the patient?

_____

_____

6. What duties does today's pharmacy technician perform that once were included as duties of the traditional pharmacist?

_____

_____

RESEARCH ACTIVITIES

Follow the instructions given in each exercise and provide a response.

1. Access the website *www.ptcb.org* and investigate the duties outlined for pharmacy technicians.

2. Access the website *http://www.bls.gov/ooh/* and investigate the duties outlined for pharmacy technicians. Do they correspond to the duties the PTCB has outlined for pharmacy technicians? In what type of pharmacy setting are most pharmacy technicians employed?

REFLECT CRITICALLY

CRITICAL THINKING

Reply to each question based on what you have learned in the chapter.

a. One of the most important aspects of a pharmacy technician's job is to gain the trust of the pharmacist. How would you, as a new technician on the job, go about gaining the trust of the pharmacist?

b. What changes have you observed in pharmacy as a consumer over the years?

5

LAB SCENARIOS

History of Pharmacy

Objective: To allow the pharmacy technician to review the history of pharmacy.

Lab Activity #1.1: Answer the following questions as they relate to the history of pharmacy.

Equipment needed:

- Internet access
- Pencil/pen

Time needed to complete this activity: 30 minutes

Access the website *https://pharmacy.wisc.edu/sites/default/files/content/american-institute-history-pharmacy/historical-sources-pharmacy-faq/timecapsule.pdf* and answer the following questions:

1. What year was the first Hepatitis B vaccine approved?
2. Which pharmaceutical company marketed the first orally active angiotensin-converting enzyme inhibitor Capoten (captopril)?
3. List the conditions Ritalin (methylphenidate) was first marketed to treat before it was found useful to treat pediatric hyperactivity or ADHD.
4. Which vitamin was successfully isolated from cod liver oil by Paul Karrer in 1931?
5. What novel by Upton Sinclair about the meat-packing industry directly led to the passing of the Pure Food and Drug Act?

Pharmacy Technician Future

Objective: To allow the pharmacy technician to gain insight into the future of pharmacy practice for pharmacy technicians.

Lab Activity #1.2: Answer the following questions about the CREST Initiative as they relate to the future of pharmacy practice for pharmacy technicians.

Equipment needed:

- Internet access
- Pencil/pen

Time needed to complete this activity: 30 minutes

Access the website *http://www.ptcb.org/about-ptcb/crest-initiative#.U4vgVnaooTA* and answer the following questions:

1. What is the main goal for the changes to the PTCB Certification Program?
2. What changes have been made in and are scheduled for the PTCB Certification Program in the years 2013 through 2020?
3. By what year will pharmacy technicians be required to complete an ASHP-accredited pharmacy technician education program to be eligible for PTCB certification?
4. Beginning in the year 2014, what must pharmacy technicians complete to qualify for PTCB recertification?
5. Beginning in the year 2015, what must pharmacy technicians complete to qualify for PTCB recertification?

2 Pharmacy Law, Ethics, and Regulatory Agencies

REINFORCE KEY CONCEPTS

TERMS AND DEFINITIONS

Select the correct term from the following list and write the corresponding letter in the blank next to the statement.

A. Act
B. Adulteration
C. Amendment
D. Barbiturate
E. Boxed Warning
F. Controlled Substance
G. Drug Diversion
H. Drug Facts and Comparisons
I. Drug Utilization Evaluation
J. Ethics
K. Legend Drug
L. Misbranding
M. Monograph
N. Morals
O. Narcotic
P. National Drug Code
Q. Negligence
R. Over-the-Counter
S. *Physicians' Desk Reference*
T. Pregnancy Category
U. Protected Health Information
V. Safety Data Sheet
W. Tort

_____ 1. Concerning or relating to what is right or wrong in human behavior

_____ 2. A process employed to ensure prescribed drugs are used appropriately; main outcome is to increase medication-related efficacy and safety

_____ 3. Reference book found in pharmacies that contains detailed information on medications

_____ 4. A legal concept that describes an action taken without the forethought that should have been taken by a reasonable person of similar competency

_____ 5. A publication that contains standards for medications, dosage forms, drug substances, excipients, medical devices, and dietary supplements

_____ 6. A term used to describe a patient's personal health data; this information is protected from being shared or distributed without permission

_____ 7. The mishandling of medication that can lead to contamination/impurity, falsification of contents, or loss of drug quality or potency; may cause injury or illness to the consumer

_____ 8. Drug that requires a prescription for dispensing

_____ 9. The intentional misuse of a drug intended for medical purposes

_____ 10. One of the many reference books of medications; this reference compiles and publishes select manufacturer-provided package inserts and prescribing information useful for health professionals

_____ 11. Any drug or other substance that is scheduled I through V and regulated by the DEA

_____ 12. Labeling of a product that is false or misleading

_____ 13. A drug derived from barbituric acid; often employed in the treatment of seizures and as sedative and hypnotic agents

_____ 14. A document providing chemical product information

_____ 15. A statutory plan passed by Congress or any legislature that is a "bill" until it is enacted and becomes law

_____ 16. A 10-digit number that indicates specifics of a prescription drug or an insulin product

_____ 17. Drug warning that is placed in the prescribing information or package insert of the product and indicates a significant risk of potentially dangerous side effects

7

_____ 18. A nonspecific term used to describe a drug that in moderate doses dulls the senses, relieves pain, and induces profound sleep but in excessive doses causes stupor, coma, or convulsions, and may lead to addiction

_____ 19. A system in use by the FDA to describe five levels of assessment of the fetal effects caused by a drug, a required section of current prescription drug labeling

_____ 20. The values and morals that are used within a profession

_____ 21. Medication that can be purchased without a prescription; nonlegend medications

_____ 22. A change in the original act or law

_____ 23. Comprehensive information on a medication's actions within that class of drugs

_____ 24. To cause harm or injury to a person intentionally or because of negligence

TRUE OR FALSE

Write T or F next to each statement.

_____ 1. The practice of pharmacy is governed by a series of laws, regulations, and rules enforced by federal, state, and local government.

_____ 2. A good understanding of pharmacy laws is not necessary to pass the Pharmacy Technician Certification Board examination.

_____ 3. Manufacturers need to prove the effectiveness of the drugs through methods such as scientific studies.

_____ 4. Two government agencies that are important with respect to pharmacy are the FDA and DEA.

_____ 5. The function of the DEA is to encourage the illegal distribution and misuse of controlled substances.

_____ 6. Only DEA Form 41 is needed by the pharmacy to dispense controlled substances.

_____ 7. The DEA requires narcotic inventory to be taken every 5 years.

_____ 8. Prescribers must be registered with the DEA to write prescriptions for controlled substances.

_____ 9. VIPPS is a label that indicates to the public that the website from which they are ordering drugs is both legitimate and licensed.

_____ 10. When federal and state law differs, the most lenient law is the one you should follow.

MULTIPLE CHOICE

Complete each question by circling the best answer.

1. Who has the authority to decide under what schedule a drug should be placed?
   A. RPh
   B. FDA
   C. Attorney general
   D. DEA

2. A C-III drug can be refilled:
   A. 0 times
   B. 2 times
   C. 5 times
   D. 6 times

3. In most states, a prescription for a C-IV drug expires after:
   A. 14 days
   B. 3 months
   C. 6 months or five refills
   D. 12 months

4. A drug monograph is:
   A. A picture of the drug
   B. Literature on the drug
   C. Literature on the manufacturer
   D. A price list for the drug

5. Methadone is a C-II controlled substance that is commonly used for:
   A. Severe depression
   B. Schizophrenia
   C. ADHD
   D. Opioid addiction

6. When prescriptions for controlled substances in C-III through C-V will be filed with other non–controlled drug prescriptions, the controlled drug prescriptions are designated in the pharmacy by stamping with a C that must appear:
   A. In red
   B. In black
   C. In green
   D. In blue

7. Which of the following numbers could be the DEA number for Dr. Green?
   A. AB5527835
   B. AG5387255
   C. AB5387255
   D. FG5378255

8. Which medication does not require a childproof cap?
   A. Amoxicillin chewable tablets
   B. Nitrostat SL tablets
   C. Mycelex troche
   D. Amoxicillin suspension

9. The highest level of a manufacturer recall, which indicates that products could cause serious harm or fatality, is a:
   A. Class 1 recall
   B. Class 2 recall
   C. Class 3 recall
   D. Class 4 recall

10. A tort is:
    A. A small fruit pie
    B. The amount of force used to inject a needle
    C. A type of instrument used in compounding
    D. Causing injury to a person intentionally or through negligence

11. To obtain a Schedule II substance from a distributor, which DEA form must be filled out?
    A. 122
    B. 222
    C. 324
    D. 306

12. Which of the following controlled substance schedule drugs can be obtained without a prescription?
    A. C-II
    B. C-III
    C. C-IV
    D. C-V

13. Invoices for C-II drugs must be kept for _____ years.
    A. 2
    B. 4
    C. 5
    D. 7

14. To destroy controlled substances, which DEA form must be used?
    A. 106
    B. 222
    C. 41
    D. 510

15. Record keeping is regulated by:
    A. Federal law
    B. State law
    C. Company policy
    D. Pharmacists

FILL IN THE BLANKS

Answer each question by completing the statement in the space provided.

1. The Pure Food and Drugs Act of 1906 is also known as the _____.

2. The drug _____ was found to cause severe birth defects, including grossly deformed limbs, when administered during pregnancy and therefore was never approved for use in the United States.

3. All addictive substances are required to be labeled with the statement "_____, _____."

4. PPPA specifies that medication should not be able to be opened by at least _____% of children under the age of 5 and that at least _____% of adults should be able to open the medication within 5 minutes.

5. The main functions of the FDA are to _____ the guidelines for manufacturers to ensure the safety and effectiveness of medications.

6. Adverse reactions should be reported to the FDA's _____ program.

7. The DEA guidelines for controlled C-II substances allow physicians to write up to _____ separate prescriptions at one time for multiple drugs, to be filled sequentially over _____ days.

8. A _____ is distributed by the pharmacy with each prescription and each prescription refill, because the information for the patient may change frequently.

9. A _____ mistake can affect a person's ability to continue to work as a technician and also may result in punitive damages.

10. Depending on the state in which the technician works, laws vary as they pertain to the _____ of the technician.

MATCHING

Matching I

Match the controlled substance designations with the correct drugs.

_____ 1. Vicodin

_____ 2. LSD

_____ 3. Lomotil

_____ 4. Demerol

_____ 5. Valium

_____ 6. Robitussin AC

_____ 7. Ritalin

_____ 8. Ativan

_____ 9. Heroin

_____ 10. Tylenol/Codeine #3

A. C-I
B. C-II
C. C-III
D. C-IV
E. C-V

Matching II

Match the pharmacy law with the correct description.

A. Federal Food and Drug Act of 1906
B. 1914 Harrison Narcotic Act
C. 1938 Food, Drug, and Cosmetic Act
D. 1951 Durham-Humphrey Amendment
E. 1962 Kefauver-Harris Amendment
F. 1970 Comprehensive Drug Abuse Prevention and Control Act
G. 1970 Poison Prevention Packaging Act
H. 1972 Drug Listing Act
I. 1983 Orphan Drug Act
J. 1987 Prescription Drug Marketing Act
K. 1990 Omnibus Budget Reconciliation Act
L. 1996 Health Insurance Portability and Accountability Act
M. 2000 Drug Addiction Treatment Act
N. 2003 Medicare Modernization Act
O. 2005 Combat Methamphetamine Epidemic Act
P. 2010 Patient Protection and Affordable Care Act
Q. 2013 Drug Quality and Security Act

_____ 1. Ensures the safety and effectiveness of all new drugs on the U.S. market

_____ 2. Addresses all areas related to manufacture of, enforcement of laws pertaining to, and sale of pseudoephedrine, which can be used to create methamphetamine

_____ 3. Encourages drug companies to develop drugs for rare diseases by providing research assistance, grants, and cost incentives to manufacturers

_____ 4. Federal act for protecting patients' rights, establishing national standards for electronic health care communication, and ensuring the security and privacy of health data

_____ 5. One of the first laws enacted to stop the sale of inaccurately labeled drugs

_____ 6. Provides a drug discount card to beneficiaries with low incomes who require pharmacy company assistance for obtaining medications

_____ 7. Helps to avoid counterfeit drugs and ingredients in the supply chain and also helps limit diversion of pharmaceutical samples and prescription drugs

_____ 8. Makes preventative care more accessible and affordable for many Americans

_____ 9. Important concepts of this act were adulteration, misbranding, and providing the legal status for the FDA.

_____ 10. Requires manufacturers and pharmacies to place all medications in containers with childproof caps or packaging, including both over-the-counter and legend drugs

Chapter **2** **Pharmacy Law, Ethics, and Regulatory Agencies**

_____ 11. Permits physicians to prescribe controlled substances (preapproved by the DEA) in schedules C-III, C-IV, or C-V to persons suffering from opioid addiction, for the purpose of maintenance or detoxification treatments

_____ 12. Added more instructions for drug companies, required the labeling "Caution: Federal law prohibits dispensing without a prescription," and made the initial distinction between legend drugs and OTC medications that do not require a physician's order

_____ 13. Gives greater oversight of bulk pharmaceutical compounding and enhances the agency's ability to track drugs through the distribution process

_____ 14. Formed the DEA to enforce the laws concerning controlled substances and their distribution and introduced a stair-step schedule of controlled substances

_____ 15. Enacted in the United States in parallel with international treaties to curb recreational use of opium

_____ 16. Requires every drug to have a unique 10-digit number divided into three segments; numbers identify the labeler, product, and trade package size

_____ 17. Congressional act that changed reimbursement limits and mandated drug utilization evaluation, pharmacy patient consultation, and educational outreach programs

SHORT ANSWER

Write a short response to each question in the space provided.

1. Explain what the letters in a DEA number represent.

_____

_____

_____

2. How do you verify that a DEA number is authentic?

_____

_____

_____

3. List five prescription drugs that can be packaged in non–child-resistant bottles.

_____

_____

_____

4. When medication from an original manufacturer's container is repackaged, list the information to be placed on each individual label.

_____

5. Name three characteristics a pharmacy technician should have to demonstrate professional ethics.

_____

_____

RESEARCH ACTIVITIES

Follow the instructions given in each exercise and provide a response.

1. Access the website *http://www.fda.gov/Safety/MedWatch/*. List two drug recalls that have occurred in the last 30 days.

2. Use the website *http://www.fda.gov/Drugs/DrugSafety/DrugSafetyPodcasts/default.htm* to listen to the FDA Drug Safety Podcasts. Listen to one podcast, list the name of the podcast, and summarize what you have learned.

REFLECT CRITICALLY

CRITICAL THINKING

Reply to each question based on what you have learned in the chapter.

1. If you could add one more law to the existing laws addressing abuse of prescription medications, what would it be?

2. Marijuana has been the subject of debate lately for possible medicinal use in patients with cancer, AIDS, and multiple sclerosis. Into which controlled substance schedule would you put marijuana if it were approved for such use?

3. Someone presents a C-II prescription in the pharmacy 31 days after it was written. Knowing that C-II drugs must be filled within 30 days of the original date written, how would you tell the patient that this prescription cannot be filled?

13

LAB SCENARIOS

Pharmacy Law

Objective: To allow the pharmacy technician to develop critical thinking skills when filling prescriptions in keeping with pharmacy laws.

Lab Activity #2.1: Answer the following questions as they relate to pharmacy practice.

Equipment needed:

■ Pencil/pen

Time needed to complete this activity: 60 minutes

1. A physician writes the following prescription:

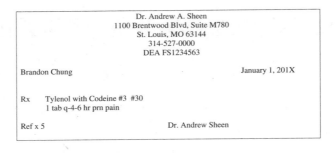

```
                            Dr. Andrew A. Sheen
                         1100 Brentwood Blvd, Suite M780
                              St. Louis, MO 63144
                                 314-527-0000
                               DEA FS1234563

Brandon Chung                                      January 1, 201X


Rx      Tylenol with Codeine #3  #30
        1 tab q-4-6 hr prn pain

Ref x 5                          Dr. Andrew Sheen
```

How many prescription refills are allowed for a Schedule III controlled substance? When must this prescription be filled before it expires?

2. A physician writes the following prescription:

```
                            Dr. Andrew A. Sheen
                         1100 Brentwood Blvd, Suite M780
                              St. Louis, MO 63144
                                 314-527-0000
                               DEA FS1234563

Brandon Chung                                      January 12, 201X


Rx      Coumadin 5 mg #30
        1 tab po qd

Ref x 5                          Dr. Andrew Sheen
```

May this prescription be filled with a generic drug? Why or why not?

3. The pharmacy receives the following prescription on a Monday:

```
                        Dr. Andrew A. Sheen
                   1100 Brentwood Blvd, Suite M780
                        St. Louis, MO 63144
                          314-527-0000
                          DEA FS1234563

Brandon Chung                                    January 12, 201X


Rx    Percocet 5 mg #30
      1 tab po q4-6 h prn pain



Ref                          Dr. Andrew Sheen
```

The pharmacy has only 20 tablets of Percocet in stock. What options does the pharmacy have in filling this prescription?

_____

_____

_____

4. A patient has the following prescription filled at a pharmacy:

```
                        Dr. Andrew A. Sheen
                   1100 Brentwood Blvd, Suite M780
                        St. Louis, MO 63144
                          314-527-0000
                          DEA FS1234563

Brandon Chung                                    January 12, 201X


Rx    Lipitor 10 mg #30
      1 tab po qd for cholesterol


Ref x 5                      Dr. Andrew Sheen
```

The patient now wishes to have the prescription filled at another pharmacy. How many times may the prescription be transferred to another pharmacy? What happens to the prescription at the original pharmacy? What information must be indicated on the original prescription?

_____

_____

_____

_____

Chapter **2** **Pharmacy Law, Ethics, and Regulatory Agencies**

5. A patient brings in the following prescription to be filled at your pharmacy:

> Dr. Andrew A. Sheen
>
> 1100 Brentwood Blvd, Suite M780
>
> St. Louis, MO 63144
>
> 314-527-0000
>
> DEA FS1234563
>
> Brandon Chung   January 12, 201X
>
> Rx   Hydrochlorothiazide 50 mg #30
>
>   1 tab po qd for fluid retention
>
> Ref prn   Dr. Andrew Sheen

When will the prescription expire?

_____

6. A patient receives the following prescription:

> Dr. Andrew A. Sheen
> 1100 Brentwood Blvd, Suite M780
> St. Louis, MO 63144
> 314-527-0000
> DEA FS1234563
>
> Brandon Chung   January 12, 201X
> Rx   Ambien 10 mg   #30
>   1 tab po q hs prn insomnia
>
> Ref x 0   Dr. Andrew Sheen

When will the prescription expire?

_____

7. A female patient brings in a new prescription for amoxicillin 500 mg. As you are entering the prescription into the system, you receive a warning showing that the patient has filled a prescription for Alesse, an oral contraceptive.

A. What should you do and why?

_____

_____

_____

B. Which pharmacy law would you be enforcing?

_____

16

C. What auxiliary labels should be applied to this prescription when dispensing?

_____

8. A 16-year-old male comes to the pharmacy counter and asks for a 10-pack of U-30 insulin syringes.

   A. How do you handle the situation and why?

   _____

   _____

   _____

   B. Why is it important to be familiar with federal and state laws and uphold them?

   _____

   _____

   _____

9. A 21-year-old male approaches the pharmacy counter and asks to buy four boxes of Sudafed tablets that are stocked behind the counter.

   A. How would you handle the situation and why?

   _____

   Which pharmacy law would you be enforcing?

   _____

10. A 16-year-old female comes to the prescription counter and asks for a 4-ounce bottle of terpin hydrate with codeine syrup.

    A. How would you handle the situation and why?

    _____

    _____

    _____

    B. Which pharmacy law would you be enforcing?

    _____

11. A. How many times in a year may a retail pharmacy request the destruction of controlled substances? What form would be used to request the destruction in a retail pharmacy?

    _____

    _____

    B. A hospital pharmacy? What form would be used to request the destruction in a hospital pharmacy?

    _____

    _____

Chapter **2** **Pharmacy Law, Ethics, and Regulatory Agencies**

12. Explain the three methods permitted for filing filled prescriptions.

_____

_____

_____

_____

13. How would you handle a patient's request to have a prescription mailed to him or her?

_____

_____

_____

14. What organization is responsible for the purity, safety, and efficacy of medications?

_____

15. What criteria must be evaluated for a medication to be considered a controlled substance?

_____

16. What do the three components of an NDC number represent?

_____

17. What organization is responsible for enforcing the Controlled Substance Act?

_____

18. A. Under what conditions may a prescription be dispensed in a non–child-resistant container?

_____

_____

_____

    B. What is an example of a medication that does not need to be placed in a child-resistant container?

_____

19. What conditions must be met for an individual to purchase an "exempt narcotic"?

_____

_____

_____

20. A. A physician calls in an "emergency" prescription for a Schedule II medication. How much time does the physician have to provide the pharmacy with a handwritten prescription?

_____

    B. According to your state laws of pharmacy, how much time does the physician have to provide the pharmacy with a handwritten prescription?

_____

2. Doug Manning, MD   MM4921739

_____

3. Tanya Smith, DDS   FS5264813

_____

4. Rick Taylor, PA   FT3814262

_____

5. Jack Jenson, DO   AJ3875245

_____

Procedural Step	Yes/No
Verified the first letter of the DEA number is either A, B, or F for primary prescribers or M for nurse practitioners and physician assistants. Marked DEA set invalid if it did not match.	
Determined if the second letter is the first letter of the prescriber's last name. Marked DEA set invalid if it did not match.	
Used the formula to add the first, third, and fifth numbers in the DEA set.	
Continued the formula by adding the second, fourth, and sixth numbers and then multiplied by 2.	
Completed the formula by adding the two sums together.	
Compared the results of the check sum. Marked DEA set valid when the last digit from the check sum matched the last number in the DEA set. Marked DEA set invalid when the last digit from the check sum did not match the last number of the DEA set.	

Role and Responsibilities of the Pharmacy Technician

Objective: To familiarize the pharmacy technician with his or her role and responsibilities as a pharmacy technician in the practice of pharmacy.

> The state board of pharmacy oversees the practice of pharmacy within a given state. The state board of pharmacy establishes requirements for an individual to be licensed as a pharmacist. In addition, the board enacts regulations that define the criteria to be met by individuals who seek to be a pharmacy technician, their role in the practice of pharmacy, and the tasks they may perform. These tasks may vary from state to state, and it is the responsibility of the pharmacy technician to become familiar with them.

Lab Activity #2.5: Refer to _http://www.nabp.net/boards-of-pharmacy/_ for the following information. Identify the tasks permitted by the board of pharmacy in your state.

Equipment needed:

- Computer with Internet access
- Pencil/pen

Time needed to complete this activity: 30 minutes

Task	Yes/No
Accept telephoned prescriptions from physician's office.	
Compound extemporaneous compounds. If yes, is additional training required?	
Counsel patients.	
Obtain refill permission from physician's office.	
Order medications.	
Prepare intravenous medications. If yes, is additional training required?	
Prepare radiopharmaceuticals. If yes, is additional training required?	
Prepare total parenteral nutrition products. If yes, is additional training required?	
Tech-check-tech If yes, is additional training required?	

Pharmacy Ethics

Objective: To identify those pharmacy situations in which a pharmacy technician will be faced with making ethical decisions.

The practice of pharmacy has established a code of ethics for both pharmacists and pharmacy technicians.

CODE OF ETHICS FOR PHARMACY TECHNICIANS

Preamble

Pharmacy technicians are health care professionals who assist pharmacists in providing the best possible care for patients. The principles of this code, which apply to pharmacy technicians working in any and all settings, are based on application and support of the moral obligations that guide the pharmacy profession in relationships with patients, health care professionals, and society.

Principles

- A pharmacy technician's first consideration is to ensure the health and safety of the patient, and to use knowledge and skills to the best of his or her ability in serving patients.
- A pharmacy technician supports and promotes honesty and integrity in the profession, which includes the duty to observe the law, maintain the highest moral and ethical conduct at all times, and uphold the ethical principles of the profession.
- A pharmacy technician assists and supports pharmacists in the safe and efficacious and cost-effective distribution of health services and health care resources.
- A pharmacy technician respects and values the abilities of pharmacists, colleagues, and other health care professionals.
- A pharmacy technician maintains competency in his or her practice and continually enhances his or her professional knowledge and expertise.
- A pharmacy technician respects and supports the patient's individuality, dignity, and confidentiality.

3 Competencies, Associations, and Settings for Technicians

REINFORCE KEY CONCEPTS

TERMS AND DEFINITIONS

Select the correct term from the following list and write the corresponding letter in the blank next to the statement.

A. Accreditation Council for Pharmacy Education (ACPE)
B. American Association of Pharmacy Technicians (AAPT)
C. American Pharmacist Association (APhA)
D. American Society of Health-System Pharmacists (ASHP)
E. ASHP Model Curriculum
F. Board of Pharmacy (BOP)
G. Certified Pharmacy Technician
H. Closed Door Pharmacy
I. Communication
J. Competency
K. Community Pharmacy
L. Continuing Education (CE)
M. Hyperalimentation
N. Inpatient Pharmacy
O. Institute for the Certification of Pharmacy Technicians (ICPT)
P. Licensed Pharmacy Technician
Q. National Association of Boards of Pharmacy (NABP)
R. National Pharmacy Technician Association (NPTA)
S. Outpatient Pharmacies
T. Parenteral Medications
U. Pharmacy Technician Certification Board (PTCB)
V. Professionalism
W. Registered Pharmacy Technician
X. Total Parenteral Nutrition (TPN)

_____ 1. A pharmacy technician who is licensed by the state board; licensing ensures that an individual has at least the minimum level of competency required by the profession

_____ 2. Pharmacies that serve patients in their communities; consumers can walk in and purchase a prescription or OTC drug

_____ 3. A pharmacy technician who is registered through the state board of pharmacy; may require a background check through the legal system

_____ 4. First pharmacy technician association; founded in 1979

_____ 5. A pharmacy in a hospital or institutional setting

_____ 6. National organization for members of state boards of pharmacy

_____ 7. Most commonly used to describe medications administered by injection, such as intravenously, intramuscularly, or subcutaneously

_____ 8. Parenteral (intravenous) nutrition for patients who are unable to eat solids or liquids

_____ 9. State-managed agency that licenses pharmacists and may either register or license pharmacy technicians to work in pharmacy

_____ 10. Large-volume intravenous nutrition administered through the central vein, which allows for a higher concentration of solutions

_____ 11. Oldest pharmacy association; founded in 1852

_____ 12. The ability to express oneself in such a way that one is readily and clearly understood

_____ 13. The capability or proficiency to perform a function

_____ 14. Pharmacy association primarily for technicians; founded in 1999

_____ 15. A pharmacy in which medications are called in from institutions such as long-term care facilities and are then delivered; not open to the public

_____ 16. Pharmacies that serve patients in community or ambulatory settings

_____ 17. This model provides details on how to meet the ASHP goals for pharmacy technician training programs

25

_____ 18. Education beyond the basic technical education, usually required for license or certification renewal

_____ 19. Conforming to the right principles of conduct (work ethics) as accepted by others in the profession

_____ 20. A technician who has passed the national certification examination; the technician can use the abbreviation CPhT after his or her name

_____ 21. National board for the certification of pharmacy technicians, which is now a part of the National Healthcareer Association (NHA)

_____ 22. Pharmacy association founded in 1942

_____ 23. National board for the certification of pharmacy technicians

_____ 24. National agency for the accreditation of professional degree programs in pharmacy and providers of continuing pharmacy education

TRUE OR FALSE

Write T or F next to each statement.

_____ 1. Job descriptions and educational requirements of pharmacy technicians are quickly changing.

_____ 2. The number of prescriptions processed per day in a pharmacy is not related to the speed and accuracy of the typist.

_____ 3. A pharmacy technician is not required to continually update and improve their computer skills.

_____ 4. Outpatient pharmacies traditionally have a wider range of stock to provide all the necessary supplies required of each department.

_____ 5. Pharmacy technicians should make sure the pharmacist has checked all drugs and/or devices before they leave the pharmacy.

_____ 6. Certified technicians must renew their certification every year and complete at least 20 hours of pharmacy-related continuing education.

_____ 7. Certified technicians must complete 1 hour of continuing education in medication safety every 2 years.

_____ 8. The ExCPT exam is the only pharmacy technician certification exam accepted in all 50 states.

_____ 9. How technicians conduct themselves in various situations reveals their professionalism and their personal maturity.

_____ 10. A pharmacy technician who has graduated from an accredited program and is nationally certified will be the preferred hire.

MULTIPLE CHOICE

Complete each question by circling the best answer.

1. The board of pharmacy:
    A. Registers pharmacists and technicians
    B. Provides a way for consumers to report complaints, problems, or illegal pharmacy actions
    C. Reviews and updates current pharmacy rules and regulations
    D. All of the above

2. The term _nondiscretionary_ means that technicians can perform:
    A. Tasks that require little or no thought
    B. Tasks in a pharmacy setting that do not require professional judgment
    C. Tasks that require interpretation of scientific studies
    D. Tasks that are unethical

3. The National Certification Examination for Pharmacy Technicians is given:
   A. 50 times a year
   B. Four times a year
   C. Daily by appointment only
   D. Three times a year

4. Which of the following is not a goal of the Pharmacy Technician Certification Board?
   A. To ensure that technicians work equally and for the same pay as pharmacists
   B. To provide improved patient care and service
   C. To create a minimum standard of knowledge
   D. To help employers determine the technician's knowledge base

5. Which of the following is not an eligibility requirement for taking the PTCB exam?
   A. High school diploma
   B. Graduate of a pharmacy technician program
   C. No convictions for a drug-related felony
   D. GED

6. What factors must be considered before a person can be a competent pharmacy technician?
   A. Job duties
   B. Communication skills
   C. Ethics
   D. All of the above

7. Which of the following is not considered professional in appearance?
   A. Wedding ring
   B. Earring
   C. Nose ring
   D. Engagement ring

8. Which of the following is *not* example of a nondiscretionary duty?
   A. Repackaging medications
   B. Counseling patients about the medications they are taking
   C. Managing inventory
   D. Filling automated dispensing machines

9. Which of the following is currently the main credential available to pharmacy technicians?
   A. CPhT
   B. CPT
   C. PhTC
   D. PT

10. Which of the following is a soft skill every employee needs?
    A. Conflict resolution
    B. Adaptability
    C. Teamwork
    D. All of the above

FILL IN THE BLANKS

Answer each question by completing the statement in the space provided.

1. Several states require _____ or _____ certification and have accepted it as their measure of the knowledge base of pharmacy technicians.

2. Technician duties focus on tasks that do not require _____ _____ but instead concentrate on their technical skills and training.

3. The _____ _____ focused on the areas Consumer Awareness, Resources, Education, State Policy, and Testing related to pharmacy technicians.

4. When state laws differ from federal laws, the _____ law should be enforced.

5. An important aspect of an inventory technician is the _____ requirements of the medications that arrive in pharmacy.

6. _____ doses are to be delivered within 15 minutes or less to the area requesting them.

7. _____ has been the leader in providing course curriculum and standards and offering students the best foundation for becoming technicians.

8. Certification is an indication of the mastery of a specific core of _____.

9. The _____ was launched as a collaborative effort by the NABP and the ACPE to provide an electronic system for pharmacists and pharmacy technicians to track their continuing pharmacy education credits.

10. Traditional settings such as the _____ or _____ pharmacy are not the only places you will find technicians working today.

MATCHING

Select the correct pharmacy job opportunity from the following list and write the corresponding letter in the blank next to the description.

A. Anticoagulant technician
B. Computer support technician
C. Chemo technician
D. Clinical technician
E. Corporate pharmacy analysis
F. Home infusion pharmacy technician
G. Insurance billing technician
H. Inventory technician
I. Nuclear pharmacy technician
J. Pharmacy business management operator
K. Pharmacy informatics analyst
L. Poison control call center operator
M. Retail technician
N. Robot filler
O. Software writer
P. Technician coordinator
Q. Technician recruiter
R. Technician trainer
S. Technician verifier

_____ 1. Trains newly hired technicians in computer programs and other skills relevant to the pharmacy

_____ 2. Receives orders and prepares all chemotherapeutic agents

_____ 3. Supports personnel by helping with automated medication dispensing systems

_____ 4. Knows the guidelines of Medicare, Blue Cross, and other insurance companies

_____ 5. Recruits technicians into outpatient or temporary agencies

_____ 6. Orders and bills all stock

_____ 7. Screens incoming calls and transfers calls to 911 operator or pharmacist; authorized to take the call if it concerns a minor issue

_____ 8. Assists the pharmacist with tracking patients' medications or compiling data for drug utilization study

_____ 9. Is trained to load mechanical dispensing equipment and keep it running smoothly

_____ 10. Hires technicians to help customers over the phone

_____ 11. Specially trained technician who performs the final verification of medication orders and identifies orders on a routine basis that need pharmacist intervention in order to improve the administration experience

_____ 12. Assists the pharmacist in the preparation of IV solutions, injectable drugs, and enteral nutrition therapy for the patient at home

_____ 13. Must have excellent communication skills, phone skills, and prescription-filling abilities

_____ 14. Assists the anticoagulant pharmacist in contacting patients when patient follow-up is necessary or the patient's anticoagulation medication or dosage needs to be changed

_____ 15. Responsible for training, regulation compliance, and scheduling of all pharmacy technician personnel

_____ 16. Specially trained technician who works with the Clinical Applications Specialists to maintain pharmacy software and computers, coordinate hardware and software updates, and work with the pharmacy informatics team

_____ 17. Assists the pharmacist with handling and preparing physicians' orders for radioactive medications used in diagnosis and treatment

_____ 18. Surveys the efficiency in all areas of the pharmacy and recommends changes to help the pharmacy operate more productively and efficiently

_____ 19. Technicians with additional computer background and/or training to prepare software services

SHORT ANSWER

Write a short response to each question in the space provided.

1. List three aspects of pharmacy technician training the _White Paper_ described as needing attention.

_____

_____

_____

2. List four responsibilities or competencies a pharmacy technician must have.

_____

_____

_____

_____

3. What are four different types of pharmacy settings in which a pharmacy technician can work?

_____

_____

_____

_____

4. What are the four different levels of pharmacy technicians?

_____

_____

_____

_____

5. What are the nine knowledge domains the PTCE assesses?

_____

_____

_____

_____

_____

RESEARCH ACTIVITIES

Follow the instructions given in each exercise and provide a response.

1. Call or visit a local retail or hospital pharmacy. Ask the lead technician or the pharmacist in charge the following questions.

   A. What qualifications do you require for technicians in your pharmacy?

   B. What duties do your technicians perform?

   C. Do you require certification?

2. Call or visit a closed door pharmacy in your area. Ask the lead technician or the pharmacist in charge the following questions.

   A. What qualifications do you require for technicians in your pharmacy?

   B. What duties do your technicians perform?

   C. Do you require certification?

CRITICAL THINKING

Reply to each question based on what you have learned in the chapter.

1. You have been asked to advise someone interested in becoming a pharmacy technician. How would you advise this person?

2. What is your definition of professionalism with regard to pharmacy technicians?

3. How long do you think new pharmacy technicians should receive training when starting a new job?

4. What does your state Practice Act require of pharmacy technicians?

5. What do you know about the pharmacy technician's scope of practice in your state?

RELATE TO PRACTICE

LAB SCENARIOS

Interviewing for a Pharmacy Technician Position

Objective: To prepare a pharmacy technician student for a pharmacy technician interview.

> After completing your pharmacy technician program, you are ready to find your first position as a pharmacy technician. This can be a very exciting time in your life. It is extremely important that you are prepared for your interview. The interview process is an opportunity for the pharmacy technician and the employer to get to know each other, to determine whether you are the right employee for the position, and for you to discern whether the pharmacy meets your requirements.
>
> It is extremely important for the pharmacy technician to be prepared for the interview. Being prepared includes wearing appropriate clothing for the interview, carrying oneself properly, answering questions asked by the interviewer, and asking questions of the interviewer. You will be assessed on what you do, what you say, and what you don't say. You will have only a few moments to impress the employer, so it is important to be prepared. Remember the saying, "Failing to prepare is preparing to fail."

Lab Activity #3.1: Mock interview

Equipment needed:

- Paper
- Pencil/pen

Time needed to complete this activity: 120 minutes

It is extremely important that you are prepared to answer any question that might be asked of you by the interviewer. Your response should be short and concise but should answer the question.

You are a pharmacy technician who has applied for a pharmacy technician position at a local pharmacy. The pharmacy has called and would like you to come in for an interview.

How would you answer the following questions?

1. Tell me about yourself.

   _____

   _____

2. Why did you decide to become a pharmacy technician?

   _____

   _____

3. Tell me about the pharmacy technician program that prepared you to become a pharmacy technician. What did you like about it? What did you dislike about it?

   _____

   _____

   _____

   _____

4. Did you have an externship? Where did you do your externship? How many hours was it?

   _____

   _____

5. Are you certified? If not, when will you be taking the test? Which test will you be taking?

   _____

   _____

6. Why will you be successful as a pharmacy technician?

   _____

   _____

7. Why do you want to work for us?

   _____

   _____

8. What do you know about our company?

_____

_____

9. Why should we hire you?

_____

_____

_____

10. What in your background prepares you for this job?

_____

_____

11. How will your job contribute to the overall goals of this company?

_____

_____

12. What type of job duties do you think you may be performing?

_____

_____

13. What do you hope to be doing in 5 years?

_____

_____

14. How do you feel about what you've accomplished so far?

_____

_____

15. How do you work under pressure? Can you give us some examples?

_____

_____

_____

16. What is your greatest strength?

_____

_____

17. What is your greatest weakness? How have you overcome your weaknesses?

_____

_____

_____

_____

18. What would your references say about you?

_____

_____

19. Who was your best boss or manager? Why?

_____

_____

20. In your last job, what tasks took most of your time?

_____

_____

21. What did you enjoy doing most in your last job? Least?

_____

_____

_____

_____

22. Why did you leave your last job?

_____

_____

23. Have you ever had your work or your suggestions criticized or attacked? How did you react?

_____

_____

24. What have you done that shows initiative?

_____

_____

25. Tell us about a time when you were completely committed.

_____

_____

26. Explain your role in a team. Tell us about something that you've accomplished working with others.

_____

_____

_____

27. Explain an event that challenged and changed you. Do you think your reaction to the event was different from others?

_____

_____

28. What types of decisions or jobs give you trouble?

_____

_____

29. What skills do you need to improve upon the most? What are you doing to remedy that situation?

_____

_____

_____

30. What coursework have you completed that applies to this job?

_____

_____

31. How do you prefer to work: by yourself or with other people?

_____

_____

During this part of the activity, act as if you are going on an interview. You will be evaluated on your professional attire, body language, and ability to answer questions. The interviewer may ask you questions from the list above, or other questions that might be relevant during an interview, and will rate your responses.

Question Being Asked by Interviewer	On a scale of 1 to 5, with 1 being the lowest and 5 being the highest, rate the potential employee's response to the question:
1.	
2.	
3.	
4.	
5.	
6.	
7.	
8.	
9.	
10.	
11.	
12.	
13.	
14.	
15.	

1. Would you hire the individual? Why or why not?

_____

_____

_____

Interview Evaluation	Yes/No
Prospective employee arrived on time for interview	
Employee introduced himself/herself to receptionist	
Completed an application legibly and did not leave questions unanswered	
Shook hands with the interviewer(s)	
Provided interviewer with a current resume	
Resume was free of spelling and grammatical errors	
Prospective employee had a neat, clean appearance	
Interviewee wore appropriate clothes for an interview	
Jewelry was appropriate for an interview	
Fragrance was subtle, not overwhelming	
Answered interview questions (behavioral and technical) appropriately	
Asked questions of the interviewer	
Thanked interviewer and shook hands as he or she was leaving	
Sent "Thank-you" note to interviewer within 24 hours	

Pharmacy Technician Certification

Objective: To introduce the pharmacy technician to the process of becoming certified as a pharmacy technician in his/her state.

Certification is the process by which a government agency grants recognition to an individual who has met predetermined qualifications specified by an agency or association. At the present moment, two pharmacy technician certification organizations are available: the Pharmacy Technician Certification Board (PTCB) and the Institute for Certification for Pharmacy Technicians (ICPT). Not all states require that a pharmacy technician is certified; however, there is a growing trend within the United States for pharmacy technicians to be certified as a prerequisite to working in a pharmacy, regardless of the setting.

Lab Activity #3.2: Visit *www.nabp.net* to obtain the website for your state board of pharmacy. After logging in to your state board of pharmacy, find out the requirements for a pharmacy technician to practice in your state. Complete the following table.

Equipment needed:

■ Computer with Internet access
■ Pencil/pen
■ Paper

Time needed to complete this activity: 30 minutes

Question	Response
Name of state	
Does your state require pharmacy technicians to be certified?	
If yes, what certification tests are approved for your state?	
What is the fee for each test approved by your state?	
Does your state require licensure of pharmacy technicians?	
Is a fee required for licensure? If so, what is the fee? How often does a pharmacy technician need to renew his or her license?	
Does your state require pharmacy technicians to register with the state board of pharmacy?	
Is a fee associated with the registration? If yes, what is the fee?	
Does your state require formal training (ASHP-accredited coursework, pharmacy technician training program)?	
Does your state allow compounding of medications, sterile and/or non-sterile? If yes, does your state require additional training or certification?	
What continuing education does your state require of pharmacy technicians? Are continuing education requirements met on a yearly basis?	
What fees are required to be paid to the state board of pharmacy for technicians?	

Lab Activity #3.3: Visit *www.ptcb.org* and *www.nationaltechexam.org* to obtain information regarding each of these examinations. Complete the following table for each examination.

Equipment needed:

■ Computer with Internet access

Time needed to complete this activity: 30 minutes

PTCB Examination	Response
What is the registration fee for the test?	
How often is the test offered?	
How many questions are included on the test?	
What is the minimum passing score for the examination?	
Where is the test offered in your area?	
If an individual does not pass the exam, when may he or she retake it?	
How long is the certification valid?	
How many continuing education units are required to renew your certification?	
Which states accept this exam?	

ExCPT Examination	Response
What is the registration fee for the test?	
How often is the test offered?	
How many questions are included on the test?	
What is the minimum passing score for the examination?	
If an individual does not pass the exam, when may he or she retake it?	
Where is the test offered in your area?	
How long is the certification valid?	
How many continuing education units are required to renew your certification?	
Which states accept this exam?	

Lab Activity #3.4: Print a copy of the content for the PTCB and ExCPT examinations. Compare and contrast the information included on each examination.

Equipment needed:

■ Computer with Internet access
■ Computer printer

Time to needed to complete this activity: 30 minutes

1. Which examination will you take and why?

_____

_____

_____

_____

_____

Lab Activity #3.5: Register for the PTCB exam or the ExCPT exam.

Equipment needed:

- Computer with Internet access
- Computer printer with paper
- Credit or debit card

Time needed to complete this activity: 30 minutes

1. When did you register?

   _____

2. When are you scheduled to take the exam?

   _____

3. Where are you to take the exam?

   _____

4. What should you bring to the exam?

   _____

Professionalism as a Pharmacy Technician

Objective: To become familiar with the professional organizations available for membership for pharmacy technicians and the resources that can be used to remain competent as a pharmacy technician.

Two of the principles of the Pharmacy Technician's Code of Ethics state the following:

- A pharmacy technician maintains competency in his or her practice, and continually enhances his or her professional knowledge and expertise.
- A pharmacy technician associates with and engages in the support of organizations that promote the profession of pharmacy through the utilization and enhancement of pharmacy technicians.

   All certified pharmacy technicians are required to maintain their competency through continuing education. Continuing education may take the form of pharmacy seminars or workshops, webinars, or reading of print materials accredited by the ACPE.

   A pharmacy technician should become involved with a pharmacy organization that will allow the pharmacy technician to develop professionally as a member of the organization. A pharmacy technician may choose to join many different types of organizations, depending on his or her interests. These organizations include the following:

- American Association of Pharmacy Technicians *(www.pharmacytechnician.com)*
- American Pharmacists Association *(www.pharmacist.com)*
- American Society of Health-System Pharmacists *(www.ashp.org)*
- National Pharmacy Technician Association *(www.pharmacytechnician.org)*
- Academy of Managed Care Pharmacy *(www.amcp.org)*

Lab Activity #3.6: Identify local, state, and national organizations that are available for membership for pharmacy technicians.

Equipment needed:

- Computer with Internet access
- Computer printer

- Paper
- Pencil/pen

Time needed to complete this activity: 20 minutes

Using the Internet, identify state and regional (local) pharmacy associations that you are eligible to join. Complete the following table.

Organization	Open to Pharmacy Technicians	Membership Fee	Continuing Education	Three Benefits of Membership	Career Opportunities
State association					
Regional association					
Academy of Managed Pharmacy (*www.amcp.org*)					
American Association of Pharmacy Technicians (*www.pharmacytechnician.com*)					
American Pharmacist Association (*www.pharmacist.com*)					
American Society of Health-System Pharmacists (*www.ashp.org*)					
National Pharmacy Technician Association (*www.pharmacytechnician.org*)					

Lab Activity #3.7: Participate in pharmacy technician continuing education.

Equipment needed:

- Computer with Internet access
- Computer printer
- Paper
- Pencil/pen

Time needed to complete this activity: 90 minutes

Using the Internet, select a pharmacy continuing education article of your choice from one of the following websites.

- *www.freece.com*
- *www.modernmedicine.com*
- *www.pharmacychoice.com*
- *www.pharmacytimes.com*
- *www.powerpak.com*
- *www.rxschool.com*
- *www.uspharmacist.com*

Read the article, take the examination, and print out the continuing education certificate. Provide the certificate to your instructor.

4 Communication and Role of the Technician with the Customer/Patient

TERMS AND DEFINITIONS

Select the correct term from the following list and write the corresponding letter in the blank next to the statement.

A. Attitude
B. Channel
C. Communication
D. Compassion
E. Diplomacy
F. Etiquette
G. Perception
H. Nonverbal Communication
I. Tact
J. Verbal Communication

_____ 1. A feeling of wanting to help someone who is sick or in trouble

_____ 2. An unwritten guideline or rule of behavior

_____ 3. A mental disposition or feeling a technician adopts in regard to customers, coworkers, or duties at work

_____ 4. The act of giving or exchanging information without using any spoken words

_____ 5. The ability to express oneself in such a way that one is understood readily and clearly

_____ 6. The way you think about or understand someone or something

_____ 7. A written message, spoken words, or body language

_____ 8. The sharing of information by individuals through using speech

_____ 9. The skill of dealing with others without causing bad feelings

_____ 10. The ability to do or say things without offending or upsetting other people

TRUE OR FALSE

Write T or F next to each statement.

_____ 1. Effective communication skills are not necessary to achieve optimal patient satisfaction and trust.

_____ 2. Not all employers require basic communication abilities as a prerequisite to hiring.

_____ 3. For pharmacy technicians to provide optimal patient care, they must have an understanding of the communication cycle.

_____ 4. Passive listening helps keep the focus on the patient.

_____ 5. It is not important for pharmacy technicians to always behave professionally.

_____ 6. A pleasant facial expression will most likely cause a patient to respond in a positive manner.

_____ 7. Talking very slowly indicates you do not know the answer.

_____ 8. Always treat customers as you would want to be treated.

_____ 9. Pharmacy technicians who speak multiple languages are in high demand.

_____ 10. The pharmacy technician is not able to influence the development of a positive atmosphere within the pharmacy setting.

Complete each question by circling the best answer:

1. Why is it important for pharmacy technicians to have good communication skills?
   A. Earn trust
   B. Achieve optimal patient satisfaction
   C. Assist with patient safety
   D. All of the above

2. The communication cycle consists of all of the following *except*:
   A. Sender
   B. Feedback
   C. Handwriting
   D. Message

3. Most people make an instant judgment of others within the first _____ of meeting.
   A. 30 seconds
   B. minute
   C. minute and a half
   D. 5 minutes

4. Which of the following could improve your vocal communication skills?
   A. Use a monotone voice all the time.
   B. Do not talk too rapidly.
   C. Talk with an extremely soft voice.
   D. Use slang.

5. Which of the following may alienate the patient and result in a loss of business?
   A. Belittling the customer's opinion
   B. Making customer feel embarrassed
   C. Causing the customer to become angry
   D. All of the above

6. When all things are equal, what is the deciding factor for customers to have their prescriptions filled at a pharmacy?
   A. Location of the pharmacy
   B. Cost of medications
   C. Pharmacy staff
   D. Generic drug availability

7. Which of the following can help optimize your communication?
   A. Use open-ended questions
   B. Provide empathetic responses
   C. Minimize distractions
   D. All of the above

8. If the call must be placed on hold, the technician should check back with the caller in _____ intervals to reassure the patient that she or he has not been forgotten.
   A. 20-second
   B. 90-second
   C. 3-minute
   D. 5-minute

9. Which of the following is not a stage that terminally ill patients experience?
   A. Regret
   B. Denial
   C. Anger
   D. Bargaining

10. _____ can help you become an effective team player.
    A. Loyalty and trust
    B. Staying informed
    C. Understanding your job duties and responsibilities
    D. All of the above

FILL IN THE BLANKS

Answer each question by completing the statement in the space provided.

1. Pharmacy technicians _____ daily with co-workers, health care professionals, and customers.

2. A _____ technician will possess excellent written and verbal communication skills.

3. The communication cycle involves two or more individuals' _____ information.

4. _____ listening is a communication technique in which the listener confirms understanding by restating or summarizing what was heard in his or her own words.

5. Rolling your eyes or sighing loudly shows _____ and a lack of _____ for the customer.

6. Exhibiting _____ body language will make your communication with the patient more effective.

7. _____ can choose where they want to fill their medication.

8. In all pharmacy settings _____ work to provide the best patient care possible.

9. _____ and _____ are key components of a successful team.

10. The first step in _____ communication barriers is to recognize they exist.

MATCHING

Select the correct form of communication and write the corresponding letter in the blank next to the correct example.

A. Nonverbal communication
B. Vocal communication
C. Verbal communication

_____ 1. Frowning at a customer

_____ 2. Smiling as a customer walks up to counter

_____ 3. Tone of voice

_____ 4. Rolling your eyes

_____ 5. Talking very fast to customers

_____ 6. Inflection of your voice

_____ 7. Folding your arms while speaking with a customer

_____ 8. Talking loudly to all customers

_____ 9. Using comforting words while talking with a patient

_____ 10. Telling a patient he or she is wrong

SHORT ANSWER

Write a short response to each question in the space provided.

1. If a customer is angry about a situation, name two things you can do to ease the person's frustration.

   _____

   _____

2. Name four nonverbal ways stress can manifest itself.

   _____

   _____

3. List four aspects of your voice that can affect the customer or person to whom you are talking.

   _____

   _____

4. List four things you can do to help improve your verbal skills.

   _____

   _____

   _____

5. List four guidelines for interacting with patients and medical personnel over the phone.

   _____

   _____

   _____

   _____

RESEARCH ACTIVITIES

Follow the instructions given in each exercise and provide a response.

1. Access the USP Pictogram Library at *http://www.usp.org/usp-healthcare-professionals/related-topics-resources/usp-pictograms*. Review the pictograms available.

   A. Do you think the pictograms would be useful for those who speak English as a second language? Why or why not?

   B. What other pictograms should be available? Draw an example of what it (they) should look like.

2. Access the website *http://www.usp.org/usp-nf/key-issues/usp-nf-general-chapter-prescription-container-labeling*. How can a standardized prescription label help with communication and reduce medication errors?

CRITICAL THINKING

Reply to each question based on what you have learned in the chapter.

1. What is a benefit of empathizing with a patient to show her or him that you can see the situation from her or his point-of-view?

2. When talking with a customer, why would using open-ended questions help prevent potential errors?

LAB SCENARIOS

Recognizing and Responding to Verbal and Nonverbal Communications

Objective: To be able to recognize and respond to verbal and nonverbal communications in a professional manner

> To be an effective communicator in the pharmacy, a pharmacy technician must be able to read nonverbal cues and control his or her own nonverbal communication cues. Additionally, pharmacy technicians must be able to communicate clearly so that the patient's message is heard and the pharmacy technician's response is understood by the patient. This will not only help improve the communications process between health care professionals, other staff members, and patients, but will also help earn their trust.

Lab Activity #4.1: Read each scenario and answer each question. With a partner, take turns role-playing each scenario. Use learned verbal and nonverbal techniques to respond to each scenario appropriately, to make sure your message is understood properly.

Equipment needed:

- Paper
- Pencil/pen

Time needed to complete this activity: 30 minutes

1. Select a classmate as a partner who will play the role of a patient for this procedure. Take turns role-playing each scenario provided and act out an appropriate response.
2. Use appropriate body language and other nonverbal skills in communicating with patients, family, and staff.
3. Demonstrate sensitivity appropriate to the message being delivered.
4. Demonstrate empathy.
5. Apply active listening skills.
6. Restate the receiver's response.
7. Analyze communications in providing appropriate responses and feedback.
   A. Scenario #1: A customer walks up to the pharmacy counter to pick up a prescription. After looking up the prescription, the pharmacy technician notices it is not ready. The pharmacy technician informs the customer she will have to wait to pick it up. The customer states "Why did I even bother to call it in ahead of time?"
   B. Scenario #2: Nurse Johnson calls the pharmacist to ask if the two drugs she is about to administer are compatible. She is in a hurry. The pharmacy technician scribbles down the question but does not get the nurse's name or telephone extension. By the time the nurse calls back to contact the pharmacist, the dose is late and the patient has been in pain while waiting for a response. The nurse asks. "Why didn't you ask the pharmacist?"

45

C. Scenario #3: A patient calls the pharmacy to ask about his medication during a busy time at the pharmacy. The patient states he is calling because his medication looks different than before and he needs to know if it's the same drug or not. The pharmacy technician asks the patient if he could be placed on hold but the patient states he is in a hurry and cannot hold.

D. Scenario #4: A patient walks up to the counter to have her prescription filled and asks whether it can be done within 5 minutes because her bus will be leaving. The pharmacy technician informs the patient that this may not be possible because of other prescriptions needing to be filled first. The patient rolls her eyes and shakes her head.

E. Scenario #5: Act out a scenario that you have been a part of during a pharmacy visit. Be sure to use nonverbal and verbal cues for your partner to pick up on and to respond to.

Procedural Step	Yes/No
Selected a classmate as a partner to play the role of a patient for this procedure.	
Took turns with partner role-playing each nonverbal cue provided.	
Used appropriate body language and other nonverbal skills in communicating with patients, family, and staff.	
Demonstrated sensitivity appropriate to the message being delivered.	
Demonstrated empathy.	
Applied active listening skills.	
Restated the patient's response.	
Determined whether the receiver understood the message correctly.	
Analyzed communications in providing appropriate responses and feedback.	

Communicating in Spanish

Objective: To be able translate prescription medication directions into Spanish

Lab Activity #4.2: Using the *Drug Topics Red Book*, translate common prescription directions into Spanish.

Equipment needed:

- Computer with Internet connection
- *Drug Topics Red Book*
- Pencil/pen

Time needed to complete this activity: 30 minutes

1. Take one tablet by mouth daily.

_____

2. Take one capsule by mouth two times a day.

_____

3. Instill three drops in the left eye four times a day.

_____

4. Put four drops in each ear three times a day.

_____

5. Take one tablespoon two times a day.

_____

6. Take one-half teaspoon three times a day.

_____

7. Do not refrigerate.

_____

8. Shake gently and keep in refrigerator.

_____

9. Use as needed.

_____

10. Apply to affected area.

_____

11. Inject forty units subcutaneously.

_____

12. Do not take at same time as other medicine.

_____

13. Do not drink alcoholic beverages while taking this medicine.

_____

14. Do not drive while taking this medicine.

_____

15. Do not use after this date.

_____

Communicating Using Sign Language

Objective: To be able translate common pharmacy terms using sign language

Lab Activity #4.3: Access the website *http://www.signingsavvy.com/* to look up common pharmacy terms in sign language. Practice using sign language for each term with a partner.

Equipment needed:

■ Computer with Internet connection

Time needed to complete this activity: 30 minutes

1. Pharmacy
2. Teaspoon
3. Tablespoon
4. Capsule
5. Ointment
6. Take pill
7. AM
8. PM
9. Twice or two times
10. Three times
11. Daily
12. Bedtime
13. With
14. At
15. At once
16. Food
17. Inject or Injection
18. Help or Help you
19. Thank you

What other signs can you find? Can you put them together to communicate a sentence?

Dosage Forms and Routes of Administration

TERMS AND DEFINITIONS

Select the correct term from the following list and write the corresponding letter in the blank next to the statement.

A. Absorption
B. Behind-the-Counter
C. Bioavailability
D. Bioequivalence
E. Distribution
F. Elimination
G. Enteral
H. First-Pass Effect
I. Half-Life
J. Instill
K. Legend Drugs
L. Metabolism
M. Over-the-Counter
N. Parenteral
O. Prodrug
P. Pharmacokinetics

_____ 1. The last step in the pharmacokinetic process; drugs or other substances exit from the body via normal body processes

_____ 2. The relationship between two drugs that have the same dosage and dosage form and that have similar bioavailability

_____ 3. To place into; instruction commonly used for ophthalmic or otic drugs

_____ 4. Nonprescription drugs that are kept behind the pharmacy counter and may have limited amounts sold or require the permission of a pharmacist to purchase

_____ 5. Drugs that require a prescription, carry the warning "Federal Law prohibits the dispensing of this medication without a prescription"

_____ 6. A route of administration by way of the intestine, such as orally, rectally, or sublingually

_____ 7. Medications that can be purchased without a prescription

_____ 8. The amount of time it takes a chemical to be decreased by one-half

_____ 9. The degree to which a drug or other substance becomes available to the target tissue after administration

_____ 10. Term used to describe a medication that is usually given by injection into a vein, skin, or muscle that bypasses the gastrointestinal system

_____ 11. The movement of a medication throughout blood, organs, and tissues after administration

_____ 12. An inactive substance that is converted to a drug within the body by the action of enzymes or other chemicals

_____ 13. The taking in of nutrients and drugs into the body from food and liquids

_____ 14. The study of the absorption, metabolism, distribution, and elimination of drugs

_____ 15. The processes by which the body breaks down or converts medications to active or inactive substances

_____ 16. Process in which a portion of the dose is metabolized before the drug has a chance to be distributed systemically

TRUE OR FALSE

Write T or F next to each statement.

_____ 1. To become proficient in the medical profession, a technician must be able to interpret orders correctly.

_____ 2. Much of the terminology used in pharmacy comes from the Latin and Greek languages.

_____ 3. It is not necessary for the pharmacy technician to learn all dosage forms and abbreviations to decipher a physician's orders.

_____ 4. The number of errors resulting from physicians' poor handwriting or from transcription of orders is of little concern.

_____ 5. A dosage form refers to the means by which a drug is available for use or the vehicle by which the drug is delivered.

_____ 6. Enteric coated tablets dissolve in the stomach.

_____ 7. Dosage forms that are especially made to release over time can be crushed or broken into pieces.

_____ 8. An emulsifier binds oil and water together in a mixture.

_____ 9. Lozenges are oral tablets that should be swallowed immediately.

_____ 10. The most common parenteral medications are given intravenously.

_____ 11. Physicians frequently use eye solutions to treat ear conditions.

_____ 12. Otic drugs (ear preparations) are always sterile.

_____ 13. If inhalers are not used properly, the medication is swallowed rather than inhaled into the lungs.

_____ 14. When the outside of a box is labeled "refrigerate or keep frozen," the contents can be left at room temperature.

_____ 15. New dosage forms are always being invented both for convenience and to achieve the best results.

MULTIPLE CHOICE

Complete each question by circling the best answer.

1. The directions for use of a medication are "ii gtts os bid." The route of administration is:
   A. Right eye
   B. Left eye
   C. Right ear
   D. Left ear

2. Which of the following is the abbreviation for "before meals"?
   A. ac
   B. pc
   C. hs
   D. au

3. The directions for use of a medication are "Tylenol 80 mg pr q6h prn." What dosage form should be dispensed?
   A. Chew tab
   B. Syrup
   C. Suppository
   D. Enema

4. The directions for use are "Nitrostat 1/200 gr sl prn." How should this be administered?
   A. In the left ear
   B. Very slowly
   C. Under the tongue
   D. Under the skin

5. When a drug is processed by the liver, this is referred to as:
   A. Absorption
   B. Distribution
   C. Metabolism
   D. Excretion

6. Which of the following dosage forms should generally be stored in the refrigerator?
   A. Suppositories
   B. Patches
   C. Enemas
   D. Tablets

7. Which route of administration has the quickest onset of action?
   A. IM
   B. PR
   C. IV
   D. PO

8. The directions for use are "i gtt od qd." The medication may be:
   A. Ear drops
   B. Eye drops
   C. Suppositories
   D. Vaginal tablets

9. The abbreviation NGT refers to:
   A. Nitroglycerin
   B. Nothing by gastrostomy tube
   C. Nasogastric
   D. Nasogastric tube

10. The pharmaceutical abbreviation CD refers to:
    A. Controlled drug
    B. Compact disk
    C. Controlled diffusion
    D. Continuous drip

11. Oral suspensions should always have which auxiliary label?
    A. Keep refrigerated
    B. Shake well
    C. For external use only
    D. May cause drowsiness

12. Tablets are often identified by:
    A. Imprint codes
    B. Shape of tablet
    C. Color of tablet
    D. All of the above

13. A positive aspect of taking tablets, capsules, or any agent by mouth is:
    A. Convenience to the patient
    B. Physicians mainly write for those forms
    C. Injectable forms are expensive
    D. Medication can be taken with water

14. Respiratory solutions are often:
    A. Refrigerated
    B. Packaged in unit dose ampules
    C. For adult use only
    D. Purchased over-the-counter

15. Patients with diabetes may be instructed to buy drug products that are:
    A. Sugar-free
    B. Alcohol-free
    C. Both A and B
    D. None of the above

MATCHING

Matching I

Match the following abbreviations with their meanings.

_____ 1. Inh
_____ 2. PV
_____ 3. SQ
_____ 4. IV
_____ 5. Top
_____ 6. BUC
_____ 7. PR
_____ 8. IM
_____ 9. PO
_____ 10. SL

A. Intravenous
B. Rectal
C. Sublingual
D. By mouth
E. Inhalant
F. Subcutaneous
G. Intramuscular
H. Vaginal
I. Topical
J. Buccal

Matching II

Match the following abbreviations with their meanings.

1. _____ tab
2. _____ elix
3. _____ lot
4. _____ dil
5. _____ cap
6. _____ tinc
7. _____ syr
8. _____ EC tab
9. _____ susp
10. _____ sup

A. Elixir
B. Tincture
C. Suppositories
D. Enteric-coated tablet
E. Suspension
F. Diluent
G. Tablet
H. Lotion
I. Syrup
J. Capsule

FILL IN THE BLANKS

Answer each question by completing the statement in the space provided.

1. Many of the top-selling drugs are available in several different _____ _____.

2. In order to substitute a different dosage form for the one ordered, the prescriber must give _____.

3. Solid agents administered enterally can be given _____, _____, _____, or _____.

4. _____ tablets are convenient for persons who have difficulty swallowing tablets and for children who are unable to swallow large tablets.

5. _____ are sterile, solid dosage forms that consist of drugs and rate-controlling excipients, and they are usually intended for insertion into a body cavity or under the skin.

6. The best approach to discarding a transdermal patch is to fold it, so the adhesive side sticks to itself, wrap it, and discard the patch in such a way that a _____ or _____ would not be able to grasp it.

7. Syrups are _____ based, and elixirs are _____ _____ _____ based.

8. Suppositories may be administered _____ and _____.

9. Oral administration is one of the _____ ways to give medication, because if too much is given there may be time to react before the drug begins to work.

10. _____ is the most commonly used sublingual tablet that treats anginal attacks.

11. Technicians need to pay close attention the _____ _____ for injectable drugs.

12. A _____ formulation can increase the amount of drug brought into the circulatory system.

13. Most of the final _____ of a drug takes place in the liver.

14. All manufactured types of _____ _____ must be approved by the Food and Drug Administration

15. Medications are packaged according to manufacturers' specifications to ensure the _____ and _____ _____ of the drug.

SHORT ANSWER

Write a short response to each question in the space provided.

1. List three classifications of drugs that describe their availability to consumers.

   _____

   _____

2. Describe the "first-pass" effect of drugs in the liver.

   _____

   _____

   _____

3. List four types of capsules.

_____

_____

4. List the common uses for transdermal patches.

_____

_____

5. List seven types of semisolids.

_____

_____

6. List four different influences than can alter drug metabolism.

_____

_____

7. List four routes of drug excretion.

_____

_____

RESEARCH ACTIVITIES

Follow the instructions given in each exercise and provide a response.

1. Visit a local pharmacy. Locate the cough and cold section. Select one brand of medication with the following dosage forms: tablet, capsule, and liquid. What are the active ingredients in all three dosage forms?

2. Visit a local pharmacy. Locate the pain management section. Select one brand of medication with the following dosage forms: tablet, capsule, and liquid. What are the active ingredients in all three dosage forms?

REFLECT CRITICALLY

CRITICAL THINKING

Reply to each question based on what you have learned in the chapter.

1. List as many dosage forms as you can. Write two advantages and two disadvantages of each.
   Example: Tablet—advantage, easy to carry; disadvantage, tastes bad

2. Interpreting prescriptions can be challenging because of the various handwriting styles of physicians. Think of three rules that can make this task easier.

3. Five-year-old Tommy refuses to take his medication for iron deficiency anemia. The pharmacist has tried to mask the taste by using various compounds, but nothing seems to work. His mother finally asks for your help. What would you use that would make Tommy want to take his medicine?

4. Compounding medications unavailable commercially is much like creating a good recipe in the kitchen. Compare and contrast the two tasks. How are they similar, and how do they differ?

RELATE TO PRATICE

LAB SCENARIOS

Medical Abbreviations

Objective: To introduce the pharmacy technician to the many abbreviations that may be encountered in the practice of pharmacy, regardless of the pharmacy setting.

Lab Activity #5.1: Write the meanings of the following medical abbreviations.

Equipment needed:

- Pencil/pen
- Medical dictionary

Time needed to complete this activity: 30 minutes

Part 1

1. BM _____

2. BPH _____

3. CAD _____

4. COPD _____

5. DDS _____

6. HA _____

7. HBP _____

8. HTN _____

9. MD _____

10. OA _____

11. SLE _____

12. Dx _____

13. TB _____

14. TIA _____

15. UC _____

16. URI _____

Part 2

1. BP _____

2. BS _____

3. CHF _____

4. CP _____

5. DJD _____

6. GERD _____

7. UTI _____

8. GI _____

9. hr _____

10. PVCs _____

11. RA _____

12. SOB _____

13. Sx _____

14. TED _____

15. TX _____

Medical Terminology

Objective: To become familiar with the meanings of prefixes, suffixes, and root words used in medical terminology.

Lab Activity #5.2: Interpreting the meanings of prefixes, suffixes, and root words that are found in medical literature associated with the practice of pharmacy.

Equipment needed:

■ Medical terminology book
■ Pencil/pen

Time needed to complete this activity: 60 minutes

Complete the following table of prefixes used in medical terminology.

Prefix	Meaning	Prefix	Meaning
a-; an-; ana-		micro-	
ab-		multi-	
ante-		neo-	
anti-		non-	
auto-		oligo-	
bi-		pan-	
brady-		para-	
carcin-		per-	
contra-		peri-	
dys-		poly-	
ect-		post-	
en-		pre-	
endo-		primi-	
epi-		retro-	
ex-		semi-	
hemi-		sub-	
hyper-		super-	
hypo-		supra-	
infra-		sym-	
inter-		syn-	
intra-		tachy-	
iso-		tri-	
macro-		uni-	
mal-		xero-	

Complete the following table of suffixes found in medical terminology.

Suffix	Meaning	Suffix	Meaning
-ac; -al; -ar; -ary		-paresis	
-algia		-pathy	
-cele		-penia	
-centesis		-pepsia	
-crine		-phagia	
-crit		-phobia	
-cyte		-phonia	

Continued

57

Suffix	Meaning	Suffix	Meaning
-cytosis		-phoresis	
-desis		-phoria	
-ectomy		-plasty	
-emesis		-plegia	
-emia		-pnea	
-genesis		-poiesis	
-globin; -globulin		-r/rhage; -r/rhagia	
-gram		-rrhea	
-graph		-rhexis	
-graphy		-scler/o	
-ia; -iac; -ic		-scope	
-ism		-scopy	
-it is		-somnia	
-lysis; -lytic		-spasm	
-malacia		-stasis	
-megaly		-sten/o	
-oid		-therapy	
-logist		-thorax	
-logy		-tocia	
-oma		-tripsy	
-osis		-trophy	
-stomy		-tropin	

Complete the following table of root words found in medical terminology.

Root Word—Combining Forms	Meaning	Root Word—Combining Forms	Meaning
Abdomen/o		mast/o	
aden/o		melan/o	
adipo/o		men/o	
amino		metacarp/o	
andr/o		metatars/o	
angi/o		morph/o	
aque/o		muc/o	
arteri/o		my/o	
arteriol/o		myc/o	
arthr/o		myel/o	
ather/o		miring/o	

Root Word—Combining Forms	Meaning	Root Word—Combining Forms	Meaning
audi/o		narc/o	
aur/o		nat/o	
bil/i		nephr/o	
blephar/o		neur/o	
bronch/o		noct/o	
bronchiol/o		nyctal/o	
bucc/o		ocul/o	
calc/i		onch/o	
capn/o		oophor/o	
carcin/o		ophthalm/o	
cardi/o		opt/o	
carp/o		or/o	
cephal/o		orch/o	
cerebr/o		orchi/o	
chol/e		orchid/o	
cholangi/o		orth/o	
cholecyst/o		oste/o	
chondr/o		ot/o	
coagul/o		ovari/o	
cochle/o		ox/o	
col/o		pachy/o	
conjunctiv/o		pancreat/o	
cor/o		par/o	
corne/o		part/o	
coron/o		patell/o	
cost/o		pector/o	
crani/o		ped/o	
cry/o		pelv/i	
cut/o		perine/o	
cutane/o		peritone/o	
cyan/o		phag/o	
cyst/o		phalang/o	
cyt/o		pharyng/o	
dacry/o		phleb/o	
dent/i		phot/o	
derm/o		phren/o	
dermat/o		pil/o	

Continued

Chapter **5 Dosage Forms and Routes of Administration**

Root Word—Combining Forms	Meaning	Root Word—Combining Forms	Meaning
dipl/o		pneum/o	
dips/o		pod/o	
duoden/o		proct/o	
dur/a		psych/o	
electr/o		pub/o	
embry/o		pulmon/o	
encephal/o		py/o	
enter/o		pyel/o	
eosin/o		quadr/i	
epis/i		radi/o	
erythr/o		rect/o	
esophag/o		ren/o	
fasci/o		retin/o	
femor/o		rhabdomy/o	
fet/o		rheumat/o	
fibul/o		rhin/o	
fund/o		salping/o	
gastr/o		sarc/o	
gingiv/o		semin/o	
glauc/o		septi	
gli/o		sial/o	
glomerul/o		sinus/o	
gloss/o		somat/o	
gluc/o		spermat/o	
glyc/o		spher/o	
gonad/o		sphygm/o	
gravid/a		spir/o	
gyn/o		splen/o	
gynec/o		spondyl/o	
hem/o		steth/o	
hemangi/o		stomat/o	
hemat/o		synovi/o	
hepat/o		tars/o	
hidr/o		ten/o	
humer/o		tendon/o	
hydr/o		test/o	
hyster/o		testicul/o	
ile/o		thorac/o	

Root Word—Combining Forms	Meaning	Root Word—Combining Forms	Meaning
ili/o		thromb/o	
immune/o		thyr/o	
is/o		trache/o	
jejun/o		tympan/o	
kal/i		ur/o	
kinesi/o		urethr/o	
lacrim/o		vas/o	
lact/o		ven/o	
lapar/o		xanth/o	
laryng/o		lip/o	
ligament/o		lumb/o	
lingu/o		mamm/o	

Dosage Forms, Routes of Administration, and Storage

Objective: To become familiar with dosage forms, routes of administration, and storage requirements for drugs commonly prescribed.

Lab Activity #5.3: Using a pharmacy reference book, find the dosage form availability, route of administration, and storage requirements for each drug listed.

Equipment needed:

■ *Drug Facts and Comparisons* or *USP DI* reference book
■ Pencil/pen

Time needed to complete this activity: 60 minutes

Complete the following table for drugs commonly prescribed.

Drug	Dosage Forms Available	Routes of Administration	Storage
acetaminophen			
albuterol			
alprazolam			
amoxicillin			
budesonide			
ciprofloxacin			
clindamycin			
clonidine			
diphenhydramine			
erythromycin			
fluticasone			
furosemide			
insulin detemir			
insulin glargine			

Continued

Drug	Dosage Forms Available	Routes of Administration	Storage
ipratropium bromide			
isosorbide mononitrate			
labetalol			
lidocaine			
lorazepam			
montelukast			
nitroglycerin			
penicillin			
promethazine			
succinylcholine			
triamcinolone			

Cleaning Nebulizer Equipment

Objective: To learn the steps to properly clean a nebulizer and its tubing in order to avoid infection.

Lab Activity #5.4: Properly explain and demonstrate, to your partner, how to clean a nebulizer kit.

Equipment needed:

- Nebulizer kit (tubing and nebulizer chamber)
- Warm water
- Soap
- Vinegar
- Paper towel

Time needed to complete this activity: 30 minutes

PROCEDURAL STEPS

1. After each treatment, rinse nebulizer cup with warm water.
2. Empty nebulizer cup of excess water and let air dry.
3. At the end of the day, wash nebulizer cup, mask, or mouthpiece in warm soapy water; rinse and allow to air dry.
4. Every third day, disinfect the equipment using a vinegar/water solution (1/2 cup white vinegar with 1½ cups water).
5. Soak for 20 minutes and rinse well under a steady stream of water.
6. Remove excess water and allow to air dry on a paper towel.
7. Make sure all equipment is completely dry before storing in a plastic zip lock bag.

Procedural Step	Yes/No
Explained and demonstrated how to rinse nebulizer cup with warm water after each treatment.	
Explained and demonstrated how to empty nebulizer cup of excess water and let air dry.	
Explained and demonstrated how to wash nebulizer cup, mask or mouthpiece in warm soapy water, rinse and allow to air dry at the end of each day.	
Explained and demonstrated how to disinfect the equipment using a vinegar/water solution (1/2 cup white vinegar with 1 ½ cups water) every third day.	
Explained and demonstrated how to soak for 20 minutes and rinse well under a steady stream of water.	
Explained and demonstrated how to remove excess water and allow to air dry on a paper towel.	
Explained and demonstrated how to make sure all equipment is completely dry before storing in a plastic zip lock bag.	

6 Conversions and Calculations

TERMS AND DEFINITIONS

Select the correct term from the following list and write the corresponding letter in the blank next to the statement.

A. Alligation
B. Apothecary System
C. Avoirdupois System
D. Conversion Factor
E. Diluent
F. Dilution
G. Drip Rate
H. Drop Factor
I. Flow Rate
J. Household System
K. International Time
L. International System of Units
M. Markup
N. Metric System
O. Retail Price
P. Volume
Q. Wholesale Cost

_____ 1. A mathematical method of solving problems that involves the mixing of two solutions or two solids possessing different percentage weights to achieve a desired third strength

_____ 2. Amount, usually a percentage, added to a wholesale price in order to make a profit

_____ 3. A fraction that is used for converting one unit to another without changing the value of the number

_____ 4. Amount of liquid enclosed within a container

_____ 5. A system of measurement once used in the practice of pharmacy to measure both volume and weight

_____ 6. Wholesale price plus markup

_____ 7. An inert product, either liquid or solid, that is added to a preparation to reduce the strength of the original product

_____ 8. 24-hour method of keeping time in which hours are not distinguished between AM and PM but are counted continuously throughout the entire day

_____ 9. The size of drops coming through the tubing; measured in gtt/mL, found on the tubing package

_____ 10. Purchase price of a product (in this case medicine), which is then marked up for resale

_____ 11. A system of measurement previously used in pharmacy for the determination of weight in ounces and pounds

_____ 12. System of measurement commonly used in the United States; measures volumes using household utensils

_____ 13. The process of adding a diluent or solvent to a compound, resulting in a product of increased volume or weight and lower concentration

_____ 14. The number of drops (gtt) administered over a specific time via an intravenous infusion, for example, gtt/min

_____ 15. System of measurement based on seven base units with prefixes that change units by multiples of 10 that are taken from the French Système International d'Unités

_____ 16. Amount of IV solution administered over a period of time, for example, mL/min, mL/hr, gtt/min

_____ 17. Approved system of measurement for pharmacy in the United States based on multiples of 10.

TRUE OR FALSE

Write T or F next to each statement.

_____ 1. The ability to manipulate conversions is a required competency of pharmacy technicians.

_____ 2. Not all transcriptions and calculations need to be checked by a pharmacist.

_____ 3. A pharmacy technician can assume that a person understands the meaning of a measurement.

_____ 4. It is important to place the proper units (mL, L, mg, or g) next to the number amount.

_____ 5. One of the most common errors made in pharmacy is placing a zero in front of a decimal.

_____ 6. A pharmacy technician should convert measurements to the metric system because it is the approved system of measurement for pharmacy in the United States.

_____ 7. Calculations should be checked at least three times before asking a pharmacist to check them.

_____ 8. The pharmacy technician should show the parent of a pediatric patient how to measure the correct dosage.

_____ 9. If you round off at each step of a calculation, your answer will be very accurate.

_____ 10. If an IM dose is calculated to be greater than 5 mL, an error has occurred in either the prescribed amount or the calculation.

MULTIPLE CHOICE

Complete each question by circling the best answer.

1. The cost of 100 g of hydrocortisone powder is $36.00. What would be the cost of 12 g?
   A. $5.42
   B. $4.32
   C. $10.60
   D. $8.94

2. A 125-pound patient weighs how many kilograms?
   A. 0.125
   B. 125,000
   C. 56.82
   D. 275

3. Convert 1200 mg to grams.
   A. 12,000
   B. 12
   C. 120
   D. 1.2

4. Of the following, volume best refers to the measurement of:
   A. Liquids
   B. Dry ingredients
   C. Distance
   D. None of the above

5. The weight of 1 grain is:
   A. 60 mg
   B. 64 mg
   C. 65 mg
   D. All of the above; different measurement systems define grains in different weights

6. There are 1000 milligrams in 1
   A. Kilogram
   B. Gram
   C. Milligram
   D. Microgram

7. A freight box that weighs 633 kg weighs how many pounds?
   A. 0.633
   B. 1392.6
   C. 287.73
   D. 28.77

8. 25 teaspoons = _____ mL.
   A. 100
   B. 250
   C. 375
   D. 125

9. A pharmacy wants to increase the price of a product by 35%. How much would an item cost with this markup if its original cost was $6.75?
   A. $6.95
   B. $8.21
   C. $12.50
   D. $9.11

10. The approximate size of a container used to dispense 120 mL of a liquid medication would be:
    A. 6 oz
    B. 4 oz
    C. 8 oz
    D. 2 oz

11. A physician orders ampicillin 0.5 g PO q6h. The medication available is ampicillin 125 mg/5 mL. What is the quantity of medication to be administered per dose?
    A. 20 mL
    B. 2 mL
    C. 0.2 mL
    D. 0.02 mL

12. The physician orders atropine 1/150 gr PO bid. The atropine available is 0.4 mg per tablet. The nurse will administer how many tablets per dose? (Use 60 mg/gr.)
    A. 0.5
    B. 0.75
    C. 1
    D. 1.5

13. A prescription is written for Pen VK 500 mg tabs PO qid for 10 days. The patient, who has throat cancer and cannot swallow, requests a liquid form. What volume of a 250 mg/5 mL suspension should be dispensed to fulfill the prescription?
    A. 40 mL
    B. 400 mL
    C. 150 mL
    D. 250 mL

14. A pharmacist dispenses 300 mL of amoxicillin 150 mg/5 mL suspension. The sig is 250 mg PO tid. How many days will the prescription last?
    A. 7
    B. 10
    C. 12
    D. 14

15. The physician's order is for Timoptic ii gtts ou bid. How many drops will the patient get in 12 days?
    A. 4
    B. 48
    C. 69
    D. 96

16. You receive an order for Kaopectate 15 mL bid prn. One dose equals how many tablespoonfuls?
    A. 2
    B. 3
    C. 1
    D. 1.5

17. Mylanta and Donnatal are to be combined in a 2:1 ratio. How many milliliters of each is required to make 120 mL of the suspension?
    A. 70 mL/50 mL
    B. 50 mL/70 mL
    C. 80 mL/40 mL
    D. 40 mL/80 mL

18. An IV solution is ordered to run at 3.5 gtts/min. It contains 875 mg in a total of 250 mL. How many milligrams will the patient receive per hour if the set is calibrated to deliver 12 gtts/mL?
    A. 0.16 mg/hr
    B. 16 mg/hr
    C. 61.25 mg/hr
    D. 610 mg/hr

19. The Roman numeral XLVIII is equivalent to:
    A. 43
    B. 48
    C. 53
    D. 68

20. Convert 12:14 AM to military (international) time.
    A. 1214
    B. 0214
    C. 0014
    D. 0140

21. The Roman numeral LVIII is equivalent to:
    A. 58
    B. 48
    C. 43
    D. 68

22. How many days will the following prescription last?
    Zoloft 100 mg #90
    Sig: 1 PO bid
    A. 55
    B. 30
    C. 45
    D. 90

23. A dose is written for 10 mg/kg every 12 hours for 1 day. The adult taking this medication weighs 165 pounds. How much drug will be needed for this order?
    A. 425 mg
    B. 950 mg
    C. 750 mg
    D. 1500 mg

24. How many tablets would be needed for the following prescription?
    Prednisone tablets 10 mg
    One qid for 6 days; one tid for 3 days; one bid for 1 day; then stop
    A. 35
    B. 15
    C. 25
    D. 45

25. Using the following DEA formula, what should be the last digit of this DEA number?
    AB461853 _____
    DEA formula: Add first+third+fifth numbers = _____
    Add second+fourth+sixth numbers = then multiply by 2 = _____
    Add the two sums together; the last digit on the right should be the last digit of the number:
    A. 7
    B. 4
    C. 2
    D. 8

26. A dosage of 0.75 g is prescribed. You have in stock 250 mg/mL. How many milliliters would be given using the dosage strength on hand?
    A. 1
    B. 15
    C. 3
    D. 500

27. How many milligrams of epinephrine is needed to prepare 3 L of a 1:30,000 solution?
    A. 0.1
    B. 1
    C. 10
    D. 100

28. How many liters of a 0.9% normal saline solution can be made from 60 g of NaCl?
    A. 6.67
    B. 66.7
    C. 667
    D. 6667

29. If 5 mL of diluent is added to a vial containing 2 g of a drug for injection, resulting in a final volume of 5.8 mL, what is the concentration in milligrams per milliliters of the drug in the reconstituted solution?
    A. 0.3 mg/mL
    B. 345 mg/mL
    C. 444 mg/mL
    D. 2035 mg/mL

30. Which prescription instructions would require 21 tablets to be dispensed?
    A. One tab PO bid for 8 d
    B. One tab ac and hs for 4 d
    C. One tab tid for 3 d; one tab bid for 3 d; one qd for 3 d
    D. Three tabs bid for 2 d; two tabs qd for 3 d; one tab qd for 3 d

Chapter 6 Conversions and Calculations

31. How many grams of potassium permanganate is required to prepare 2 quarts of a 1:750 solution of potassium permanganate?
   A. 1.28
   B. 3
   C. 2.56
   D. 5

32. If the dosage of a drug is 35 mg/kg/day in six divided doses, how much would be given in each dose to a 38-pound child?
   A. 17.3 mg
   B. 60.4 mg
   C. 101 mg
   D. 604 mg

33. To make 300 mL of a 5% dextrose solution, using 10% dextrose solution and water, how much of each do you need?
   A. 150 mL dextrose 10% solution and 150 mL water
   B. 175 mL dextrose 10% solution and 125 mL water
   C. 180 mL dextrose 10% solution and 120 mL water
   D. 200 mL dextrose 10% solution and 100 mL water

34. How many capsules, each containing 1.5 gr of a drug, can be filled completely from a 28 g bottle of the drug? (Use 60 mg/gr.)
   A. 24
   B. 32
   C. 311
   D. 431

35. An IV solution containing 20,000 units of heparin in 500 mL of 0.45% NaCl solution is to be infused to provide 1000 units of heparin per hour. Roughly how many drops per minute should be infused to deliver the desired dose if the IV set calibrates at 15 gtt/mL?
   A. 0.42 gtt/min
   B. 6.3 gtt/min
   C. 0.16 gtt/min
   D. 44.4 gtt/min

FILL IN THE BLANKS

Conversions

Convert the following measurements:

1. 8 ounces = _____ mL

2. 90 mL = _____ oz

3. 3 kg = _____ g

4. 2 pints = _____ cups

5. 3.5 = _____ %

6. 0.25 = _____ %

7. 1.5 gr = _____ mg

8. 55 lb = _____ kg

9. 125 kg = _____ lb

10. 2500 mL = _____ L

11. 0.15 mg = _____ mcg

12. 3600 mL = _____ pts

13. 78 mg = _____ gr

14. 33% = _____ decimal

15. 40% = _____ decimal

Roman numerals and Arabic numbers

Interpret the following:

1. XV _____

2. XCIV _____

3. 250 _____

4. 49 _____

5. MDX _____

6. XXXIII _____

7. 125 _____

8. 60 _____

9. IX _____

10. CC _____

International Time

Convert each time to either international or standard time:

1. 0330 = _____

2. 4:45 PM = _____

3. 1430 = _____

4. 1715 = _____

5. 8:20 PM = _____

6. 9:40 AM = _____

7. 2300 = _____

8. 9:10 PM = _____

9. 1925 = _____

10. 11:30 AM = _____

Temperature

Convert to Fahrenheit or Celsius as appropriate:

1. 212° F = _____ ° C

2. 32° C = _____ ° F

3. 66° C = _____ ° F

4. 104° F = _____ ° C

5. 32° F = _____ ° C

6. 2° C = _____ ° F

7. 8° C = _____ ° F

8. 48° F = _____ ° C

9. 25° C = _____ ° F

10. 85° F = _____ ° C

MATCHING

Match the conversion factors with their correct equivalents.

A. 5 mL
B. 15 mL
C. 30 mL
D. 480 mL
E. 3840 mL
F. 454 g
G. 1 ounce
H. 8 ounces
I. 2.2 lb

_____ 1. 1 gallon

_____ 2. 30 grams

_____ 3. 1 tablespoon

_____ 4. 1 pint

_____ 5. 1 cup

_____ 6. 1 kg

_____ 7. 1 teaspoon

_____ 8. 1 fluid ounce

_____ 9. 1 pound

SHORT ANSWER

Write a short response to each question in the space provided.

1. Give the units used in the metric system for the following:

A. Volume

_____

B. Weight

_____

2. Give the units used in the household system for the following:

   A. Volume

   _____

   B. Weight

   _____

3. Give the units used in the apothecary system for the following:

   A. Liquids

   _____

   B. Dry weights

   _____

4. Give the units used in the avoirdupois system for the following:

   A. Liquids

   _____

   B. Weights

   _____

RESEARCH ACTIVITIES

Follow the instructions given in each exercise and provide a response.

1. Access the website *http://www.medcalc.com/body.html*. Use the BSA calculator to determine the BSA of the following:

   A. Patient: length 62 inches; weight 59 kg

      BSA = _____

   B. Patient: length 65 inches; weight 145 lb

      BSA = _____

   C. Patient: length 21 inches; weight 7 lb

      BSA = _____

   D. Patient: length 48 inches; weight 20 kg

      BSA = _____

   E. Patient: length 68 inches; weight 170 lb

      BSA = _____

2. Access one of the continuing education websites for pharmacy technicians listed in Chapter 3 and find a continuing education course on pharmacy calculations.

   A. Where was the continuing education course found?

   B. Is the continuing education course for both pharmacists and pharmacy technicians?

   C. Does the continuing education course cover topics not mentioned in this chapter? If so, which topics?

   D. Is the continuing education course a good review of the calculations pharmacy technicians should know?

   E. Complete the continuing education course and turn in results to your instructor.

REFLECT CRITICALLY

CRITICAL THINKING

Reply to each question based on what you have learned in the chapter.

1. Bobbi is a second semester pharmacy technician student. She is having difficulty with her calculations course. Although the instructor assures her it is necessary to have a solid working knowledge of pharmacy math, she is not sure she will really ever have to use it on the job. How would you convince Bobbi of the importance of a strong calculations foundation?

2. Proper decimal notation is crucial in pharmacy calculations, and technicians cannot afford to misread a prescription. What would be the outcome if a pharmacy technician mistook 5 mcg for 5 mg and the pharmacist did not catch the error?

3. A compounding pharmacy receives an order for a 1% ointment. The technician weighs out 2 g of the active ingredient. What is the final weight of the correctly compounded prescription?

4. A technician is filling a medication for a 4-year-old child. The average adult dose is 250 mg. How much medication should the child receive?

RELATE TO PRACTICE

LAB SCENARIOS

Pharmacy Conversions

Objective: To introduce and review various pharmacy math conversions with the pharmacy technician.

Prescribers write prescriptions and medication orders using a variety of measurement systems, which include metric, household, apothecary, and avoirdupois systems. Two advantages of the metric system are (1) that its tables are simple to understand because they are based on the decimal system, and (2) that the greater of two consecutive denominations is always ten times the lesser amount.

The basic units of measurements of the metric system are as follows:

- The meter for length
- The liter for volume
- The gram for weight

The metric system is the official system of the United States Pharmacopeia (USP). However, the pharmacy technician must be familiar with the other systems of measurement when interpreting prescription and medication orders.

Lab Activity #6.1: Identify the meaning of the following metric prefixes.

Equipment needed:

- Pencil/pen

Time needed to complete this activity: 5 minutes

1. micro- _____
2. milli- _____
3. centi- _____
4. deci- _____
5. deca- _____
6. hecto- _____
7. kilo- _____

Lab Activity #6.2: Convert the following measurements. Make sure to use decimals with the metric system! It is common practice to use fractions with household measurements.

Equipment needed:
- Pencil/pen
- Calculator

Time needed to complete this activity: 30 minutes

1. 250 mcg = _____ mg

2. 100 mg = _____ g

3. 10 g = _____ mg

4. 12 fl oz = _____ pt

5. 2 pt = _____ gal

6. 2500 g = _____ kg

7. 10 tbsp = _____ fl oz

8. 480 mL = _____ qt

9. 5 kg = _____ g

10. 12 tsp = _____ tbsp

11. 3 gr = _____ mg

12. 144 tsp = _____ gal

13. 6 tbsp = _____ mL

14. 1500 mcg = _____ g

15. 30 mL = _____ tsp

16. 6 fl oz = _____ tsp

17. 12 fl oz = _____ cup

18. 0.4 kg = _____ mg

19. 360 mL = _____ cup

20. 0.5g = _____ mcg

21. 480 mL = _____ gal

22. 8 tsp = _____ mL

23. 0.1 mg = _____ mcg

24. 1 pt = _____ tsp

25. 12 tsp = _____ cup

26. 720 mL = _____ pt

27. 32 fl oz = _____ qt

28. 325 mg = _____ gr

29. 48 tsp = _____ pt

30. 1 cup = _____ pt

31. 12 tbsp = _____ tsp

32. 120 mL = _____ fl oz

33. 4 cup = _____ gal

34. 24 tsp = _____ fl oz

35. 4 pt = _____ qt

36. 24 tbsp = _____ cup

37. 4 fl oz = _____ mL

38. 90 mL = _____ tbsp

39. 8 fl oz = _____ tbsp

40. 0.5 kg = _____ mcg

41. 64 fl oz = _____ gal

42. 2 cup = _____ mL

43. 1/2 gal = _____ pt

44. 1/2 cup = _____ tbsp

45. 1 qt = _____ fl oz

46. 1 cup = _____ fl oz

47. 96 tbsp = _____ qt

48. 1/4 gal = _____ fl oz

49. 2 cup = _____ qt

50. 96 tsp = _____ qt

51. 2 pt = _____ mL

52. 1 pt = _____ fl oz

53. 1 cup = _____ tsp

54. 2 pt = _____ cup

55. 2 gal = _____ cup

56. 2 qt = _____ mL

57. 1½ qt = _____ tsp

58. 1 qt = _____ tbsp

59. 2 qt = _____ pt

60. 1 qt = _____ gal

61. 2 gal = _____ mL

62. 1/4 gal = _____ tsp

63. 1 gal = _____ tbsp

64. 8 pt = _____ tbsp

65. 48 tbsp = _____ pt

66. 1 gal = _____ qt

Reducing and Enlarging a Formula

Objective: To introduce and review with the pharmacy technician the steps needed to enlarge or reduce a prescription.

A pharmacy technician may receive a prescription or medication order that requires enlargement or reduction of the formula for a compound. The technician may be required to calculate the quantity of each ingredient in the compound. A ratio and proportion may be expressed in specific quantities for each ingredient or in parts. To enlarge or reduce a formula using specific quantities, the following formula may be used:

$$\frac{Quantity\ of\ ingredient\ in\ original\ formula}{Total\ quantity\ of\ original\ formula} = \frac{Quantity\ of\ ingredient\ desired}{Total\ quantity\ desired}$$

Normally this will be solved with X as the unknown *quantity of ingredient desired* to make a reduced or increased amount of medication.

If the order is written using parts, the following formula can be used:

$$\frac{Number\ of\ parts\ of\ ingredient\ in\ original\ formula}{Total\ number\ of\ parts\ in\ original\ formula} = \frac{Number\ of\ parts\ of\ ingredient\ desired}{Total\ number\ of\ parts\ desired}$$

Normally this will be solved with X as the unknown *number of parts of ingredients desired*.

Chapter **6** **Conversions and Calculations**

Lab Activity #6.3: Reducing and enlarging a prescription. Calculate the correct quantities of each ingredient needed to prepare the following compounds.

Equipment needed:

- Pencil/pen
- Calculator

Time needed to complete this activity: 30 min

1. Following is the formula to compound 1000 g of Yellow Ointment, USP:

Yellow Wax	50 g
Petrolatum	950 g

How much of each ingredient should be used to prepare 2 ounces of Yellow Ointment, USP?

Yellow Wax _____

Petrolatum _____

2. Following is the formula for Calamine Lotion:

Calamine	80 g
Zinc Oxide	80 g
Glycerin	20 g
Bentonite Magma	250 mL
Calcium Hydroxide qs	1000 mL

How much of each ingredient should be used to prepare 8 fluid ounces of Calamine Lotion?

Calamine _____

Zinc Oxide _____

Glycerin _____

Bentonite Magma _____

Calcium Hydroxide qs _____

3. Following is the formula for Benzoin Tincture Compound:

Benzoin	100 g
Aloe	20 g
Storax	80 g
Tolu Balsam	40 g
Alcohol qs	1000 mL

How much of each ingredient should be used in this preparation to make one quart of Benzoin Tincture Compound?

Benzoin _____

Aloe _____

Storax _____

Tolu Balsam _____

Alcohol qs _____

4. Following is the formula for Coal Tar Ointment:

Coal Tar	5 parts
Zinc Oxide	10 parts
Hydrophilic Ointment	50 parts

How much of each ingredient should be used to make one pound of Coal Tar Ointment?

Coal Tar _____

Zinc Oxide _____

Hydrophilic Ointment _____

5. Following is the formula to prepare 1000 g of Hydrophilic Petrolatum, USP:

Cholesterol	30 g
Stearyl Alcohol	30 g
White Wax	80 g
White Petrolatum	860 g

How much of each ingredient should be used to prepare ½ pound of Hydrophilic Petrolatum, USP?

Cholesterol _____

Stearyl Alcohol _____

White Wax _____

White Petrolatum _____

6. Following is the formula to prepare about 1000 g of Hydrophilic Ointment, USP:

Methylparaben	0.25 g
Propylparaben	0.15 g
Sodium Lauryl Sulfate	10 g
Propylene Glycol	120 g
Stearyl Alcohol	250 g
White Petrolatum	250 g
Purified Water	370 g

How much of each ingredient should be used to prepare 4 oz of Hydrophilic Ointment, USP?

Methylparaben _____

Propylparaben _____

Sodium Lauryl Sulfate _____

Propylene Glycol _____

Stearyl Alcohol _____

White Petrolatum _____

Purified Water _____

7. Following is the formula to prepare 1000 mL of Benzyl Benzoate Lotion:

Benzyl Benzoate	250 mL
Triethanolamine	5 mL
Oleic Acid	20 mL
Purified Water qs	1000 mL

How much of each ingredient should be used to prepare one pint of Benzyl Benzoate Lotion?

Benzyl Benzoate _____

Triethanolamine _____

Oleic Acid _____

Purified Water qs _____

8. Following is the formula to prepare 1000 mL of Phenobarbital Elixir:

Phenobarbital	4 g
Orange Oil	0.25 mL
Certified Red Color	qs
Alcohol	200 mL
Propylene Glycol	100 mL
Sorbitol Solution	600 mL
Water qs	1000 mL

How much of each ingredient should be used to prepare 2 gallons of Phenobarbital Elixir?

Phenobarbital _____

Orange Oil _____

Certified Red Color _____

Alcohol _____

Propylene Glycol _____

Sorbitol Solution _____

Water qs _____

9. Following is the formula to prepare 1 liter of White Lotion, USP:

Zinc Sulfate	40 g
Sulfurated Potash	40 g
Purified Water qsad	1000 mL

How much of each ingredient should be used to prepare 1 cup of White Lotion, USP?

Zinc Sulfate _____

Sulfurated Potash _____

Purified Water qsad _____

10. Following is the formula to prepare 1 liter of Iodine Topical Solution, USP:

Iodine	20 g
Sodium Iodide	24 g
Purified Water qsad	1000 mL

How much of each ingredient should be used to prepare sixty 15-mL bottles of Iodine Topical Solution, USP?

Iodine _____

Sodium Iodide _____

Purified Water qsad _____

Medication Concentrations (Strengths)

Objective: To become familiar with the concepts of percent weight-weight, weight-volume, and volume-volume.

A medication's concentration (strength) can be expressed mathematically in several different manners, which include a fraction, a ratio, or a percent. The term *percent* or its corresponding sign (%) means "by the hundred," and percentage means "rate per 100." A percent may also be expressed as a ratio represented as a common or decimal fraction. Percents are usually changed to equivalent decimal fractions.

A medication expressed as a percent can be a solid dissolved in another solid, a solid dissolved in a liquid, or a liquid dissolved in another liquid.

- w/w% is defined as the number of grams of solute dissolved in 100 grams of vehicle base.
- w/v% is defined as the number of grams of solute dissolved in 100 milliliters of vehicle base.
- v/v% is defined as the number of milliliters of solute dissolved in 100 milliliters of vehicle base.

The following formula can be used in calculating the amount of solute, the total amount of vehicle base, or its percent.

$$\frac{amount\ of\ solute}{amount\ of\ vehicle\ base} = \frac{x}{100}$$

$$x = \%\ strength$$

The concentration of a weak solution or liquid preparation is frequently expressed in terms of ratio strength. Because all percentages represent a ratio of parts per hundred, ratio strength is another way of expressing the percentage strength of solutions or liquid preparations. For example, 10% means 10 parts per 100 or 10:100. Although 10 parts per 100 designates a ratio strength, it is customary to translate the designation; therefore, 10:100 : 1:10.

When a ratio strength is used to designate a concentration, it is *always* expressed in the form of 1:x.

For example, the ratio strength 1:1000 is to be interpreted as the following:

- For solids in liquids : 1 g of solute in 1000 mL of solution or liquid preparation
- For liquids in liquids : 1 mL of solute in 1000 mL of solution or liquid preparation
- For solids in solids : 1 g of solute in 1000 g of mixture

The following formula can be used to calculate the number of parts, the total number of parts, or the percent of a ratio strength problem:

$$\frac{\#\ parts}{total\ parts} = \frac{x}{100}$$

$$x = \%\ strength$$

Lab Activity #6.4: In the following table, convert the percent strength to ratio strength and ratio strength to percent strength.

Equipment needed:

- Calculator
- Pencil/pen

Time needed to complete this activity: 15 minutes

Percent Strength	Ratio Strength
25%	
	1:200
15%	
	1:400
50%	
	1:150
4%	
	1:500
2%	
	1:175

Lab Activity #6.5: Solve the following problems involving percent strength and ratio strength.

Equipment needed:

- Calculator
- Pencil/pen
- Paper

Time needed to complete this activity: 45 minutes

1. How many grams of antipyrine should be used in preparing the prescription?

   _____

   Rx:
   Antipyrine   5%
   Glycerin   qsad 90 mL
   Sig: gtt v in right ear tid

2. How many grams of resin of podophyllum should be used in preparing the prescription?

   _____

   Rx:
   Resin of Podophyllum   25%
   Compound Benzoin Tincture   qsad 60 mL
   Sig: Apply to papillomas tid

3. How many grams of potassium iodide and ephedrine sulfate should be used in preparing the prescription?

_____

_____

Rx:
Potassium Iodide Solution   10%
Ephedrine Sulfate Solution   3%   aa 45 mL
Sig: Place five drops in water as directed

4. What is the percentage strength (w/w) each of iodochlorhydroxyquin and hydrocortisone in the prescription?

_____

_____

Rx:
Iodochlorhydroxyquin   1.8 g
Hydrocortisone   0.3 g
Cream Base   qsad   60 g
Sig: Apply to the affected areas of skin once a day.

5. How many milligrams of methylparaben are needed to prepare 16 fluid ounces of a solution containing 0.12% (w/v) of methylparaben?

_____

6. A formula for a mouth rinse contains 1/10% (w/v) of zinc chloride. How many grams of zinc chloride should be used in preparing 20 liters of the mouth rinse?

_____

7. If 425 g of sucrose is dissolved in enough water to make 500 mL, what is the percentage strength (w/v) of the solution?

_____

8. How many milliliters of 0.9% (w/v) sodium chloride solution can be made from 1 lb of sodium chloride?

_____

9. One gallon of a certain lotion contains 946 mL of benzyl benzoate. Calculate the percentage (v/v) of benzyl benzoate in the lotion.

_____

10. A liniment contains 15% of methyl salicylate. How many milliliters of the liniment can be made from 1 quart of methyl salicylate?

_____

11. How many grams each of resorcinol and hexachlorophene should be used in preparing 2 pounds of an acne ointment that is to contain 2% resorcinol and 0.25% of hexachlorophene?

_____

_____

12. How many milligrams of procaine hydrochloride should be used in preparing 60 suppositories, each weighing 2 grams and containing 1/4% of procaine hydrochloride?

_____

13. If a topical cream contains 1.8% (w/w) of hydrocortisone, how many milligrams of hydrocortisone should be used in preparing 1 ounce of the cream?

_____

14. A pharmacist incorporates 6 grams of coal tar into 120 grams of a 6% coal tar ointment. Calculate the percentage (w/w) of coal tar in the finished product.

_____

15. Express each of the following concentrations as a ratio strength:

A. 2 mg of active ingredient in mL of solution _____

B. 0.125 mg of active ingredient in 5 mL of solution _____

C. 2 g of active ingredient in 500 mL of solution _____

D. 100 mg of active ingredient in 100 mL of solution _____

16. A vaginal cream contains 0.01% (w/v) of dienestrol. Express this concentration as a ratio strength.

_____

17. How many milligrams each of menthol and hexachlorophene should be used in compounding the prescription?

_____

_____

Rx:
Menthol   1:500
Hexachlorophene   1:800
Hydrophilic Ointment Base   qsad 60 g
Sig: Apply to hands bid

18. Hepatitis B Virus Vaccine Inactivated is inactivated with 1:4000 (w/v) of formalin. Express this ratio strength as a percentage strength.

_____

19. Versed Injection contains 5 mg of midazolam per milliliter of injection. Calculate the ratio strength of midazolam in the injection.

_____

20. A sample of white petrolatum contains 10 mg of tocopherol per kilogram as a preservative. Express the amount of tocopherol as a ratio strength.

_____

Dilution Calculations

Objective: To become familiar with calculations used in the dilution of a product.

A pharmacy may receive a prescription for a medication in which the prescribed concentration is less than what is currently stocked in the pharmacy. The concentration may be written in the form of a percent, fraction, or ratio. In a dilution problem, the initial strength (the stock strength) is greater than the final strength (the desired strength). A diluent (an inert substance that does not have strength—such as water or petrolatum) is added to the initial volume or weight to make the final volume or weight. In other words, the amount of diluent can be calculated by using the following formula:

Final volume (weight) − Initial volume (weight) = Amount of diluent to be added

A dilution problem may be solved using the following formula:

(Initial volume) (Initial strength) = (Final volume) (Final strength)

or

(Initial weight) (Initial strength) = (Final weight) (Final strength)

It is important to remember that both initial and final strengths must be expressed in the same unit of concentration, and that initial and final volumes (weight) must be expressed in the same unit of measurement. It is easiest to change all strengths to percents before solving dilution problems so you may see the equations written as:

(Stock volume/weight) (Stock percent) = (Desired volume/weight) (Desired percent) or

$$SV \cdot SP = DV \cdot DP \quad \text{where amount of diluent needed} = DV - SV$$

$$SW \cdot SP = DW \cdot DP \quad \text{where amount of diluent needed} = DW - SW$$

Lab Activity #6.6: Calculate the quantity of the ingredient needed to prepare the following prescriptions.

Equipment needed:

- Calculator
- Pencil/pen
- Paper

Time to complete this activity: 45 minutes

1. Rx 1:

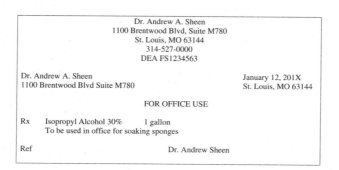

Dr. Andrew A. Sheen
1100 Brentwood Blvd, Suite M780
St. Louis, MO 63144
314-527-0000
DEA FS1234563

Dr. Andrew A. Sheen   January 12, 201X
1100 Brentwood Blvd Suite M780   St. Louis, MO 63144

FOR OFFICE USE

Rx   Isopropyl Alcohol 30%   1 gallon
           To be used in office for soaking sponges

Ref   Dr. Andrew Sheen

The pharmacy has in stock 70% Isopropyl alcohol. How much of the 70% concentration and diluent is needed to prepare this prescription?

Isopropyl Alcohol 70%: _____

Diluent: _____

2. Rx 2:

```
                        Dr. Andrew A. Sheen
                    1100 Brentwood Blvd, Suite M780
                        St. Louis, MO 63144
                           314-527-0000
                          DEA FS1234563

Dr. Andrew A. Sheen                              January 12, 201X
1100 Brentwood Blvd Suite M780                   St. Louis, MO 63144

                         FOR OFFICE USE

Rx      Zephiran 7.5%        1 gallon
        For office use

Ref                                  Dr. Andrew Sheen
```

The pharmacy has in stock Zephiran Chloride 20%. How much of the 20% Zephiran Chloride and diluent is needed to prepare this prescription?

Zephiran Chloride 20%: _____

Diluent: _____

3. Rx 3:

```
                        Dr. Andrew A. Sheen
                    1100 Brentwood Blvd, Suite M780
                        St. Louis, MO 63144
                           314-527-0000
                          DEA FS1234563

Dr. Andrew A. Sheen                              January 12, 201X
1100 Brentwood Blvd Suite M780                   St. Louis, MO 63144

                         FOR OFFICE USE

Rx      Hypochlorous acid 1:10    4 liters
        For office use

Ref                                  Dr. Andrew Sheen
```

The pharmacy has in stock 25% Hypochlorous Acid. How much of the 25% Hypochlorous Acid and diluent is needed to prepare this order?

Hypochlorous Acid 25%: _____

Diluent: _____

4. How many milliliters of a ½% solution of gentian violet should be used in preparing the prescription?

   _____

   Rx   Gentian Violet Solution   1:100,000   500 mL
   Sig: Use as a mouthwash

5. How many milliliters of a 17% solution of benzalkonium chloride should be used in preparing the prescription?

   _____

   Rx   Benzalkonium Chloride Solution   240 mL
   Make a solution such that 10 mL diluted to a liter equals a 1:5000 solution.
   Sig: 10 mL diluted to a liter for external use

6. How many milliliters of a 1:50 (w/v) boric acid solution can be prepared from 500 mL of a 5% (w/v) boric acid solution?

_____

7. How many milliliters of water must be added to 250 mL of a 25% (w/v) stock solution of sodium chloride to prepare a 0.9% (w/v) sodium chloride solution?

_____

8. How many milliliters of a 1% (w/v) solution of phenyl mercuric nitrate may be used in preparing a 100-mL prescription requiring 1:50,000 (w/v) of phenyl mercuric nitrate as a preservative?

_____

9. How many milliliters of water should be added to 1gallon of 70% isopropyl alcohol to prepare a 30% solution for soaking sponges?

_____

10. How many milliliters of water should be added to a liter of 1:3000 (w/v) solution to make a 1:8000 (w/v) solution?

_____

11. How many milliliters of water for injection must be added to 10 liters of a 50% (w/v) dextrose injection to reduce the concentration to 30% (w/v)?

_____

12. A physician orders 1 pint of 10% ethyl alcohol. The stock solution is 200 mL of 95% ethyl alcohol. How many milliliters of the 95% stock solution would be necessary to prepare the 10% solution?

_____

13. The pharmacy has 300 mL of a 50% solution. 200 mL is added to this solution to reduce the concentration. How many grams of active ingredient would be included in 4 fluid ounces of the diluted solution?

_____

14. How many grams of salicylic acid should be added to 75 g of a polyethylene glycol ointment to prepare an ointment containing 6% (w/w) of salicylic acid?

_____

15. How many grams of petrolatum (diluent) should be added to 250 g of ichthammol ointment to make a 5% ointment?

_____

Lab Activity #6.7: Calculate the final strength of the compound to appear on the prescription label from the following prescription.

Equipment needed:

- Calculator
- Pencil/pen
- Paper

Time needed to complete this activity: 30 minutes

1. If 250 mL of a 1/800 (v/v) solution is diluted to 1 liter, what will be the ratio strength (v/v)?

    _____

2. Aluminum acetate topical solution contains 5% (w/v) of aluminum acetate. When 100 mL is diluted to a 0.5 liter, what will be the resulting ratio strength?

    _____

3. If 500 mL of a 10% (w/v) solution is diluted to 2 liters, what will be the ratio strength (w/v)?

    _____

4. If 2 tablespoonfuls of povidone-iodine solution (10% w/v) is diluted to 1 quart with purified water, what is the ratio strength of the dilution?

    _____

5. If 400 mL of a 20% (w/v) solution is diluted to 2 liters, what will be the ratio strength?

    _____

6. If a 0.067% (w/v) methylbenzethonium chloride lotion is diluted with an equal volume of water, what will be the ratio strength (w/v) of the dilution?

    _____

7. In preparing a solution for a wet dressing, two 0.3-g tablets of potassium permanganate are dissolved in 1 gallon of purified water. What will be the percentage strength (w/v) of the solution?

    _____

8. If 150 mL of a 17% (w/v) concentrate of benzalkonium chloride is diluted to 5 gallons, what will be the ratio strength?

    _____

9. If a pharmacy technician adds 3 g of hydrocortisone to 60 g of a 5% (w/w) hydrocortisone cream, what is the final percentage strength of hydrocortisone in the product?

    _____

10. If 20 mL of a 2% (w/v) solution is diluted with water to 8 pints, what is the ratio strength (w/v) of the solution?

    _____

Alligation Calculations

Objective: Perform pharmacy calculations using both alligation medial and alligation alternate in compounding prescriptions with multiple strengths of a medication.

Alligation medial is a method by which the "weighted average" percentage strength of a mixture of *two or more* substances of known quantity and concentration may be easily calculated. By this method, the percentage strength of each component expressed as a decimal fraction is multiplied by its corresponding quantity (volume or weight); then the sum of the products is placed over the total quantity and a ratio and proportion is solved to find the amount per 100 or the percent strength. Alligation medial can be used with both solids and liquids.

For example, consider the following problem. What is the percentage strength in a mixture of 300 mL of a 40% (v/v) alcohol, 100 mL of a 60% (v/v) alcohol, and 100 mL of a 70% alcohol?

$$0.4 \times 300 \text{ mL} = 120 \text{ mL}$$

$$0.6 \times 100 \text{ mL} = 60 \text{ mL}$$

$$0.7 \times 100 \text{ mL} = 70 \text{ mL}$$

500 mL total quantity and 250 mL alcohol

$$250 \text{ mL}/500 \text{ mL} = x/100$$

x = 50 so the resultant solution is 50% strength

Alligation alternate, which uses a tic-tac-toe style, is a method by which we calculate the number of parts of *two* components of a given strength needed to prepare a mixture of a different desired strength. The desired strength of the compound must be between the strengths of the two medications on hand. This method is demonstrated in detail in the textbook.

Lab Activity #6.8: Practice pharmacy calculations using alligation medial and alligation alternate.

Equipment needed:

- Calculator
- Pencil/pen
- Paper

Time needed to complete this activity: 45 minutes

1. Four equal amounts of belladonna extract, containing 1.15%, 1.3%, 1.35%, and 1.2% of alkaloids, respectively, were mixed. What was the percentage strength of the mixture?

   _____

2. What is the percentage of alcohol in a mixture containing 150 mL of witch hazel (14% alcohol), 200 mL of glycerin, and 500 mL of 50% alcohol?

   _____

3. A pharmacy technician mixes 20 g of 10% ichthammol ointment, 45 g of 5% ichthammol ointment, and 100 g of petrolatum (diluent). What is the percentage of ichthammol in the finished compound?

   _____

4. Calculate the percentage of alcohol in the lotion.

_____

Rx   Coal Tar Solution (85% alcohol)   80 mL
     Glycerin   160 mL
     Alcohol (95% alcohol)   500 mL
     Boric Acid qs   1000 mL
     Sig: Use as a medicated lotion once a day.

5. A manufacturing pharmacy has four lots of ichthammol ointment, containing 50%, 25%, 10%, and 5% ichthammol. How many grams of each should be used in preparing 1 pound of 20% ichthammol ointment? (Hint: There are 4 possible combinations using alligation alternate.)

_____

_____

_____

_____

6. How much 95% and 30% alcohol should be mixed to make 1 pint of 70% alcohol?

_____

_____

7. How many grams of 5% and 1% hydrocortisone should be mixed to make 1 pound of 2½% hydrocortisone ointment?

_____

_____

8. Prepare 1 liter of 0.75% sodium chloride solution from normal saline (0.9%) and half-normal saline (0.45%). How much of each strength would be required to fill this order?

_____

_____

9. Prepare 1 liter of $D_{10}W$ using both D_5W and $D_{20}W$. How much of each is required to fill this order?

_____

_____

10. Prepare 1 pound of 20% ointment using both 10% and 30% of the ointment. How much of each should be used?

_____

_____

IV Drip Rate Calculations

Objective: Calculate the flow rates or the amount of drug found in intravenous fluid administered to a patient.

Small-volume parenterals are generally considered to be 100 mL or less in volume. Some are injected into the body site slowly using a handheld syringe and needle. The medication is drawn into a syringe from a single dose ampule or a multidose vial. Some syringes are packaged prefilled by the manufacturer or hospital pharmacist or pharmacy technician. Other small volume doses are piggybacked through a large-volume IV.

Large-volume parenterals for continuous administration are hung at the patient's bed and are allowed to drip slowly into a vein by gravity flow or through the use of electrical or battery-operated volumetric infusion pumps. Some of these pumps can be calibrated to deliver "micro infusion" volumes such as 0.1 mL per hour or up to 2000 mL per hour, depending on the drug and the requirements. Solutions of additive drugs can be placed directly into large-volume parenterals or small-volume parenterals (minibags) containing the additive drug that may be hung piggyback and allowed to enter the tubing of the primary intravenous fluid and then enter the patient at a controlled rate. In either situation, the physician specifies the rate of flow of intravenous fluids as milliliters per minute, drops per minute, or total volume to be delivered over a number of hours.

In a hospital, the pharmacy is responsible for preparing fluids to be injected intravenously into a patient. The pharmacy technician may be required to calculate the flow or drip rate of an intravenous solution. The rate that a volume is infused per hour can be calculated by setting the following information equal to x mL/hr and solving for x:

$$\frac{\text{Volume (milliliters)}}{\text{Time (hours)}}$$

At times, a pharmacy technician may be required to calculate the number of drops per minute that a patient is to receive. In this situation, the technician will need to know the flow rate and drop factor (number of drops per milliliter of the substance that the tubing delivers) and must use a conversion factor to convert hours to minutes. This can be done using the following formula:

$$\text{Drops/min} = (\text{Drop factor})\ (\text{Flow rate})\ (\text{Conversion factor})$$

or

$$\text{gtt/min} = (\text{gtt/mL})\ (\text{mL/hr})\ (1\ \text{hr/60 min})$$

At other times, the pharmacy technician may need to calculate the amount of drug delivered over a specified period of time. This can be done using the following formula:

$$(\text{amount of drug in IV/total volume}) \cdot \text{rate of administration}$$

A conversion factor for time may be needed depending on whether the rate is given per hour or per minute and a conversion factor may be needed for weight depending on how it is given (example: mg or g).

Lab Activity #6.9: Complete the following questions.

Equipment needed:

- Calculator
- Pencil/pen
- Paper

Time needed to complete this activity: 30 minutes

1. 500 mL of a 2% sterile solution is to be administered by intravenous infusion over a period of 4 hours; how many milliliters will be administered over 1 hour?

2. A physician orders 1 liter of normal saline infused over 24 hours; how many milliliters of the intravenous solution will the patient receive after 8 hours?

_____

3. How many mL are delivered per hour in question #2?

_____

4. A physician prescribes 1 liter of $D_{20}W$ to be administered over 8 hours using an infusion kit with a drop factor of 10 gtt/mL. What will be the number of drops per minute?

_____

5. A physician writes a medication order for $D_{10}W$. The drop factor is set at 60 gtt/mL and the flow rate is 50 mL/hr. How many liters of fluid would be required to fill this order for 1 day?

_____

6. A physician prescribes 1 liter of 1/2 NS to be infused at 6 mL/min and the drop factor is 20 gtt/mL. How many drops per minute will the patient receive?

_____

7. A physician prescribes 1000 mL of lactated Ringer's solution to be infused over 8 hours using a drop factor of 20 gtt/mL. How many gtt/min will the patient receive?

_____

8. A physician orders a 2-g vial of a drug to be added to 500 mL of D_5W (5% dextrose in water for injection). If the administration rate is set at 125 mL per hour, how many milligrams of the drug will a patient receive per minute?

_____

9. A certain hyperalimentation fluid measures 1 liter. If the solution is to be administered over 8 hours and if the administration set is calibrated at 25 drops/mL, at what rate should the set be calibrated to administer the solution during the designated time interval?

_____

10. Five hundred (500) milliliters of an intravenous solution contains 0.2% of succinylcholine chloride in sodium chloride injection. At what rate should the infusion be administered to provide 2.5 mg of succinylcholine chloride per minute?

_____

Special Dosing Calculations

Objective: Calculate doses using Clark's Rule, Young's Rule, BSA, and body weight.
Lab Activity #6.10: Complete the following questions about individualized doses.

Equipment needed:

- Calculator
- Pencil/pen
- Paper

Time needed to complete this activity: 30 minutes

1. Drug Y has a recommended dose of 5 mg/kg of body weight given as a single daily dose. How many milligrams should this patient take daily if the patient weighs 120 pounds?

_____

2. The dose of a drug is 500 mcg per kg of body weight. How many milligrams should be given to a child weighing 40 lb?

_____

3. The dose of gentamicin sulfate is 1.7 mg per kg of body weight every 8 hours. How many milliliters of an injectable solution containing 40 mg of gentamicin per mL should be administered per dose to a person weighing 176 lb?

_____

4. If the adult dose of a drug is 5 gr, what is the dose in mg for a child who weighs 50 lb and is 8 years old?

   A. Use Young's Rule to calculate the dose.

   B. Use Clark's Rule to calculate the dose.

5. The adult dose of a medication is 500 mg. What is the dose for a 3-year-old who weighs 32 lb?

   A. Use Young's Rule to calculate the dose.

   B. Use Clark's Rule to calculate the dose.

6. The adult dose of a medication is 200 mg, three times a day. What would be the daily dose for a 5-year-old child who weighs 55 lb?

   A. Use Young's Rule to calculate the dose.

   B. Use Clark's Rule to calculate the dose.

7. The pediatric dose is 25mg/m². What would be the dose if the child is 18 kg, 36 inches, and has a BSA of 0.65m²?

_____

8. The adult dose is 150mg/m². What would be the dose if the adult is 100 kg, 73 inches, and has a BSA of 2.24m²?

_____

9. The adult dose of a drug is 250 mg/m². If the drug is available as 150 mg/mL, what would be the dose in mL if the adult is 67 inches, 175 lb, and has a BSA of 1.91m²?

_____

10. The adult dose of a drug is 100 mg/m². If the drug is available as 50 mg/mL, what would be the dose in mL if the adult has a BSA of 1.8m²?

_____

Business Calculations

Objective: Calculate retail prices.

Lab Activity #6.11: Complete the following questions about retail pricing.

Equipment needed:

- Calculator
- Pencil/pen
- Paper

Time needed to complete this activity: 15 minutes

1. You order 6 cases of anti-itch cream. Each case has 12 tubes of cream and costs $14.50 per case. Your drug wholesaler will give you a discount of 20% if the invoice is paid within 2 weeks. What would be the total paid for this order if the invoice is paid within 2 weeks?

_____

2. Your pharmacy is having a 15%-off sale for all antihistamines. Calculate the cost of each of the following items:

   A. Benadryl Allergy, $6.50 _____

   B. Children's Allegra, $9.99 _____

   C. Claritin, $18.99 _____

   D. Zyrtec, $21.99 _____

   E. Alavert, $8.49 _____

3. Your pharmacy has Ben-Gay cream on sale at 10% off the price of $5.89 per tube. How much will the customer save?

_____

4. All new customers are being given 25% off new prescriptions. What is the dollar amount lost by the pharmacy if all the new prescriptions for the day added up to $1,327.27?

_____

5. Your pharmacy received an order of 10 cases of cough medicine. Each case contains 15 bottles and costs $20 per case. If each bottle is sold for $5.50, what is the percent markup?

_____

TERMS AND DEFINITIONS

Select the correct term from the following list and write the corresponding letter in the blank next to the statement.

A. Brand Name
B. Chemical Structure
C. Drug Classification
D. Formulary
E. Generic Name
F. Monograph
G. Non-formulary
H. Package Insert

_____ 1. Categorization based on various characteristics, including the chemical structure of a drug, the action of a drug, and/or the therapeutic or anatomic use of a drug

_____ 2. The official prescribing information for a prescription drug

_____ 3. Name assigned to a medication or nonproprietary name of a drug

_____ 4. Trademark of a drug or device held by the originating manufacturing company

_____ 5. Comprehensive information on a medication's actions within that class of drugs

_____ 6. The makeup of a chemical, including the elements, the shape, the bonding types, the molecular configurations, charges, etc.

_____ 7. Drugs not included in the drug list approved for reimbursement by the health care plans

_____ 8. A list of approved drugs to be stocked by the pharmacy; also a list of drugs covered by an insurance company

TRUE OR FALSE

Write T or F next to each statement.

_____ 1. Pharmacy reference books are used by pharmacy personnel only.

_____ 2. Pharmacists rely on drug information references to give correct information to health care workers.

_____ 3. Manufacturers give a drug a name based on its chemical attributes.

_____ 4. Finding websites at universities and through publishing companies is a good way to look for information.

_____ 5. Contraindications list the main conditions for which the drug is used.

_____ 6. All technicians should carry a *Facts and Comparisons* in their pocket.

_____ 7. Most generic drug names typically begin with J or W

_____ 8. It is important for technicians to carry a good pocket guide.

_____ 9. Electronic devices such as smartphones and tablets are becoming more popular but are not economical.

_____ 10. Employees are not supposed to have their phones out during work.

MULTIPLE CHOICE

Complete each question by circling the best answer.

1. A reference text familiar to most pharmacists and available in hardback, loose-leaf hardback, pocket-sized, or by electronic subscription is:
   A. *Drug Facts and Comparisons*
   B. *Physicians' Desk Reference*
   C. *The Red Book*
   D. *United States Pharmacopeia*

2. The section of *Drug Facts and Comparisons* that shows in color 250 of the most frequently used drugs is the:
   A. Index
   B. Drug monograph
   C. Drug identification
   D. Appendix

3. This book is a compilation of package inserts (official labels) provided by manufacturers who have paid a fee for inclusion into the reference.
   A. *Pharmacists' Drug Reference*
   B. *Physicians' Desk Reference*
   C. *Pharmacists' Desk Reference*
   D. *Pharmacy Dosage Regulations*

4. The PDR contains which of the following?
   A. Manufacturers' addresses and phone numbers
   B. Manufacturer-provided package inserts for select FDA-approved drugs
   C. Products listed by classification or method of action
   D. All of the above

5. The diagnostic product information section of the PDR contains:
   A. A key to controlled substances
   B. A key to FDA pregnancy ratings
   C. An FDA telephone directory
   D. Information on drug products used as diagnostic agents

6. If a technician must know the upper limit price and rules or the billing units for each type of drug under state AIDS drug assistance programs, he or she would use:
   A. *Drug Facts and Comparisons*
   B. *Physicians' Desk Reference*
   C. *Drug Topics Red Book*
   D. *Orange Book Code*

7. A patient has taken a drug in tablet form but does not know what it is; the technician might use which reference to find out what the drug is?
   A. *American Hospital Formulary Service Drug Information*
   B. *United States Pharmacopeia Drug Information*
   C. *Ident-A-Drug*
   D. *The Injectable Drug Handbook*

8. The book used to reference the compatibility of various parenteral agents is:
   A. *American Hospital Formulary Service Drug Information*
   B. *United States Pharmacopeia Drug Information*
   C. *Ident-A-Drug*
   D. *The Injectable Drug Handbook*

9. *Drug Facts and Comparisons* in book form is updated:
   A. Monthly
   B. Yearly
   C. A and B
   D. None of the above

10. Pharmacy journals contain information about:
    A. New drugs
    B. The future of pharmacy
    C. Legislative changes
    D. All of the above

11. Which section of the *Drug Topics Red Book* will list drugs that cannot be crushed?
    A. Clinical reference guide
    B. Practice management and professional development
    C. Drug reimbursement information
    D. Prescription product listings

12. Of the sources listed here, which would be best for finding a recommendation for a sugar-free and alcohol-free cough syrup?
    A. *Physicians' Desk Reference*
    B. *Drug Topic Red Book*
    C. *Facts and Comparisons*
    D. *Ident-A-Drug*

13. Clinical Pharmacology is an electronic drug compendium used in:
    A. Retail pharmacies
    B. Hospital pharmacies
    C. Physicians' offices
    D. All of the above

14. Clinical Xpert provides online and mobile applications used by:
    A. Pharmacists and technicians
    B. Physicians and nurses
    C. Both A and B
    D. None of the above

15. _____ offers basic free drug information that can be downloaded onto a personal computer or handheld device.
    A. *Epocrates*
    B. *Remington's Pharmaceutical Sciences*
    C. *American Drug Index*
    D. *Red Book*

FILL IN THE BLANKS

Answer each question by completing the statement in the space provided.

1. Pharmacy organizations have _____ on the Internet.

2. Many _____ _____ have weekly news boards that reference important information concerning pharmacy.

3. _____ should not be limited to books alone.

4. Many websites provide _____ _____ in the form of _____ _____ and _____ _____ _____.

5. Another way to attain new drug information is to join an _____.

6. Becoming familiar with various _____ and understanding the _____ are essential for becoming a competent pharmacy technician.

7. _____ and continuing education _____, provided by pharmacy associations, are sometimes sponsored by drug companies and are another good source of information on drug topics.

8. Knowing the proper book to reference is important not only for finding the correct information, but also for saving _____ and avoiding _____.

9. Avoid books that only reference _____ _____ one way because their use can become time consuming.

10. Most drugs have many _____, depending on the drug company that manufactures them.

MATCHING

Matching I

Match the controlled substance designations with the correct drugs.

_____ 1. UPC

_____ 2. AWP

_____ 3. NDC

_____ 4. DP

_____ 5. OBC

A. Average Wholesale Price
B. Orange Book Code
C. Direct Price
D. Universal Product Code
E. National Drug Code

Matching II

Match the following drug reference books with their correct description.

A. *Drug Facts and Comparisons*
B. *Physicians' Desk Reference*
C. *Drug Topics Red Book*
D. *Orange Book*
E. *American Hospital Formulary Service Drug Information*
F. *USP–NF*
G. *United States Pharmacists' Pharmacopeia*
H. *Clinical Pharmacology*
I. *Ident-A-Drug*
J. *Micromedex Healthcare Evidence*
K. *Handbook on Injectable Drugs*
L. *American Drug Index*
M. *Goodman & Gilman's The Pharmacological Basis of Therapeutics, Pharmacogenomics, and Principles of Therapeutics in All Areas of the Body System*
N. *Handbook of Nonprescription Drugs*
O. *Martindale's The Complete Drug Reference*
P. *Remington's Pharmaceutical Sciences: The Science and Practice of Pharmacy*
Q. *Pediatric and Neonatal Dosage Handbook*
R. *Geriatric Dosage Handbook*

_____ 1. Provides access to official standards of the FDA

_____ 2. A good source of information pertaining to average and wholesale drug costs and prices

_____ 3. Lists pharmacokinetics and pharmacodynamics, drug transport/drug transporters, drug metabolism

_____ 4. A comprehensive compilation of information on compounding products and ingredients and their safety as well as products used to treat specific medical conditions

_____ 5. Provides information on suggested current dosages for pediatric patients

_____ 6. Contains quick and accurate reference and drug comparison and is the most frequently used book by pharmacists

_____ 7. Provides an online and mobile application that can be used by physicians, pharmacists, and nurses within a health care facility through several different software programs that can be purchased

_____ 8. Provides self-care options for nonprescription medications, nutritional supplements, medical foods, and complementary and alternative therapies to name a few

_____ 9. An electronic drug compendium commonly encountered in retail and health system pharmacy settings and an officially recognized compendium by the Centers for Medicare & Medicaid Services

_____ 10. A compilation of package inserts with a complete description of each drug, including its chemical structure and study results

_____ 11. Provides information on suggested current dosages for geriatric patients

_____ 12. A well-known reference used for information on parenteral agents; used mostly in the hospital setting

_____ 13. Includes more than 38,000 listings of tablet and capsule identifications

_____ 14. Covers the entire scope of pharmacy, from the history of pharmacy and ethics to the specifics of industrial pharmacy and pharmacy practice

_____ 15. A comprehensive listing used to determinate whether a generic drug is the same as a brand drug

_____ 16. Provides drug monographs that list drug information; used mainly by hospitals

_____ 17. Provides information on drugs in clinical use worldwide

_____ 18. Contains information for both prescription and OTC products; covers pronunciation of drugs, active ingredients, dosage forms, and packaging, to name a few

SHORT ANSWER

Write a short response to each question in the space provided.

1. List the five sections of the _Drug Facts and Comparisons._

    A. _____

    B. _____

    C. _____

    D. _____

    E. _____

2. List the six sections of the PDR.

    A. _____

    B. _____

    C. _____

    D. _____

    E. _____

    F. _____

3. List the 10 sections of the _Red Book._

    A. _____

    B. _____

    C. _____

    D. _____

    E. _____

F. _____

G. _____

H. _____

I. _____

J. _____

4. List five components of drug information included in the *American Drug Index*.

_____

_____

_____

_____

_____

5. List five self-care options in the *Handbook of Nonprescription Drugs*.

_____

_____

_____

_____

_____

RESEARCH ACTIVITIES

Follow the instructions given in each exercise and provide a response.

1. Access the websites listed in Table 7-6 of the textbook. Describe the type of information provided on each website.

2. Access the websites listed in Table 7-7 of the textbook. Describe the type of information provided on each website.

REFLECT CRITICALLY

CRITICAL THINKING

Reply to each question based on what you have learned in the chapter.

1. Of all the reference books discussed in this chapter, which one seems to be the easiest to use and understand?

2. Think of some of the magazines you have read or glanced through lately. How many of them included some sort of medical, drug, or health-related article or information? Did the articles spark your interest? If so, why? Were any of them written by professionals in the field?

3. List drug information resources that can be accessed without purchasing a book.

RELATE TO PRACTICE

LAB SCENARIOS

Reference Materials

Objective: To familiarize the pharmacy technician with various forms of reference materials and the terminology associated with each.

> Each pharmacy regardless of the setting is required by state boards of pharmacy to maintain a library relevant to its practice. State boards of pharmacy require that a pharmacy maintain a current edition of the *USP-NF* (the official compendium in the United States) and a copy of the United States Controlled Substance Act.
>
> A pharmacy technician must be familiar with proper usage of these reference materials, which may consist of books, journals, and pharmacy magazines. In many situations, these materials may be found in an electronic format.

Lab Activity #7.1: Use the *Physicians' Desk Reference (PDR)* or *Drug Facts and Comparisons* to define the terms found in these reference materials.

Equipment needed:

- *Physicians' Desk Reference (PDR)* or *Drug Facts and Comparisons*
- Pencil/pen

Time needed to complete this activity: 15 minutes

Define the following terms used in pharmacy reference materials.

1. Adverse reactions

_____

2. Clinical pharmacology

_____

3. Contraindication

_____

4. Description

_____

5. Dosage and administration

_____

100

6. How supplied

_____

7. Indication

_____

8. Mechanism of action

_____

9. Monograph

_____

10. Pharmacokinetics

_____

11. Precautions

_____

12. Teratogenic effects

_____

13. Warnings

_____

Lab Activity #7.2: Use *Approved Drug Products with Therapeutic Equivalence Evaluations (Orange Book)* to define the following terms found in drug monographs.

Equipment needed:

■ Computer with Internet connection (*www.fda.gov*)
■ Pencil/pen

Time needed to complete this activity: 10 minutes

Define the following terms.

1. Pharmaceutical equivalents

_____

2. Pharmaceutical alternatives

_____

3. Therapeutic equivalent

_____

4. Bioavailability

_____

5. Bioequivalent drug products

_____

Lab Activity #7.3: Use *Approved Drug Products with Therapeutic Equivalence Evaluations (Orange Book)* to define the following therapeutic equivalent evaluation codes.

Equipment needed:

- Computer with Internet connection (*www.fda.gov*) to access *Approved Drug Products with Therapeutic Evaluations (Orange Book)*
- Pencil/pen

Time needed to complete this activity: 30 minutes

Define the following therapeutic equivalent evaluation codes.

1. A

_____

2. AA

_____

3. AB

_____

4. AN

_____

5. AO

_____

6. AP

_____

7. AT

_____

8. B

_____

9. BC

_____

10. BD

_____

11. BE

_____

12. BN

_____

13. BP

_____

14. BR

_____

15. BS

_____

16. BT

_____

17. BX

_____

Lab Activity #7.4: Use *Approved Drug Products with Therapeutic Equivalence Evaluations (Orange Book)* to determine the following therapeutic equivalent evaluation codes.

Equipment needed:

- Computer with Internet connection (*www.fda.gov*) to access *Approved Drug Products with Therapeutic Evaluations (Orange Book)*
- Pencil/pen

Time needed to complete this activity: 30 minutes

1. Atorvastatin 10-mg tablet

_____

2. Mirtazapine 45-mg ODT

_____

3. Amoxicillin 250-mg capsule

_____

4. Montelukast 5-mg chewable tablet

_____

5. Zolpidem Extended Release 6.25-mg tablet

_____

6. Furosemide 10-mg/mL injection

_____

7. Lorazepam 2-mg/mL oral solution

_____

8. Clotrimazole 1% topical solution

_____

9. Fluoxetine hydrochloride 20-mg capsule

_____

10. Carisoprodol 350-mg tablet

_____

11. Clindamycin phosphate/tretinoin 1.2%/0.025% topical gel

_____

12. Nebivolol 20-mg tablet

_____

13. Indomethacin sodium 1-mg base/vial injection

_____

14. Diclofenac sodium 0.1% ophthalmic solution

_____

15. Verapamil hydrochloride Extended Release 180-mg tablet (Covera-HS)

_____

Lab Activity #7.5: Use *RxList Pill Identification Tool* to determine the following drugs from their description.

Equipment needed:

■ Computer with Internet connection (*http://www.rxlist.com/pill-identification-tool/article.htm*) to access *RxList Pill Identification Tool.*
■ Pencil/pen

Time needed to complete this activity: 30 minutes

1. This drug is a yellow, oval, scored tablet imprinted with "A CJ."

_____

2. This drug is a pink, round, scored tablet imprinted with "A CL" and "032."

_____

3. This drug is a white, oblong tablet imprinted with "ADG" and "375."

_____

4. This drug is a white, oblong, film-coated tablet imprinted with "XR 150."

_____

5. This drug is a white, round, scored, film-coated tablet imprinted with "A ms."

_____

6. This drug is a pink, oval, film-coated tablet imprinted with "2788."

   _____

7. This drug is a pink, oblong capsule imprinted with "TPV 250."

   _____

8. This drug is a white, oblong capsule imprinted with "FL" and "20."

   _____

9. This drug is a light blue, oblong capsule imprinted with "G" and "M."

   _____

10. This drug is a dark orange, oblong capsule imprinted with "R50."

    _____

8 Community Pharmacy Practice

TERMS AND DEFINITIONS

Select the correct term from the following list and write the corresponding letter in the blank next to the statement.

A. Adjudication
B. Auxiliary Label
C. Behind-the-Counter
D. Bank Identification Number
E. Brand Name
F. Chain Pharmacy
G. DAW Code
H. Drug Utilization Evaluation
I. e-Prescribing
J. Federal Legend
K. Franchise
L. Generic Name
M. Help Desk
N. Inscription
O. National Provider Number
P. NDC Number
Q. Prescription
R. Refill
S. Repackaging
T. Signa
U. Sole Proprietorship
V. Subscription
W. Superscription
X. Therapeutic Alliance

_____ 1. Provides supplementary information regarding proper and safe administration, use, or storage of a medication

_____ 2. Nonproprietary name assigned to a drug

_____ 3. Unique 10- or 11-digit number, composed of three segments, that is assigned to a medication

_____ 4. Corporate-owned group of pharmacies that share a brand name and central management and usually have standardized business methods and practices

_____ 5. A trust relationship between a health care professional and a patient, incorporating patient perceptions of the acceptability of interventions and mutually agreed upon goals for treatment

_____ 6. Numerical set of codes, created by the NCPDP, which are used when filling prescriptions; they can affect reimbursement amounts by insurance companies

_____ 7. An order for medication issued by a physician, dentist, or other properly licensed practitioner such as a physician assistant or nurse practitioner

_____ 8. Classification of medications that are kept behind the pharmacy counter that requires a pharmacist's intervention before selling the medication to a patient

_____ 9. Heading of a prescription represented by the Latin symbol Rx meaning "take thou" or "you take"

_____ 10. A 24/7 toll-free hotline to an insurance company for pharmacists that can address specific questions relating to insurance claims and coverage, as well as pharmacy-specific inquiries

_____ 11. Act of reducing the amount of medication taken from a bulk bottle

_____ 12. Authorized, structured, ongoing review of health care provider prescribing, pharmacist dispensing, and patient use of medication

_____ 13. Name, dosage form, strength, and quantity of the medication being prescribed

_____ 14. Statement, "Federal law prohibits the dispensing of this drug without a prescription," which is found on the labeling of all prescription medications

_____ 15. Six-digit number, found on a prescription drug card, which is used for routing and identification in order to process a prescription claim

_____ 16. Form of business organization in which a firm that already has a successful product or service enters into a continuing contractual relationship with other businesses operating under the franchisor's trade name and usually with the franchisor's guidance, in exchange for a fee

_____ 17. Directions on a prescription that explain how the patient is to take the prescribed medication; a Latin expression meaning to "write on label"

_____ 18. Trademark name under which a drug product is marketed

_____ 19. Unincorporated business owned by one person

_____ 20. Process by which a prescription is submitted electronically to a third-party payer for the pharmacy to be reimbursed for the medication dispensed

_____ 21. Permission by a prescriber to replenish a prescription

_____ 22. Computer-to-computer transfer of prescription data among pharmacies, prescribers, and payers

_____ 23. Unique 10-digit identification number for covered health care providers that is issued by the Centers for Medicare and Medicaid Services

_____ 24. Part of the prescription that provides specific instructions to the pharmacist on how to compound the prescription

TRUE OR FALSE

Write T or F next to each statement.

_____ 1. The success of a community pharmacy is very dependent on the knowledge and training of its pharmacy technicians.

_____ 2. If technicians cannot interpret the information on a prescription, they should quickly make an educated guess.

_____ 3. The Pure Food and Drug Act requires that every ambulatory pharmacy maintain patient profiles.

_____ 4. The Metric System is the official system of measurement for weights and volumes in the United States.

_____ 5. The pharmacist is responsible for inputting the patient's information into the pharmacy's computer information system.

_____ 6. Submitting a prescription claim using the incorrect DAW code will not affect the pharmacy being reimbursed properly for the medication that was dispensed.

_____ 7. State laws require that patient product information (PPI) be provided to the patient when specific medications are dispensed.

_____ 8. The technician should check the medication against the script and the label when selecting medication from the shelf.

_____ 9. Controlled substance inventory should be done twice yearly and when there is a change of the pharmacist-in-charge.

_____ 10. When the prescription is being picked up, the pharmacy technician will ask the patient if he or she has any questions for the pharmacist.

MULTIPLE CHOICE

Complete each question by circling the best answer.

1. When taking in a prescription, neither the technician nor the pharmacist can decipher the physician's writing; therefore:
   A. The technician should guess what to fill
   B. The technician should ask the patient
   C. The pharmacist should call the physician
   D. The technician should tell the patient to go back to the doctor and get a prescription that can be read

2. Which of the following is *not* the duty of a technician upon taking in a prescription?
   A. Translating the prescription
   B. Entering information into the database
   C. Filling the prescription
   D. Providing patient consultation

3. When a new prescription is called in to the pharmacy, who can take the prescription over the phone?
   A. Pharmacy clerk
   B. Pharmacy technician
   C. Pharmacist
   D. Pharmacy custodian

4. If a prescription is for a controlled substance, the technician must make sure the prescription includes the physician's:
   A. FDA number
   B. DEA number
   C. HMO number
   D. NABP number

5. Which of the following is *not* an exception to the safety lid law?
   A. Nitroglycerin
   B. Patient's request
   C. Oral contraceptives
   D. Technician's opinion that the patient looks too weak to open a safety lid

6. Which of the following is *not* printed on a prescription label as required by law?
   A. Address and phone number of prescriber
   B. Prescription number
   C. Drug, strength, and dosage form
   D. Refill information

7. Which of the following is not a common auxiliary label for NSAIDs?
   A. May cause drowsiness
   B. May cause sensitivity to light
   C. May cause dizziness
   D. Take with food

8. The law states that all prescriptions must be kept on file for at least
   A. 6 months
   B. 1 year
   C. 2 years
   D. 5 years

9. Prescriptions that have a red "C" stamped on the right side when filed in the pharmacy indicate that the prescription is:
   A. A controlled substance
   B. A cough medication
   C. A drug containing codeine
   D. A cardiac medication

10. Pharmacy technicians must be capable of:
    A. Interpreting and transcribing prescriptions
    B. Filling prescriptions quickly and accurately
    C. Following proper billing practices
    D. All of the above

11. According to federal law, when should a patient receive counseling?
    A. At the last refill of the patient's medication
    B. Only when the patient asks for it
    C. When a new prescription is filled
    D. When a Medicaid patient receives a new prescription

12. Most boards of pharmacy prefer to allow transfer of prescriptions only _____ time(s).
    A. One
    B. Two
    C. Three
    D. Zero

13. If the medication has to be counted or measured:
    A. Have the pharmacist check measurements
    B. Put medication into a bottle of appropriate size
    C. Place into the refrigerator
    D. None of the above

14. Which of the following is *not* an advantage of e-prescribing?
    A. Linking information from a patient's medical file to a patient's prescription file
    B. Expediting refills
    C. Notifying the prescriber if a drug product is covered by the patient's insurance plan when the order is being generated rather than when it is presented at the pharmacy
    D. Increasing errors associated with illegible handwriting

15. Which of the following is *not* a form of nonverbal communication?
    A. Eye rolling
    B. Smiling at a customer
    C. Saying hello to each customer
    D. Crossing your arms when talking with a customer

FILL IN THE BLANKS

Answer each question by completing the statement in the space provided.

1. A _____ designates a specific medication and dosage to be administered to a particular patient at a specific time.

2. A _____ _____ is a tool that can assist in helping eliminate medication errors.

3. The _____ symbol represents prescription and the pharmacy.

4. The _____ is responsible for reducing medication errors and drug-related illnesses.

5. Scanning prescriptions is a quality assurance tool used to _____ medication errors.

6. To prevent _____ of tablets and capsules, the counting tray should be wiped clean after each use, as powder from tablets may remain on the tray.

7. A retail pharmacy will have a _____ _____ to ensure that Schedule II medications are kept secure at all times.

8. Every patient should be treated with the same _____ that is due to him or her.

9. Your _____ can have a direct effect on whether or not a pharmacy customer comes back and can also alter your image as a technician.

10. _____ _____ _____ is medical care provided by pharmacists whose aim is to optimize drug therapy and improve therapeutic outcomes for patients.

MATCHING

Matching I

Match the pharmacy abbreviations with the correct meaning.

A. ac
B. subcut
C. gtts
D. ut dict
E. qd
F. as
G. tsp
H. ung
I. os
J. qid
K. stat
L. tsbp

_____ 1. Teaspoonful

_____ 2. Left eye

_____ 3. Subcutaneously

_____ 4. Left ear

_____ 5. Immediately

_____ 6. As directed

_____ 7. Drops

_____ 8. Every day

_____ 9. Ointment

_____ 10. Before meals

_____ 11. Four times a day

_____ 12. Tablespoonful

Matching II

Match the pharmacy abbreviations with the correct meaning.

A. aa
B. ad
C. prn
D. tid
E. WA
F. po
G. ou
H. bid
I. od
J. au
K. pc
L. hs

_____ 1. Both ears

_____ 2. Three times a day

_____ 3. Both eyes

_____ 4. At bedtime

_____ 5. By mouth

_____ 6. Right ear

_____ 7. As needed

_____ 8. Twice a day

_____ 9. After meals

_____ 10. Right eye

_____ 11. Of each

_____ 12. While awake

SHORT ANSWER

Write a short response to each question in the space provided.

1. List the five rights of the patient to medication safety.

A. _____

B. _____

C. _____

D. _____

E. _____

2. List the two options for filing filled prescriptions.

A. _____

B. _____

3. List four different ways a new prescription can be received in a community pharmacy.

A. _____

B. _____

C. _____

D. _____

4. List the required information every prescription is required to contain.

_____

_____

RESEARCH ACTIVITIES

Follow the instructions given in each exercise and provide a response.

1. Access the website *http://www.mckesson.com/pharmacies/pharmacies/*.

A. List one product/solution available to community pharmacies.

B. How can this product/solution help the community pharmacy?

2. Access the website *https://www.nabp.net/boards-of-pharmacy* to access your state board of pharmacy website.

A. Does your pharmacy state law allow pharmacists to administer immunizations?

B. If so, which immunizations may a pharmacist administer in a community pharmacy setting?

C. How can a pharmacy technician be helpful to an immunizing pharmacist in a community pharmacy setting?

CRITICAL THINKING

Reply to each question based on what you have learned in the chapter.

1. When you check the label against the script, for what are you checking?

2. Why would elderly patients want non-safety lids on their medications?

3. Why should technicians initial any prescriptions that they fill?

4. Many computer systems have a labeling system. What information is printed on one sheet?

5. When labeling prescription bottles, a technician should remember professionalism. Why is this important?

6. You have received a faxed prescription from a doctor's office. You are not sure what the drug is on the prescription so you consult the pharmacist. After some discussion, the two of you decide what the drug is and the order is prepared. Who else would be able to verify that this is the correct medication before it is dispensed to the patient?

7. After filling about 25 prescriptions on a very busy morning in the pharmacy, you realize that you might have made a mistake on the last one. It is time to go to lunch, so you decide to let it go, believing that the pharmacist will catch it. Unfortunately, the pharmacist checks the prescription hurriedly, trusting that you did your job correctly, and the prescription goes home with the patient.

   A. What should you have done to prevent this medication error?

   B. Whose fault is it that the prescription was dispensed as is?

C. What can you do to remedy the situation before the patient is harmed by your mistake?

LAB SCENARIOS

The Patient Profile

Objective: To familiarize the pharmacy technician with the information required for a patient profile.

The patient profile is a full list of patient prescriptions and all related information for the prescriptions including the original date of fill, refill dates, and the prescribing practitioner.

A complete patient profile will also include the following information:

- Full name
- Home address—number, street, city, state, and zip code
- Telephone numbers—home, mobile, and work
- Birth date
- Gender
- Allergies—drug and food
- Physical and medical conditions
- Generic preference
- Prescription insurance information—group number, member number, and relationship to the cardholder
- Non–child-resistant container preference
- List of over-the-counter medications and herbal supplements being taken

This information is used to develop a patient profile for the patient and should be reviewed for accuracy each time a patient fills a prescription at the pharmacy. A thorough and accurate patient profile can help eliminate possible adverse drug events and medication errors.

Lab Activity #8.1: Identify what is missing from the following patient profiles.

Equipment needed:

- Pencil/pen

Time needed to complete this activity: 30 minutes

1. Patient Profile 1

Patient Profile

Name: _____ Sandy Smith _____

Address: _____ 125 N. Main Street _____

City: _____ Anywhere _____ State: _____ WI _____ Zip code _____

Gender: ☐ M ☒ F Birthdate: _____

Home Ph: _____ 212-555-5476 _____ Cell Ph: _____

Email: _____

Prescription insurance provider: _____ Cigna _____

ID Number: _____ U52428 _____ Group Number: _____ 1X854 _____

Relationship to Cardholder ☐ Self ☒ Spouse ☐ Child ☐ Other

Allergies to Medications: _____ none _____

Medical Conditions: _____

List any OTC products, herbal supplements, or other medications: _____

_____

_____

Would you like child-resistant containers? ☒ Yes ☐ No

Would you like generic drugs when available? ☒ Yes ☐ No

What I have provided is true and correct. If my medical conditions change or if I have a drug or food reaction, I will inform the pharmacy.

Signature: _____ *Sandy Smith* _____ Date: _____ 01-13-1X _____

What is missing from this patient profile?

_____

2. Patient Profile 2

Patient Profile

Name: _____ Andrew Rodriguez _____

Address: _____ 145 S 1st _____

City: _____ Austin _____ State: ____ TX _____ Zip code __ 78748 _____

Gender: ☒ M   ☐ F   Birthdate: __ 7-14-70 _____

Home Ph: ____ 512-555-1154 _____ Cell Ph: _____

Email: _____

Prescription insurance provider: __ TXBC _____

ID Number: _____ Group Number: _____

Relationship to Cardholder   ☒ Self   ☐ Spouse   ☐ Child   ☐ Other

Allergies to Medications: _____

Medical Conditions: _____ High blood pressure _____

List any OTC products, herbal supplements, or other medications: __ none _____

_____

_____

Would you like child-resistant containers?   ☒ Yes   ☐ No

Would you like generic drugs when available?   ☒ Yes   ☐ No

What I have provided is true and correct. If my medical conditions change or if I have a drug or food reaction, I will inform the pharmacy.

Signature: _Andrew Rodriguez_____ Date: _2-1-1X_____

What is missing from this patient profile?

_____

3. Patient Profile 3

Patient Profile

Name: _____

Address: _____55 North Main_____

City: _____Yonder_____ State: __NM__ Zip code __87004_____

Gender: ☒ M ☐ F Birthdate: __6-1-82_____

Home Ph: _____ Cell Ph: __215-555-0789_____

Email: _____

Prescription insurance provider: _____

ID Number: _____ Group Number: _____

Relationship to Cardholder ☐ Self ☐ Spouse ☐ Child ☐ Other

Allergies to Medications: ____Penicillin_____

Medical Conditions: ____none_____

List any OTC products, herbal supplements, or other medications: ___none_____

_____

_____

Would you like child-resistant containers? ☐ Yes ☐ No

Would you like generic drugs when available? ☐ Yes ☐ No

What I have provided is true and correct. If my medical conditions change or if I have a drug or food reaction, I will inform the pharmacy.

Signature: _____ Date: __1-4-1X_____

What is missing from this patient profile?

_____

4. Patient Profile 4

Patient Profile

Name: _____Megan Morris_____

Address: _____8978 West Parkway_____

City: _____Park_____ State: ____NY____ Zip code ___17352_____

Gender: ☐ M   ☒ F   Birthdate: _____

Home Ph: _____ Cell Ph: ____212-555-8952_____

Email: _____

Prescription insurance provider: ___BCBS_____

ID Number: ___Y5238_____ Group Number: ___52138_____

Relationship to Cardholder   ☐ Self   ☐ Spouse   ☒ Child   ☐ Other

Allergies to Medications: ___none_____

Medical Conditions: ____none_____

List any OTC products, herbal supplements, or other medications: _____

_____

_____

Would you like child-resistant containers?   ☒ Yes   ☐ No

Would you like generic drugs when available?   ☐ Yes   ☐ No

What I have provided is true and correct. If my medical conditions change or if I have a drug or food reaction, I will inform the pharmacy.

Signature: _Megan Morris_____ Date: __8-14-1X_____

What is missing from this patient profile?

_____

5. Patient Profile 5

Patient Profile

Name: _____ David Castro _____

Address: _____ 9634 East 29th Ave _____

City: _____ Park City _____ State: _____ UT _____ Zip code ___ 84060 _____

Gender: ☒ M ☐ F Birthdate: _____

Home Ph: _____ Cell Ph: _____

Email: _____

Prescription insurance provider: ___ BCBS _____

ID Number: _____ Group Number: _____

Relationship to Cardholder ☒ Self ☐ Spouse ☐ Child ☐ Other

Allergies to Medications: ___ Sulfa _____

Medical Conditions: _____ none _____

List any OTC products, herbal supplements, or other medications: _____
_____
_____

Would you like child-resistant containers? ☒ Yes ☐ No

Would you like generic drugs when available? ☒ Yes ☐ No

What I have provided is true and correct. If my medical conditions change or if I have a drug or food reaction, I will inform the pharmacy.

Signature: _____ Date: _____

What is missing from this patient profile?

_____

6. Patient Profile 6

```
┌─────────────────────────────────────────────────────────────────────┐
│                         Patient Profile                              │
│                                                                       │
│   Name:        Kristie Adams                                          │
│                                                                       │
│   Address:     5247 Train Ave                                         │
│                                                                       │
│   City:        Railroad              State:    OK    Zip code  73002  │
│                                                                       │
│   Gender:      ☐ M        ☐ F               Birthdate: _____  │
│                                                                       │
│   Home Ph: _____ Cell Ph: ___405-555-8474_____   │
│                                                                       │
│   Email:       kadams@email.com                                      │
│                                                                       │
│   Prescription insurance provider:    Aetna                          │
│                                                                       │
│   ID Number:   T854569               Group Number:    03289          │
│                                                                       │
│   Relationship to Cardholder    ☒ Self    ☒ Spouse   ☐ Child   ☐ Other│
│                                                                       │
│   Allergies to Medications:    Biaxin                                │
│                                                                       │
│   Medical Conditions: _____ │
│                                                                       │
│   List any OTC products, herbal supplements, or other medications: none│
│                                                                       │
│   Would you like child-resistant containers?       ☒ Yes     ☐ No    │
│                                                                       │
│   Would you like generic drugs when available?     ☒ Yes     ☐ No    │
│                                                                       │
│   What I have provided is true and correct. If my medical conditions  │
│   change or if I have a drug or food reaction,                        │
│   I will inform the pharmacy.                                         │
│                                                                       │
│   Signature:   Kristie Adams            Date:    9-19-1X              │
└─────────────────────────────────────────────────────────────────────┘
```

What is missing from this patient profile?

_____

7. Patient Profile 7

```
┌─────────────────────────────────────────────────────────────────────────────┐
│                             Patient Profile                                   │
│                                                                               │
│   Name: _____ Brian Norris _____   │
│                                                                               │
│   Address: _____ 2367 Treetop Drive _____   │
│                                                                               │
│   City: _____ Forrest City _____ State: ___ AR ___ Zip code __ 72335 _  │
│                                                                               │
│   Gender:      ☐ M        ☐ F              Birthdate: _____       │
│                                                                               │
│   Home Ph: __ 870-555-7458 _____ Cell Ph: ___ 870-555-2147 ____   │
│                                                                               │
│   Email: _____ brian.norris@email.net _____   │
│                                                                               │
│   Prescription insurance provider: ___ Cigna _____    │
│                                                                               │
│   ID Number: ___ U85469 _____ Group Number: ___ 20135 _____     │
│                                                                               │
│   Relationship to Cardholder   ☒ Self   ☐ Spouse   ☐ Child   ☐ Other          │
│                                                                               │
│   Allergies to Medications: ___ Codeine _____    │
│                                                                               │
│   Medical Conditions: _____    │
│                                                                               │
│   List any OTC products, herbal supplements, or other medications: __ St. John's Wort __ │
│                                                                               │
│   _____   │
│                                                                               │
│   _____   │
│                                                                               │
│   Would you like child-resistant containers?        ☒ Yes        ☒ No         │
│                                                                               │
│   Would you like generic drugs when available?      ☒ Yes        ☐ No         │
│                                                                               │
│   What I have provided is true and correct. If my medical conditions change or if I have a drug or food reaction, │
│   I will inform the pharmacy.                                                  │
│                                                                               │
│   Signature: __ Brian Norris _____ Date: _____ 5-2-1X _____     │
│                                                                               │
└─────────────────────────────────────────────────────────────────────────────┘
```

What is missing from this patient profile?

_____

8. Patient Profile 8

Patient Profile

Name: _____ Danielle Davila _____

Address: _____ 7156 Long Road _____

City: _____ Long Beach _____ State: ___ NY ___ Zip code ___ 11561 _____

Gender: ☐ M   ☒ F   Birthdate: __ 4-23-85 _____

Home Ph: __ 512-555-5871 _____ Cell Ph: ___ 516-555-1934 _____

Email: _____ d.davila@email.com _____

Prescription insurance provider: ___ Caremark _____

ID Number: __ X13570 _____ Group Number: ___ 87014 _____

Relationship to Cardholder   ☐ Self   ☒ Spouse   ☐ Child   ☐ Other

Allergies to Medications: ___ none _____

Medical Conditions: ___ none _____

List any OTC products, herbal supplements, or other medications: ___ Claritin _____
_____
_____

Would you like child-resistant containers?   ☒ Yes   ☐ No

Would you like generic drugs when available?   ☒ Yes   ☐ No

What I have provided is true and correct. If my medical conditions change or if I have a drug or food reaction, I will inform the pharmacy.

Signature: _____ Danielle Davila _____ Date: _____ 3-18-1X _____

What is missing from this patient profile?

_____

9. Patient Profile 9

Patient Profile

Name: Percy Parson

Address:

City: State: Zip code

Gender: ☐ M ☒ F Birthdate: 11-12-65

Home Ph: Cell Ph: 505-555-0231

Email:

Prescription insurance provider: Express Scripts

ID Number: T14320 Group Number: 019732

Relationship to Cardholder ☒ Self ☐ Spouse ☐ Child ☐ Other

Allergies to Medications: none

Medical Conditions: diabetes

List any OTC products, herbal supplements, or other medications: cinnamon capsules

Would you like child-resistant containers? ☒ Yes ☐ No

Would you like generic drugs when available? ☒ Yes ☐ No

What I have provided is true and correct. If my medical conditions change or if I have a drug or food reaction, I will inform the pharmacy.

Signature: Percy Parsons Date: 9-8-1X

What is missing from this patient profile?

_____

10. Patient Profile 10

Patient Profile

Name: _____Nikki_____

Address: _____321 Lane Street_____

City: _____ State: _____ Zip code _____

Gender: ☐ M   ☒ F   Birthdate: __4-21-77_____

Home Ph: _____ Cell Ph: ___854-555-0354_____

Email: _____Nikki30@email.net_____

Prescription insurance provider: ___Meridian Rx_____

ID Number: ___Z46217_____ Group Number: ___013978_____

Relationship to Cardholder   ☐ Self   ☒ Spouse   ☐ Child   ☐ Other

Allergies to Medications: ___Tylenol_____

Medical Conditions: ___none_____

List any OTC products, herbal supplements, or other medications: __Vitamin D_____

_____

_____

Would you like child-resistant containers?   ☒ Yes   ☐ No

Would you like generic drugs when available?   ☐ Yes   ☒ No

What I have provided is true and correct. If my medical conditions change or if I have a drug or food reaction, I will inform the pharmacy.

Signature: ___*Nikki*_____ Date: _____8-17-1X_____

What is missing from this patient profile?

_____

The Prescription

Objective: To familiarize the pharmacy technician with the information required in a legal prescription.

Every day, retail pharmacies receive prescriptions for patients. A prescription is an order for a specific medication prescribed by a physician or other health care professional such as a physician assistant or a nurse practitioner, who is permitted by state law to prescribe medications. Each prescription must contain specific information if the pharmacy is to fill the order.

Information required on a prescription includes the following:

- Prescriber information: name, office address, office telephone number, NPI number, and DEA number if the prescription is a controlled substance
- Patient information: patient's name, birth date, and home address. A pharmacy will attempt to obtain a telephone number for the patient.
- Date: the date on which the prescription was written. This date may be different from the date the prescription is filled.
- Rx symbol: a symbol for a Latin word meaning "recipe" or "take this drug"
- Inscription: medication prescribed, which may be listed under the brand or generic name, and the strength and quantity of the drug to be dispensed
- Subscription: instructions to the pharmacist on dispensing the medication
- Signa (sig): directions for the patient to follow
- Additional filling information, such as refills permitted or generic substitution
- Prescriber's signature

Lab Activity #8.2: Identify what is missing from the following prescriptions.

Equipment needed:

- Pencil/pen

Time needed to complete this activity: 30 minutes

1. Rx 1:

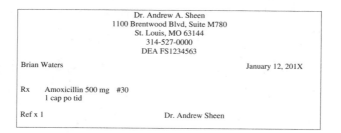

Dr. Andrew A. Sheen
1100 Brentwood Blvd, Suite M780
St. Louis, MO 63144
314-527-0000
DEA FS1234563

Brian Waters   January 12, 201X

Rx   Amoxicillin 500 mg #30
       1 cap po tid

Ref x 1   Dr. Andrew Sheen

What is missing on this prescription?

_____

2. Rx 2:

Dr. Andrew A. Sheen
1100 Brentwood Blvd, Suite M780
St. Louis, MO 63144
314-527-0000
DEA FS1234563

Brian Waters   January 12, 201X
4433 Simon Blvd, Apt 321, St. Louis, MO 63144

Rx   Naprosyn 375 mg   #30
     1 tab po tid prn back pain

Ref x 2

What is missing on this prescription?

_____

3. Rx 3:

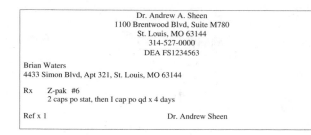

Dr. Andrew A. Sheen
1100 Brentwood Blvd, Suite M780
St. Louis, MO 63144
314-527-0000
DEA FS1234563

Brian Waters
4433 Simon Blvd, Apt 321, St. Louis, MO 63144

Rx   Z-pak #6
        2 caps po stat, then 1 cap po qd x 4 days

Ref x 1   Dr. Andrew Sheen

What is missing on this prescription?

_____

4. Rx 4:

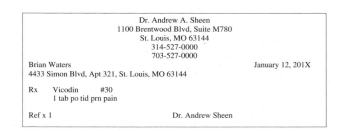

Dr. Andrew A. Sheen
1100 Brentwood Blvd, Suite M780
St. Louis, MO 63144
314-527-0000
DEA FS1234563

Brian Waters   January 12, 201X
4433 Simon Blvd, Apt 321, St. Louis, MO 63144

Rx   Lotrisone Cream
        Apply to the affected rash on arm twice a day

Ref x 1   Dr. Andrew Sheen

What is missing on this prescription?

_____

5. Rx 5:

Dr. Andrew A. Sheen
1100 Brentwood Blvd, Suite M780
St. Louis, MO 63144
314-527-0000
703-527-0000

Brian Waters   January 12, 201X
4433 Simon Blvd, Apt 321, St. Louis, MO 63144

Rx   Vicodin   #30
        1 tab po tid prn pain

Ref x 1   Dr. Andrew Sheen

What is missing on this prescription?

_____

6. Rx 6:

```
                    Dr. Andrew A. Sheen
                1100 Brentwood Blvd, Suite M780
                    St. Louis, MO 63144
                       314-527-0000
                      DEA FS1234563

Brian Waters                                    January 12, 201X
4433 Simon Blvd, Apt 321, St. Louis, MO 63144

Rx      Flexeril       #30
        1 tab po tid prn muscle spasms

Ref x 1                         Dr. Andrew Sheen
```

What is missing on this prescription?

_____

7. Rx 7:

```
                    Dr. Andrew A. Sheen
                1100 Brentwood Blvd, Suite M780
                    St. Louis, MO 63144
                       314-527-0000
                      DEA FS1234563

Brian Waters                                    January 12, 201X
4433 Simon Blvd, Apt 321, St. Louis, MO 63144

Rx      Xalantan eye drops    1 bottle
        UD

Ref x 1                         Dr. Andrew Sheen
```

What is missing on this prescription?

_____

8. Rx 8:

```
                    Dr. Andrew A. Sheen
                1100 Brentwood Blvd, Suite M780
                    St. Louis, MO 63144
                       314-527-0000
                      DEA FS1234563
Brian Waters                                    January 12, 201X
4433 Simon Blvd, Apt 321, St. Louis, MO 63144

Rx      Synthroid 0.15 mg    #30
        1 tab po qd

Ref x 6                         Dr. Andrew Sheen
```

What is missing on this prescription?

_____

9. Rx 9:

> Dr. Andrew A. Sheen
> 1100 Brentwood Blvd, Suite M780
> St. Louis, MO 63144
> 314-527-0000
> DEA FS1234563
>
> January 12, 201X
>
> 4433 Simon Blvd, Apt 321, St. Louis, MO 63144
>
> Rx   Xanax 0.5 mg   #60
>   1 tab po tid prn anxiety
>
> Ref x 5   Dr. Andrew Sheen

What is missing on this prescription?

_____

10. Rx 10:

> Dr. Andrew A. Sheen
> 1100 Brentwood Blvd, Suite M780
> St. Louis, MO 63144
> 314-527-0000
> DEA FS1234563
>
> Brian Waters   January 12, 201X
> 4433 Simon Blvd, Apt 321, St. Louis, MO 63144
>
> Rx   Coreg
>   1 tab po tid
>
> Ref x 1   Dr. Andrew Sheen

What is missing on this prescription?

_____

Lab Activity #8.3: View the following DEA numbers and determine whether each is valid. If a number is not a valid DEA number, explain why.

Equipment needed:

- Pencil/pen
- Calculator

Time needed to complete this activity: 15 minutes

1. Dr. Andrew Shedlock   AS123987

_____

2. Dr. William Dagit   BD7643219

_____

3. Dr. Jerry Kraisinger   JK1234563

_____

4. Dr. Richard Kunze   RK5555555

_____

5. Dr. Bruce Fisher   BF1236579

_____

6. Dr. Clark Andersen   FD4596328

___

Interpreting a Prescription

Objective: To properly identify the specific information that must be entered into a pharmacy's computer for processing and reimbursement for the prescription.

In a community pharmacy setting, the pharmacy technician may be asked to enter the information from the prescription into the pharmacy's computer (information) system. The computer system prompts the technician to enter information in a particular sequence. Although each organization's system is unique, the information requested is the same.

The technician will be asked to enter the quantity of the medication being dispensed in metric terms, unless it is just the number of tablets or capsules. If an ointment or cream is prescribed, it will be dispensed in grams, and if a liquid is prescribed, it will be dispensed in milliliters.

The days' supply can be calculated by dividing the quantity dispensed by the total amount taken during the day.

The prescriber must indicate the number of refills permitted on the prescription. If no refills are indicated, the technician would indicate "0." Some physicians may indicate "prn" refills on a prescription. Depending on state board of pharmacy regulations, most states will permit a "prn" refill to be valid for 1 year from the date the prescription is written.

The pharmacy technician will be required to select the appropriate DAW code. Before selecting the DAW code, the pharmacy technician must determine whether the prescriber will permit a generic drug to be dispensed. A pharmacy will dispense a generic medication unless the physician writes in his or her own handwriting one of the following: "Brand Name Medically Necessary," "Dispense as Written," or "DAW." Most state boards of pharmacy no longer recognize the checking of boxes to indicate whether a generic can be dispensed. If in doubt, refer to your state board of pharmacy's regulations involving generic substitution.

The following are approved DAW codes:

DAW 0: no product selection indicated
DAW 1: substitution not allowed by provider
DAW 2: substitution allowed: patient requested product dispensed
DAW 3: substitution allowed: pharmacist selected product dispensed
DAW 4: substitution allowed: generic drug not in stock
DAW 5: substitution allowed: brand drug dispensed as generic
DAW 6: override
DAW 7: substitution not allowed: brand drug mandated by law
DAW 8: substitution allowed: generic drug not available in marketplace
DAW 9: other

If a pharmacy technician selects the incorrect DAW code, the pharmacy may not be properly reimbursed by a third-party provider.

___

Lab Activity #8.4: Answer the questions based on the prescription orders for each question.

Equipment needed:

- *Physicians' Desk Reference* or *Drug Facts and Comparisons*
- Pencil/pen
- Calculator

Time needed to complete this activity: 45 minutes

1. Rx 1:

   Augmentin 250 mg #30
   1 tab PO tid $\bar{c}$ yogurt
   Ref ×1

   A. How much will be dispensed?

___

B. How many days will the medication last?

_____

C. How many refills are permitted on the prescription?

_____

D. What DAW code will be used?

_____

E. Write the directions as they would appear on the medication label.

_____

_____

_____

F. What auxiliary label(s) should be affixed to the medication label?

_____

_____

2. Rx 2:
Ampicillin 250 mg/tsp 200 mL
1 tsp PO qid ac and hs
Ref ×2

A. How much will be dispensed (use metric quantities)?

_____

B. How many days will the medication last?

_____

C. How many refills are permitted on the prescription?

_____

D. What DAW code will be used?

_____

E. Write the directions as they would appear on the medication label.

_____

_____

_____

F. What auxiliary label(s) should be affixed to the medication label?

_____

_____

3. Rx 3:

Zithromax 250 mg #6
2 caps PO stat, then 1 cap qd × 4 days

A. How much will be dispensed?

_____

B. How many days will the medication last?

_____

C. How many refills are permitted on the prescription?

_____

D. What DAW code will be used?

_____

E. Write the directions as they would appear on the medication label.

_____

_____

_____

F. What auxiliary label(s) should be affixed to the medication label?

_____

_____

4. Rx 4:

Cortisporin Otic Soln 7.5 mL
gtts V in left ear q6h
Ref ×2

A. How much will be dispensed (use metric quantities)?

_____

B. How many days will the medication last?

_____

C. How many refills are permitted on the prescription?

_____

D. What DAW code will be used?

_____

E. Write the directions as they would appear on the medication label.

_____

_____

_____

F. What auxiliary label(s) should be affixed to the medication label?

_____

_____

5. Rx 5:
   Doxycycline 100 mg 1 month supply
   1 cap PO qd
   Ref ×6

   A. How much will be dispensed?

   _____

   B. How many days will the medication last?

   _____

   C. How many refills are permitted on the prescription?

   _____

   D. What DAW code will be used?

   _____

   E. Write the directions as they would appear on the medication label.

   _____

   _____

   _____

   F. What auxiliary label(s) should be affixed to the medication label?

   _____

   _____

6. Rx 6:
   Tylenol #3 #30 (Hint: Controlled Substance Schedule III)
   1-2 tab PO q4-6h prn pain
   Ref × ii

   A. How much will be dispensed?

   _____

   B. How many days will the medication last?

   _____

   C. How many refills are permitted on the prescription?

   _____

   D. What DAW code will be used?

   _____

E. Write the directions as they would appear on the medication label.

_____

_____

_____

F. What auxiliary label(s) should be affixed to the medication label?

_____

_____

7. Rx 7:

Flonase Nasal Spray 14.2 mL (120 sprays)
2 spr to each nost bid
Ref × 6

A. How much will be dispensed (use metric quantities)?

_____

B. How many days will the medication last?

_____

C. How many refills are permitted on the prescription?

_____

D. What DAW code will be used?

_____

E. Write the directions as they would appear on the medication label.

_____

_____

_____

F. What auxiliary label(s) should be affixed to the medication label?

_____

_____

8. Rx 8:

Viscous Xylocaine 100 mL
1 tsp PO swish and spit qid

A. How much will be dispensed (use metric quantities)?

_____

B. How many days will the medication last?

_____

C. How many refills are permitted on the prescription?

_____

D. What DAW code will be used?

_____

E. Write the directions as they would appear on the medication label.

_____

_____

_____

F. What auxiliary label(s) should be affixed to the medication label?

_____

_____

9. Rx 9:
Naprosyn 375 mg #30
1 tab PO tid c food

A. How much will be dispensed?

_____

B. How many days will the medication last?

_____

C. How many refills are permitted on the prescription?

_____

D. What DAW code will be used?

_____

E. Write the directions as they would appear on the medication label.

_____

_____

_____

F. What auxiliary label(s) should be affixed to the medication label?

_____

_____

133

10. Rx 10:

Prednisone 5 mg

ii tab PO qd × 5 d; i tab qd × 5d. Take with milk.

A. How much will be dispensed?

_____

B. How many days will the medication last?

_____

C. How many refills are permitted on the prescription?

_____

D. What DAW code will be used?

_____

E. Write the directions as they would appear on the medication label.

_____

_____

_____

F. What auxiliary label(s) should be affixed to the medication label?

_____

_____

11. Rx 11:

Terazol 3 Vag supp 1 box of 3

1 supp pv q hs

Ref ×1

A. How much will be dispensed?

_____

B. How many days will the medication last?

_____

C. How many refills are permitted on the prescription?

_____

D. What DAW code will be used?

_____

E. Write the directions as they would appear on the medication label.

_____

_____

_____

F. What auxiliary label(s) should be affixed to the medication label?

_____

_____

12. Rx 12:

Sporanox 200 mg #7
1 cap PO qd c̄ food for 7 d, skip 21 d and resume
Ref ×6

A. How much will be dispensed?

_____

B. How many days will the medication last?

_____

C. How many refills are permitted on the prescription?

_____

D. What DAW code will be used?

_____

E. Write the directions as they would appear on the medication label.

_____

_____

_____

F. What auxiliary label(s) should be affixed to the medication label?

_____

_____

13. Rx 13:

Flagyl 250 mg 14-day supply
1 tab PO qid for patient for 14 days. No alcohol.
Brand name medically necessary

A. How much will be dispensed?

_____

B. How many days will the medication last?

_____

C. How many refills are permitted on the prescription?

_____

D. What DAW code will be used?

_____

E. Write the directions as they would appear on the medication label.

_____

_____

_____

F. What auxiliary label(s) should be affixed to the medication label?

_____

_____

14. Rx 14:

Proventil HFA Inhaler (200 sprays) #ii inhalers
1-2 inhalations q4-6h prn asthma and 15 min before exercise
Ref ×6

A. How much will be dispensed?

_____

B. How many days will the medication last?

_____

C. How many refills are permitted on the prescription?

_____

D. What DAW code will be used?

_____

E. Write the directions as they would appear on the medication label.

_____

_____

_____

F. What auxiliary label(s) should be affixed to the medication label?

_____

_____

15. Rx 15:

Coumadin 5 mg #45
1 tab PO odd numbered days, 2 tab PO even numbered days
DAW
Ref prn

A. How much will be dispensed?

_____

B. How many days will the medication last?

_____

C. How many refills are permitted on the prescription?

_____

D. What DAW code will be used?

_____

E. Write the directions as they would appear on the medication label.

_____

_____

_____

F. What auxiliary label(s) should be affixed to the medication label?

_____

_____

16. Rx 16:
    Dilantin 100 mg #120
    1 cap PO qid ac and hs
    Dispense as written
    Ref ×6

    A. How much will be dispensed?

    _____

    B. How many days will the medication last?

    _____

    C. How many refills are permitted on the prescription?

    _____

    D. What DAW code will be used?

    _____

    E. Write the directions as they would appear on the medication label.

    _____

    _____

    F. What auxiliary label(s) should be affixed to the medication label?

    _____

    _____

17. Rx 17:

    Synthroid 0.1 mg #30
    1 tab PO qd
    Brand name medically necessary
    Ref ×3

    A. How much will be dispensed?

    _____

    B. How many days will the medication last?

    _____

    C. How many refills are permitted on the prescription?

    _____

    D. What DAW code will be used?

    _____

    E. Write the directions as they would appear on the medication label.

    _____

    _____

    _____

    F. What auxiliary label(s) should be affixed to the medication label?

    _____

    _____

18. Rx 18:

    Zoloft 100 mg #30
    1 tab PO q am
    Ref ×3

    A. How much will be dispensed?

    _____

    B. How many days will the medication last?

    _____

    C. How many refills are permitted on the prescription?

    _____

    D. What DAW code will be used?

    _____

E. Write the directions as they would appear on the medication label.

_____

_____

_____

F. What auxiliary label(s) should be affixed to the medication label?

_____

_____

19. Rx 19:

Zovirax 200 mg #25
1 cap PO q4h (5 times per day)
Ref ×2

A. How much will be dispensed?

_____

B. How many days will the medication last?

_____

C. How many refills are permitted on the prescription?

_____

D. What DAW code will be used?

_____

E. Write the directions as they would appear on the medication label.

_____

_____

_____

F. What auxiliary label(s) should be affixed to the medication label?

_____

_____

20. Rx 20:

Cephulac Syrup 1 pint
1 tbsp PO bid prn constipation
Ref ×6

A. How much will be dispensed (use metric quantities)?

_____

B. How many days will the medication last?

_____

C. How many refills are permitted on the prescription?

_____

D. What DAW code will be used?

_____

E. Write the directions as they would appear on the medication label.

_____

_____

F. What auxiliary labels should be affixed to the medication label?

_____

Reviewing the Prescription

Objective: To demonstrate the importance of multiple checks during the prescription filling process.

During the prescription filling process, a pharmacy technician should check the prescription at least three times.

Lab Activity #8.5: Identify the error that appears on the prescription label.

Equipment needed:

- Pencil/pen
- List of pharmacy abbreviations

Time needed to complete this activity: 15 minutes

1. Rx 1:

Dr. Andrew A. Sheen
1100 Brentwood Blvd, Suite M780
St. Louis, MO 63144
314-527-0000
DEA FS1234563

Brian Waters   January 12, 201X
4433 Simon Blvd, Apt 321, St. Louis, MO 63144
DOB 12/2/1956

Rx   Amoxicillin   500 mg   #30
          1 cap po tid

Ref x 1   Dr. Andrew Sheen

Prescription label:

Your Friendly Pharmacy
1234 Park Avenue
Arlington, VA 22209
703-243-0036; Fax 703-243-0037

Rx 1001   Date 1/13/201X
Brian Waters   Dr. Shedlock
DOB: 12/2/1956

4433 Simon Blvd, Apt 321, St. Louis, MO 63144
Amoxicillin 500 mg   #30
Take one capsule by mouth four times a day.
Refills: 1

Identify the error on the prescription label and indicate how it should be corrected.

_____

_____

_____

2. Rx 2:

Dr. Andrew A. Sheen
1100 Brentwood Blvd, Suite M780
St. Louis, MO 63144
314-527-0000
DEA FS1234563

Brian Waters   January 12, 201X
4433 Simon Blvd, Apt 321, St. Louis, MO 63144
DOB: 12/2/1956

Rx   Warfarin   5 mg   #60
             1 tab po bid

Ref x 3   Dr. Andrew Sheen

Prescription label:

Your Friendly Pharmacy
1234 Park Avenue
Arlington, VA 22209
703-243-0036; Fax 703-243-0037

Rx 1002
Brian Waters   Dr. Shedlock
DOB: 12/2/1956

4433 Simon Blvd, Apt 321, St. Louis, MO 63144
Warfarin   5 mg   #60
Take one tablet by mouth two times a day.
Refills: 3

Identify the error on the prescription label and indicate how it should be corrected.

_____

_____

_____

3. Rx 3:

Dr. Andrew A. Sheen
1100 Brentwood Blvd, Suite M780
St. Louis, MO 63144
314-527-0000
DEA FS1234563

Brian Waters   January 12, 201X
4433 Simon Blvd, Apt 321, St. Louis, MO 63144
DOB: 12/2/1956

Rx   Lipitor   10 mg   #30
             1 tab po with evening meal

Ref x 5   Dr. Andrew Sheen

Prescription label:

Your Friendly Pharmacy
1234 Park Avenue
Arlington, VA 22209
703-243-0036; Fax 703-243-0037

Rx 1003   Date 1/13/201X
Brian Waters   Dr.Shedlock
DOB: 12/2/1956

4433 Simon Blvd, Apt 321, St. Louis, MO 63144
Lipitor   10 mg   #30
Take one tablet by mouth with evening meal

Refills: 5

Identify the error on the prescription label and indicate how it should be corrected.

_____

_____

_____

4. Rx 4:

Dr. Andrew A. Sheen
1100 Brentwood Blvd, Suite M780
St. Louis, MO 63144
314-527-0000
DEA FS1234563

Brian Waters   January 12, 201X
4433 Simon Blvd, Apt 321, St. Louis, MO 63144
DOB: 12/2/1956

Rx   Furosemide   40 mg   #30
          1 tab po q am

Ref x 11   Dr. Andrew Sheen

Prescription label:

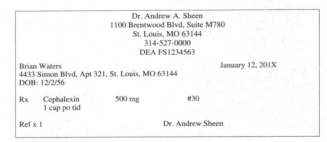

Your Friendly Pharmacy
1234 Park Avenue
Arlington, VA 22209
703-243-0036; Fax 703-243-0037

Rx 1004   Date 1/13/201X
Brian Waters   Dr. Shedlock
DOB: 12/2/1956

4433 Simon Blvd, Apt 321, St. Louis, MO 63144
Furosemide 40 mg   #30
Take one tablet by mouth every morning.

Refills: 10

Identify the error on the prescription label and indicate how it should be corrected.

_____

_____

_____

5. Rx 5:

Dr. Andrew A. Sheen
1100 Brentwood Blvd, Suite M780
St. Louis, MO 63144
314-527-0000
DEA FS1234563

Brian Waters   January 12, 201X
4433 Simon Blvd, Apt 321, St. Louis, MO 63144
DOB: 12/2/56

Rx   Cephalexin   500 mg   #30
          1 cap po tid

Ref x 1   Dr. Andrew Sheen

Prescription label:

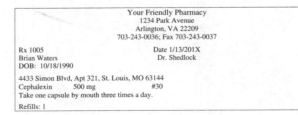

Your Friendly Pharmacy
1234 Park Avenue
Arlington, VA 22209
703-243-0036; Fax 703-243-0037

Rx 1005   Date 1/13/201X
Brian Waters   Dr. Shedlock
DOB: 10/18/1990

4433 Simon Blvd, Apt 321, St. Louis, MO 63144
Cephalexin   500 mg   #30
Take one capsule by mouth three times a day.
Refills: 1

Identify the error on the prescription label and indicate how it should be corrected.

_____

_____

_____

6. Rx 6:

> Dr. Andrew A. Sheen
> 1100 Brentwood Blvd, Suite M780
> St. Louis, MO 63144
> 314-527-0000
> DEA FS1234563
>
> Brian Waters   January 12, 201X
> 4433 Simon Blvd, Apt 321, St. Louis, MO 63144
> DOB: 12/2/1956
>
> Rx   Albuterol Inhaler   17 g   #1
>   1 spray to each nost q 4-6 hr prn asthma
>
> Ref x 11   Dr. Andrew Sheen

Prescription label:

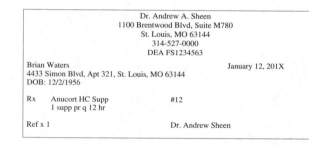

> Your Friendly Pharmacy
> 1234 Park Avenue
> Arlington, VA 22209
> 703-243-0036; Fax 703-243-0037
>
> Rx 1006   Date 1/13/201X
> Brian Waters   Dr. Shedlock
> DOB: 12/2/1956
>
> 4433 Simon Blvd, Apt 321, St. Louis, MO 63144
> Albuterol Inhaler 17 g   #1
> One spray to one nostril every 6-8 hours as needed for asthma.
>
> Refills: 11

Identify the error on the prescription label and indicate how it should be corrected.

_____

_____

_____

7. Rx 7:

> Dr. Andrew A. Sheen
> 1100 Brentwood Blvd, Suite M780
> St. Louis, MO 63144
> 314-527-0000
> DEA FS1234563
>
> Brian Waters   January 12, 201X
> 4433 Simon Blvd, Apt 321, St. Louis, MO 63144
> DOB: 12/2/1956
>
> Rx   Anucort HC Supp   #12
>   1 supp pr q 12 hr
>
> Ref x 1   Dr. Andrew Sheen

Prescription label:

> Your Friendly Pharmacy
> 1234 Park Avenue
> Arlington, VA 22209
> 703-243-0036; Fax 703-243-0037
>
> Rx 1007   Date 1/13/201X
> Brian Waters   Dr. Shedlock
> DOB: 12/2/1956
>
> 4433 Simon Blvd, Apt 321, St. Louis, MO 63144
> Anucort HC Supp   #12
> Take one suppository by mouth every 12 hours.
>
> Refills: 1

Identify the error on the prescription label and indicate how it should be corrected.

_____

_____

_____

8. Rx 8:

```
                    Dr. Andrew A. Sheen
                  1100 Brentwood Blvd, Suite M780
                      St. Louis, MO 63144
                         314-527-0000
                        DEA FS1234563

Brian Waters                                   January 12, 201X
4433 Simon Blvd, Apt 321, St. Louis, MO 63144
DOB: 12/2/1956

Rx      Levothyroxine      0.1 mg        #30
          1 tab po q am

Ref x 5                          Dr. Andrew Sheen
```

Prescription label:

```
                    Your Friendly Pharmacy
                      1234 Park Avenue
                      Arlington, VA 22209
                  703-243-0036; Fax 703-243-0037

Rx 1008                          Date 1/13/201X
Brian Waters                         Dr. Shedlock
DOB:  12/2/1956

4433 Simon Blvd, Apt 321, St. Louis, MO 63144
Levothyroxine    0.1 mg               #30
1 tab po q am.

Refills: 5
```

Identify the error on the prescription label and indicate how it should be corrected.

_____

_____

_____

9. Rx 9:

```
                    Dr. Andrew A. Sheen
                  1100 Brentwood Blvd, Suite M780
                      St. Louis, MO 63144
                         314-527-0000
                        DEA FS1234563

Brian Waters                                   January 12, 201X
4433 Simon Blvd, Apt 321, St. Louis, MO 63144
DOB: 12/2/1956

Rx      Nitrostat      1/150 gr     #25
          1 tab sl prn angina attack, may repeat every 5 minutes up to 5 times per attack

Ref x prn                          Dr. Andrew Sheen
```

Prescription label:

```
                    Your Friendly Pharmacy
                      1234 Park Avenue
                      Arlington, VA 22209
                  703-243-0036; Fax 703-243-0037

Rx 1009                          12/13/201X
Brian Waters                         Dr. Shedlock
DOB: 12/2/1956

4433 Simon Blvd, Apt 321, St. Louis, MO 63144
Nitrostat        1/150              #25
Take one tablet by mouth as needed for angina attack; may repeat every 5 minutes up to 5 times per attack.

Refills: prn
```

Identify the error on the prescription label and indicate how it should be corrected.

_____

_____

_____

10. Rx 10:

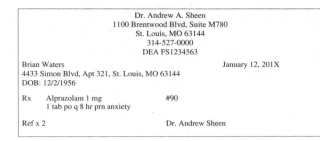

Dr. Andrew A. Sheen
1100 Brentwood Blvd, Suite M780
St. Louis, MO 63144
314-527-0000
DEA FS1234563

Brian Waters   January 12, 201X
4433 Simon Blvd, Apt 321, St. Louis, MO 63144
DOB: 12/2/1956

Rx   Alprazolam 1 mg   #90
          1 tab po q 8 hr prn anxiety

Ref x 2   Dr. Andrew Sheen

Prescription label:

Your Friendly Pharmacy
1234 Park Avenue
Arlington, VA 22209
703-243-0036; Fax 703-243-0037

Rx 1010   Date 8/3/201X
Brian Waters
DOB: 12/2/1956

4433 Simon Blvd, Apt 321, St. Louis, MO 63144
Alprazolam   1 mg   #90
Take one tablet by mouth three times a day as needed for anxiety.

Refills: 2

Identify the error on the prescription label and indicate how it should be corrected.

_____

_____

_____

Customer Service

Objective: To emphasize the importance of customer service in the practice of pharmacy.

> The pharmacist and the pharmacy technician assist patients in their treatment. During their interaction with the patient, it is vital that they listen carefully to the patient. They must be able to explain things to the patient in words the patient can understand. In addition to the words that are used, the pharmacist and the pharmacy technician must be aware of their body language and what it conveys to the patient. Empathy should be conveyed to the patient.
>
> Customer service issues occur every day. Many of these issues could have been avoided if the customer had been acknowledged in a timely manner and treated properly. Common complaints by the patient include the wait time for a prescription to be processed, being out of stock of a medication, and issues caused through billing of their prescription to their third-party prescription carrier. A pharmacy technician must be able to assist in finding solutions to problems that arise in the practice of pharmacy.

Lab Activity #8.6: Read each of the following scenarios. Explain how you would resolve the issue and why you made that decision.

Equipment needed:

■ Paper
■ Pencil/pen

Time needed to complete this activity: 45 minutes

1. Kathy Kraisinger brings her empty prescription bottle of hydrochlorothiazide 5 mg into the pharmacy for a refill on Saturday afternoon at 4 PM. No refills are indicated on the bottle. You call the physician's office for a refill, but the office has closed for the day and will not reopen until Monday morning at 8 AM. What will you do and why?

_____

_____

_____

_____

_____

2. You are entering a patient's prescription into your computer system and have submitted the prescription to the patient's prescription provider. The prescription is rejected by the prescription provider with the following explanation "INVALID ID NUMBER/INVALID GROUP NUMBER." How would you handle the situation?

_____

_____

_____

_____

_____

3. Bill Kunze is picking up his prescription at Preston's Pharmacy. The pharmacy technician notices that a prescription for Bill's wife has been filled and is in the prescription bins. What will you do and why?

_____

_____

_____

_____

_____

4. Tom Dagit brings in a prescription for Dilaudid 2 mg #30. The pharmacy technician checks for the amount of Dilaudid 2 mg on hand and notices that the pharmacy is temporarily out of stock. What will you do and why?

_____

_____

_____

_____

_____

5. You are processing a prescription for a patient, and the prescription is rejected by the prescription provider with the following explanation "REFILL TOO SOON." You inform the patient of the situation, and he tells you he is leaving on vacation tomorrow for 3 weeks. How would you handle this situation?

_____

_____

_____

_____

_____

6. A patient comes to the pharmacy counter and asks you where she can find a bottle of ibuprofen to purchase. What will you do and why?

_____

_____

_____

_____

_____

7. What will you say when you are answering the pharmacy's telephone?

_____

_____

_____

_____

_____

8. A patient comes to the pharmacy and asks you to recommend an allergy medication. What would you do and why?

_____

_____

_____

_____

_____

9. You are the only technician working with the pharmacist today. The pharmacist has asked you to accept patients' prescriptions at the drug counter. A patient approaches the drug counter at the same time the telephone begins to ring. How will you handle this situation?

_____

_____

_____

_____

10. A Hispanic patient brings in a new prescription to be filled at the pharmacy. When you ask the patient for his address and insurance information, you learn that he does not speak English. Neither the pharmacist nor you are able to speak Spanish. How would you handle this situation?

_____

_____

_____

_____

147

11. You are filling a prescription for a patient and receive the following rejection message from the prescription provider: "DRUG NOT ON FORMULARY." How would you handle the situation?

_____

_____

_____

_____

_____

12. It is Friday afternoon at 4 PM, and you are ringing up customers' prescriptions at the cash register. A total of 11 people are waiting in line to drop off or pick up their prescriptions. How would you handle the situation? Why?

_____

_____

_____

_____

_____

13. A woman found a prescription for penicillin for her boyfriend from the community's sexually transmitted disease clinic. The prescription was filled at the pharmacy 2 days ago, and she would like to know what it is used to treat. What would you tell her?

_____

_____

_____

_____

_____

14. A mother is dropping off a prescription at the pharmacy with her sixth-grade son. As they are waiting for the prescription to be filled, the son asks you what the difference is between prescription and over-the-counter medications. How would you explain this to him?

_____

_____

_____

_____

_____

15. A patient comes to the pharmacy and asks for a box of pseudoephedrine that is kept at the pharmacy. You ask to see his driver's license as a form of identification. The patient becomes extremely upset with your request and states that at other pharmacies they do not have this requirement. How would you handle the situation?

_____

_____

_____

_____

_____

16. A patient appears to be upset as she hands you a prescription for a terminal illness for which she has been diagnosed. Would you demonstrate sympathy or empathy toward the patient? Why?

_____

_____

_____

_____

_____

9 Institutional Pharmacy Practice

TERMS AND DEFINITIONS

Select the correct term from the following list and write the corresponding letter in the blank next to the statement.

A. ASAP Order
B. Aseptic Technique
C. Automated Dispensing System
D. Computerized Physician Order Entry (CPOE)
E. Crash Carts
F. Electronic Medication Administration Record (eMAR)
G. Floor Stock
H. Formulary
I. Institutional Pharmacy
J. Investigational Drug
K. Medication Order
L. Non-Formulary Medications
M. PAR
N. Parenteral Medication
O. Protocol
P. Pyxis
Q. Satellite Pharmacy
R. Standing Order
S. Stat Order
T. The Joint Commission
U. Unit Dose
V. USP-797

_____ 1. A prescription written for administration in a hospital or institutional setting

_____ 2. Computerized cabinets that control inventory on nursing floors, emergency departments, surgical suites, and other patient care areas

_____ 3. Written protocols for drugs or treatments that are to be used in specific situations

_____ 4. An independent nonprofit organization that accredits hospitals and other health care organizations in the United States; accreditation is required in order to accept Medicare and Medicaid payment

_____ 5. Technology that automatically documents the administration of medication into certified electronic health record (EHR) systems.

_____ 6. Medication that bypasses the digestive system but is intended for systemic action

_____ 7. A medication order that must be filled immediately—as quickly as is safely possible to prepare the dose, usually within 5 to 15 minutes

_____ 8. A drug that has not been approved by the FDA for marketing but is in clinical trials or an FDA-approved drug that is seeking a new indication for use

_____ 9. Techniques used in the sterile compounding of hazardous and non-hazardous materials to minimize the introduction of microbes or unwanted debris that could cause contamination of the preparation

_____ 10. Guidelines enforceable for the safe preparation of sterile products

_____ 11. A set of standards and guidelines within which a facility operates

_____ 12. A list of drugs that has been approved for use in hospitals by the pharmacy and therapeutics' committee of the institution and become the standard stock carried by the pharmacy and other departments

_____ 13. Drugs that are not approved for use within the institution unless specific exceptions are filed and accepted by the institutional protocols

_____ 14. Computerized order entry

_____ 15. Individualized packaged doses used in institutional practice settings

_____ 16. Drugs not labeled for a specific patient and maintained at a nursing station or other department of the institution (excluding the pharmacy) for the purpose of administration to a patient of the facility

_____ 17. A medications order to be filled as soon as possible but not an emergency

_____ 18. An automated dispensing system often used in hospitals

_____ 19. A pharmacy in which patients receive care on-site such as hospitals, extended-living homes, long-term care, and hospice facilities

_____ 20. A specialty pharmacy located away from the central pharmacy

_____ 21. Moveable carts containing trays of medications, administration sets, oxygen, and other materials that are used in life-threatening situations such as cardiac arrest

_____ 22. Periodic automatic replenishment; a set level of certain medications kept on hospital floors

TRUE OR FALSE

Write T or F next to each statement.

_____ 1. A hospital pharmacy is one of the most challenging areas in which a pharmacy technician can work.

_____ 2. Hospital pharmacies have more job openings than community pharmacies.

_____ 3. Large hospitals may have a central pharmacy and smaller satellite pharmacies throughout the hospital.

_____ 4. Satellite pharmacies stock specific medications for the ward they service to speed up the turnaround time on medication orders.

_____ 5. All hospitals must meet only state guidelines to be reimbursed for patients who have Medicare or Medicaid.

_____ 6. The board of pharmacy has the authority to impose fines and close down pharmacies.

_____ 7. Technicians must have scheduling flexibility because they will need to work all shifts, including weekends and holidays.

_____ 8. All medications are delivered to the patient floors using one cart that is rotated daily.

_____ 9. A hospital pharmacy must stock a wide variety of medications in many dosage forms.

_____ 10. When nurses call the pharmacy, the most common question is, "Where are the meds I ordered?"

_____ 11. Automated systems used in hospitals are replacing technicians.

_____ 12. A hospital pharmacy technician should be able to work in all areas of the pharmacy as needed.

_____ 13. When unit dose medications are prepared, the final check is always done by the lead technician.

_____ 14. The Joint Commission now requires hospitals to make all medications patient-dose specific.

_____ 15. The task of counting and tracking controlled substances is a critical job that requires perfection.

MULTIPLE CHOICE

Complete each question by circling the best answer.

1. The policies and procedures handbook contains information about:
   A. Mandatory training
   B. Cafeteria menus
   C. Physicians' orders
   D. All of the above

2. Factors that differentiate hospitals include:
   A. Outpatient services
   B. Diagnostic capabilities
   C. Surgical procedures
   D. All of the above

3. One of the agencies that governs the operation of hospitals is the:
   A. HFC
   B. HCFA
   C. RPH
   D. ICU

4. All necessary information included on a patient's admitting record to ensure that orders are filled correctly is provided by:
   A. A physician or nurse
   B. A unit clerk
   C. Both A and B
   D. Pharmacy staff

5. When patients with the same last name end up on the same floor, which auxiliary label should be used?
   A. Take as directed
   B. Name alert
   C. May cause drowsiness
   D. Shake well

6. IV medication order labels show the:
   A. Drug name, strength, and dosage form
   B. Route of administration and scheduled dosing time
   C. Patient's name, medical record number, and room number
   D. All of the above

7. The technician responsible for stocking the intravenous room with all of the supplies needed for the day is the:
   A. IV technician
   B. Satellite technician
   C. Unit dose cart fill technician
   D. Floor stock technician

8. Which of the following is *not* an automated hospital system?
   A. PYXIS
   B. SureMed
   C. Robot RX
   D. TJC

9. Point of entry systems provide electronic access to:
   A. Medical and drug information data
   B. Secure entry into the pharmacy
   C. Pyxis machine
   D. Hospital supply room

10. Using the computerized prescriber order entry, a _____ can enter all labs, dietary requirements, medications, and special notes into the computer.
    A. Nurse
    B. Physician
    C. Unit clerk
    D. Pharmacy technician

11. Enforceable regulations for IV preparations have been provided by the:
    A. Joint Commission
    B. Board of Pharmacy
    C. United States Pharmacopeia-797
    D. *Physicians' Desk Reference*

FILL IN THE BLANKS

Answer each question by completing the statement in the space provided.

1. _____ are small specialty pharmacies that supply a clinic, such as the emergency department or an entire floor of a hospital.

2. _____ _____ _____ outline the rules of the facility and procedures and explain how, when, and/or why the policies are to be executed.

3. Nurses are the pharmacy's _____ _____ and should be provided with the highest level of support.

4. All controlled substances are counted two or three times _____ depending on the length of a nursing shift.

5. A pharmacy technician and a _____ must observe the addition or return of controlled substance stock.

6. Only specially trained and properly garbed pharmacy personnel are allowed into the _____ _____.

7. All _____ must be labeled before they leave the pharmacy.

8. All _____ _____ medications should always be placed in the tray in the same order.

9. _____ areas of a hospital can include areas that a patient never sees or those areas that are used as temporary patient care areas.

10. The technician that has experience in many different settings and a broad knowledge base about pharmacy practice and will be in _____ _____.

MATCHING

Match the following primary unit acronyms with their correct meaning.

A. CCU
B. ED
C. ICU
D. L&D
E. NICU
F. NSY
G. OR
H. ORTHO
I. PACU
J. PED

_____ 1. Neonatal intensive care unit

_____ 2. Post anesthesia care unit

_____ 3. Emergency department

_____ 4. Operating room

_____ 5. Labor and delivery

_____ 6. Intensive care unit

_____ 7. Pediatrics

_____ 8. Nursery

_____ 9. Coronary care unit

_____ 10. Orthopedics unit

SHORT ANSWER

Write a short response to each question in the space provided.

1. List three duties of the inventory control technician.

_____

_____

_____

2. What three specialty departments in an institution (hospital) stock many drugs in injectable forms, as well as a variety of oral and injectable controlled substances?

_____

_____

_____

3. List three types of stat trays stocked for code carts by hospital pharmacies.

_____

_____

_____

4. For what are the following governmental agencies responsible?

A. TJC _____

B. CMS _____

C. BOP _____

D. HHS _____

E. DPH _____

RESEARCH ACTIVITIES

Follow the instructions given in each exercise and provide a response.

1. Access *http://www.nabp.net/boards-of-pharmacy* and look up the duties of a hospital technician in your state.

2. Visit or call a local hospital pharmacy and interview the following hospital technicians: IV therapy, chemotherapy, UD fill, and controlled substance technicians. Ask the following questions:

A. What are your job duties?

B. What training did you receive?

C. What is the most satisfying part of your job?

CRITICAL THINKING

Reply to each question based on what you have learned in the chapter.

1. Many technicians work in inpatient hospital pharmacies because the pay scale is higher than that found in retail or community pharmacies. What are some other reasons a technician might want to work in an inpatient hospital pharmacy?

2. The job descriptions of inpatient pharmacy technicians are changing because of the various automated systems coming into use to fill medication carts. Outline a job description for an automated dispensing technician.

3. The relationship between nursing and pharmacy staffs can be tumultuous at times. How can you, as a technician, foster a better relationship between these two groups of professionals?

RELATE TO PRACTICE

LAB SCENARIOS

Hospital Pharmacy

Objective: To learn about the various manufacturers of automated dispensing systems and the benefits of each.

> Automated dispensing systems are used in hospital pharmacies and result in improved patient care. Automation speeds up the dispensing process, resulting in fewer medication errors and improved patient outcomes. Computer dispensing systems allow for improved inventory management by the institution, resulting in fewer dollars invested in the pharmacy's inventory. Many of the tasks previously performed in the pharmacy by an individual were time consuming and had a high potential for error. Technology enables the role of both the pharmacist and the pharmacy technician to continue to evolve.

Lab Activity #9.1: Identify manufacturers of pharmacy automation using *www.rxinsider.com.*

Equipment needed:

- Computer with Internet connection
- Pencil/pen
- Paper

Time needed to complete this activity: 45 minutes

1. Identify five manufacturers of each of the following products/systems.

   A. Automated dispensing cabinets

      1. _____

      2. _____

      3. _____

155

4. _____

5. _____

B. Automation/robotics

1. _____

2. _____

3. _____

4. _____

5. _____

C. Bar code supplies/systems

1. _____

2. _____

3. _____

4. _____

5. _____

D. E-prescribing systems

1. _____

2. _____

3. _____

4. _____

5. _____

E. Hoods/clean rooms/glove boxes

1. _____

2. _____

3. _____

4. _____

5. _____

F. Pneumatic tubes

1. _____

2. _____

3. _____

4. _____

5. _____

G. Tablet/capsule counters

1. _____

2. _____

3. _____

4. _____

5. _____

Lab Activity #9.2: Research automated dispensing systems

Equipment needed:

- Computer with Internet connection
- Computer printer
- Computer paper

Time needed to complete this activity: 45 minutes

Using the Internet, collect information about automated dispensing systems from the following websites:

- *www.omnicell.com*
- *www.carefusion.com*
- *www.mckesson.com*
- *www.parata.com*
- *www.swisslog.com*

1. Complete the following table.

Manufacturer	System	Features of the System	Benefits of the System
Omnicell	Pharmacy Workflow System		
	Controlled Substance Management		
	Medication Order Management		
Pyxis	Pyxis Cubie System		
	Pyxis PARx System		
	Pyxis CII Safe		
	Pyxis Connect System		
	Pyxis MedStation System		
	Pyxis Remote Manager		
	Pyxis Specialty Station System		
McKesson	Fulfill-Rx		
	Bar Code Medication Packaging Solution		
	PACMED		
Parata	Parata Max		
	Parata Mini		
Swisslog	ATP High-Speed Tablet Packager		
	PillPick		
	BoxPicker		

Inventory

Objective: To learn the procedures for maintaining inventory in the institutional pharmacy.

Lab Activity #9.3: Order up-to quantity

Equipment needed:

- Calculator
- Pencil/Pen

Time needed to complete this activity: 15 minutes

1. Calculate the number of full bottles of medication you would order to meet the order up-to quantity of each medication.

Medication	Package Size	Quantity on Hand (Bottles)	Desired Quantity (Bottles)	Number of Bottles Ordered
Albuterol inhaler (200 sprays)	1	45	75	
Alprazolam 0.5 mg	1000	1	2.5	
Amitriptyline 50 mg	500	1.75	2	
Amlodipine 10 mg	500	3	2	
Amoxicillin 500 mg	500	2.5	4.25	
Cephalexin 500 mg	500	3.25	3.75	
Furosemide 40 mg	1000	2.75	4	
Hydrochlorothiazide 50 mg	1000	0.75	3.5	
Hydrocodone 5 mg/ acetaminophen 500 mg	500	1	2	
Levothyroxine 0.1 mg	1000	2.75	3.25	
Lexapro 10 mg	90	3.05	4.25	
Lisinopril 10 mg	1000	0.95	1.8	
Metoprolol 50 mg	1000	0.25	2.75	
Potassium chloride 8 mEq	500	2	3.5	
Propranolol 40 mg	1000	3	5.5	
Serevent inhaler (120 sprays)	1	34	52	
Simvastatin 40 mg	1000	1.75	2.8	
Singulair 10 mg	8000	0.75	1.25	
Warfarin 5 mg	1000	3.25	4.5	
Zolpidem 5 mg	500	0.75	1.25	

Lab Activity #9.4: Perpetual inventory of controlled substances

Equipment needed:

- Calculator
- Pencil/pen
- Paper

Time needed to complete this activity: 15 minutes

The hospital pharmacy has received the following orders for alprazolam 0.5 mg to be delivered to the narcotics cart in various parts of the hospital on the following dates:

- February 1, 2013: dispensed 100 tablets to the emergency room
- February 3, 2014: received 1000 tablets from wholesaler on invoice 0202201108
- February 3, 2014: dispensed 50 tablets to ICU
- February 4, 2014: received 10 outdated tablets from crash cart
- February 4, 2014: dispensed 30 tablets to crash cart
- February 5, 2014: dispensed 100 tablets cardiac care unit
- February 6, 2014: dispensed 200 tablets to the emergency room

1. Based on the above information, complete the following log.

Date	Dispensed	Received	Invoice Number	On-Hand Quantity
January 31, 2013	X	X	X	475

Crash Cart

Objective: To learn the procedures for preparing crash cart trays.
Lab Activity #9.5: Crash Cart Fill

Equipment needed:

- Crash cart
- Medications as listed
- Pen

Time needed to complete this activity: 20 minutes

1. Fill the following medications into the assigned crash cart drawers.
2. List the soonest expiration date for each drug placed in the crash cart.
3. Have pharmacist verify medications, quantity, expiration date, and placement of items.

Item	PAR Level	Drawer #	Expiration Date
Alcohol swabs	6	1	
Amiodarone 150 mg 3 mL vial	2	1	
Atropine 1 mg/10 mL syringe	3	1	
Calcium chloride 1 g/10 mL syringe	2	1	
Dextrose 50% (0.5 mg/mL) 50 mL syringe	1	1	
Dopamine 400 mg/250 mL IV bag	1	1	
Epinephrine 1 mg/10 mL (1:10,000) syringe	6	1	

Continued

Item	PAR Level	Drawer #	Expiration Date
Lidocaine 100 mg, 5 mL syringes	4	1	
Lidocaine 2 g/250 mL IV bag	1	1	
Povidone-iodide swab stick	2	1	
Sodium bicarbonate 50 mEq/50 mL syringe	3	1	
Sodium chloride 0.9% 10 mL vial	2	1	
Sterile water for injection 20 mL vial	2	1	
Vasopressin 20 units/mL, 1 mL vial	2	2	
Dextrose 5% 250 mL IV bag	2	2	
Sodium chloride 0.9% 100 mL IV bag	2	2	
Sodium chloride 0.9% 1000 mL IV bag	2	2	
Atropine 0.5 mg/5 mL syringe	3	3	
Sodium bicarbonate 10 mEq/10 mL (8.4%) syringe	4	3	
Saline flush syringes	5	3	
Sodium chloride 0.9% 10 mL flush syringe	5	3	

Task	Yes/No
Pulled the correct medications/items	
Pulled the correct amount of medications/items needed	
Placed medications/items in the correct drawer	
Listed the correct expiration date for each medication/item	

Automated Dispensing System

Objective: To learn the procedures for refilling the automated dispensing machine.

Lab Activity #9.6: Automated Dispensing Machine Fill

Equipment needed:

- Automated dispensing system
- Medications as listed
- Pencil/pen

Time needed to complete this activity: 30 minutes

1. List the quantity of each medication needed to fill the ADS to the indicated PAR level.
2. Pull each of the medications needed to fill the ADS to PAR level.
3. Have the pharmacist verify medications and quantity.
4. Place the medications in the ADS.

ADS	Medication	PAR Level	Quantity Available	Quantity to Fill
Med/Surg #1	Mevacor 20 mg tab	5	1	
Med/Surg #1	Fluoxetine 20 mg tab	4	0	
Med/Surg #1	Gabapentin 300 mg cap	6	2	
Med/Surg #1	Diltiazem 30 mg tab	4	1	
Med/Surg #1	Atenolol 50 mg tab	6	2	
Med/Surg #2	Benztropine 1 mg tab	4	1	

ADS	Medication	PAR Level	Quantity Available	Quantity to Fill
Med/Surg #2	Acetaminophen 325 mg tab	6	2	
Med/Surg #2	Methotrexate 2.5 mg tab	4	1	
Med/Surg #2	Sertraline 50 mg	4	0	
Med/Surg #2	Glyburide 2.5 mg	4	2	
Med/Surg #2	Amitriptyline 10 mg	4	1	
ICU	Furosemide 20 mg tab	5	2	
ICU	Digoxin 0.125 mg tab	4	1	
ICU	Aspirin 81 mg	5	2	
ED #1	Cefaclor 250 mg cap	4	1	
ED #1	Metronidazole 500 mg tab	4	0	
ED #1	Aspirin 325 mg	6	2	
ED #1	Diphenhydramine 50 mg tab	5	1	
ED #2	Metoprolol 50 mg	3	1	
ED #2	Acetaminophen 325 mg tab	6	3	
ED #2	Promethazine 25 mg supp	4	1	
ED #2	Ranitidine 150 mg tab	3	1	
ED #2	Augmentin 500 mg tab	4	0	
L&D	Ibuprofen 600 mg tab	8	3	
L&D	Acetaminophen 325 mg	6	2	

Narcotic Fill List:

    5. List the quantity of each medication needed to fill the ADS to the indicated PAR level.
    6. Pull each of the medications needed to fill the ADS to PAR level.
    7. Have the pharmacist verify medications and quantity.
    8. With a nurse, verify the current quantity of each controlled substance medication listed in the ADS.
    9. With a nurse, place the controlled substance medications in the ADS.

ADS	Medication	PAR Level	Quantity Available	Quantity to Fill	Nurse's Initials
Med/Surg #1	Alprazolam 0.5 mg tab	4	1		
Med/Surg #1	Diazepam 5 mg tab	4	2		
Med/Surg #2	Lorazepam 2 mg/mL, 1 mL vial	6	2		
Med/Surg #2	Oxycodone 5 mg tab	4	3		
Med/Surg #2	Zolpidem 5 mg tab	5	2		
ICU	Diazepam 5 mg tab	5	1		
ICU	Lorazepam 2 mg/mL, 1 mL vial	8	3		
ICU	Hydromorphone 4 mg tab	4	1		
ED #1	Hydrocodone 5 mg/APAP 325 mg	5	2		
ED #2	Carisoprodol 350 mg tab	5	1		
ED #2	Diazepam 5 mg tab	5	2		
L&D	Hydrocodone 5 mg/APAP 325 mg	8	2		
L&D	Oxycodone 5 mg tab	5	2		

Task	Yes/No
Correctly calculated quantity needed for each medication to fill to PAR level	
Pulled the correct medication in the correct quantity	
Had pharmacist verify medication and quantity	
Placed medication in the correct ADS in the correct quantity	
Had nurse verify controlled substance medications placed in ADS	

Medication Cart Fill

Objective: To learn the procedures for preparing daily medication cart fill.
Lab Activity #9.7: 24-Hour Medication Cart Fill

Equipment needed:

- Medication cart
- Medications as listed
- Pencil/pen

Time needed to complete this activity: 30 minutes

1. Fill the medication orders for each patient as listed for a 24-hour period.
2. Pull each of the medications needed for each patient room.
3. Have pharmacist verify medications and quantity.
4. Place the medications in the correct patient drawer.

Patient Room	Medication	Directions	Quantity to Fill for 24 Hours
201	Augmentin 250 mg tab	1 cap po qid	
	Promethazine 25 mg tab	1 po ac & hs	
203	Quinapril 40 mg tab	1 po bid	
	Simvastatin 20 mg tab	1 po qd	
205	Theophylline 450 mg	1 po qd	
206	Verapamil ER 120 mg cap	1 po bid	
	Mevacor 20 mg tab	1 po qpm	
210	Finasteride 5 mg	1 po qam	
302	Isosorbide dinitrate 40 mg tab	1 po q6h	
304	Benzonatate 100 mg cap	1 po q12h	
	Fexofenadine 60 mg tab	1 po q6h	
305	Glipizide ER 5 mg tab	1 po 30 min ac	
306	Lansoprazole 30 mg cap	1 po bid	
	Potassium chloride 20 mEq tab	1 po q6h	
310	Metoclopramide 10 mg tab	1 po ac & hs	
	Nifedipine 60 mg tab	1 po bid	
401	Ondansetron 8 mg tab	1 po q8h	
402	Gabapentin 800 mg cap	1 po tid	
404	Amoxicillin 875 mg cap	1 po qid	
	Hydroxyzine 25 mg tab	1 po hs	

Patient Room	Medication	Directions	Quantity to Fill for 24 Hours
406	Levofloxacin 500 mg tab	1 po bid	
408	Hydrochlorothiazide 25 mg tab	1 po q6h	
	Enalapril 5 mg	1 po bid	
410	Dicyclomine 20 mg	1 po q8h	
	Famotidine 20 mg	1 po ac & hs	

Task	Yes/No
Correctly calculated quantity needed for each medication to fill	
Pulled the correct medication in the correct quantity	
Had pharmacist verify medication and quantity	
Placed medication in the correct patient drawer in the correct quantity	

Personnel Cleansing and Garbing Order

Objective: To learn the steps required to cleanse and don PPE in order to properly prepare compounded sterile preparations.

Lab Activity #9.8: Personnel Cleansing and Garbing Order

Equipment needed:

- Antiseptic hand cleanser
- Surgical scrub
- Shoe cover
- Head and facial hair cover
- Face mask or eye shield
- Non-shedding gown
- Sterile powder-free gloves
- Sink with hot and cold running water

Procedure

1. Remove all personal outer garments
2. Remove all cosmetics, visible jewelry, watches, and objects up to the elbow.
3. Wash hands thoroughly with soap and water.
4. Pull shoe cover over the toe of the shoe first, around the bottom of the shoe, and finally over the heel of the shoe. Please note that shoe covers are not designated as left and right but are interchangeable.
5. Apply foam alcohol to the palm of one hand and rub hands thoroughly. Allow hands to air dry.
6. Put on hair cover by gathering loose hair and placing it into the back of the hair cover. Pull front of hair cover over forehead. No hair should be outside of the hair cover.
7. Apply foam alcohol to the palm of one hand, and rub hands thoroughly. Allow hands to air dry.
8. Slip on face mask by situating the top of the mask at the bridge of the nose. Pull the two top ties of the face mask and attach them together. Attach the two lower ties behind the neck. The mask should cover the nose, mouth, and chin.
9. Turn on water faucets with a paper towel if not foot operated.
10. Make sure water temperature is lukewarm.
11. Avoid unnecessary splashing during washing process.
12. Use a nailbrush to clean under every fingertip.
13. Apply sufficient disinfecting/cleansing agent to hands in a circular motion, holding the fingertips downward.
14. Clean all four surfaces of each finger, and rub well between the fingers.
15. Clean all surfaces of hands, wrists, and arms up to the elbows in a circular motion.
16. Rinse well.
17. Repeat the scrubbing process a second time and rinse.

18. Dry hands with paper towels.
19. Do not touch the sink, faucet, or other objects that could contaminate hands.
20. Turn off the water using a paper towel.
21. Discard paper towels in biohazard waste container.
22. Open the package of the sterile gown. The gown should never make contact with any surface.
23. Slip one arm into the sleeve of the sterile gown, and pull it up to the shoulder. Repeat this procedure with the other arm. Tie the neck strings behind the neck, and repeat with the waist strings.
24. Apply foam alcohol to the palm of one hand, and rub hands thoroughly. Allow hands to air dry.
25. Open package containing sterile latex (or latex-free) gloves. Remove glove from package and maintain fingers within the cup of the gown. Place glove on palm of hand with the thumb side of the glove toward the palm. Pull the glove's cuff so that it covers the gown's cuff. Unfold the glove's cuff so that it covers the cuff of the gown. Take hold of the glove and gown at waist level. Pull glove onto the hand and work fingers into the glove. Repeat procedure for the other glove.

Time needed to complete this activity: 15 minutes

Evaluation of Personnel Cleansing and Garbing Order	Yes/No
Removed all cosmetics, visible jewelry, watches, and objects up to the elbow	
Was not wearing acrylic nails or nail polish	
Washed hands before donning PPE	
Shoe covers put on	
Applied foam alcohol to hands and allowed to air dry	
Hair cover(s) put on properly	
Applied foam alcohol to hands and allowed to air dry	
Face mask put on properly	
Started water and adjusted to the correct temperature	
Avoided unnecessary splashing during process	
Used a nailbrush to clean under every fingertip	
Used sufficient disinfecting agent/cleanser	
Cleaned all four surfaces of each finger	
Cleaned all surfaces of hands, wrists, and arms up to the elbows in a circular motion	
Did not touch the sink, faucet, or other objects that could contaminate the hands	
Rinsed off all soap residue	
Rinsed hands, holding them upright and allowing water to drip to the elbow	
Repeated the scrubbing process a second time and rinsed hands, holding them upright and allowing water to drip to the elbow	
Did not turn off water until hands were completely dry	
Turned water off with a clean, dry, lint-free paper towel	
Did not touch the faucet while turning off the water	
Sterile gown put on properly	
Foam alcohol applied	
Sterile gloves put on properly	

10 Additional Pharmacy Practice Settings

TERMS AND DEFINITIONS

Select the correct term from the following list and write the corresponding letter in the blank next to the statement.

A. Managed Care
B. Medication Reconciliation
C. Pharmacy Benefit Management (PBM)
D. Telepharmacy

_____ 1. The development and management of broad and cost efficient prescription drug benefits for a large group of patient populations

_____ 2. An organized health care delivery system designed to improve both the quality and the accessibility of health care, including pharmaceutical care, while containing costs

_____ 3. The provision of pharmaceutical care through the use of telecommunications and information technologies to patients at a distance

_____ 4. The process of comparing a patient's medication orders with all of the medications that the patient has taken prior to admission to the hospital

TRUE OR FALSE

Write T or F next to each statement

_____ 1. Most pharmacies require the pharmacy purchasing agent to have up to 6 months of experience as a pharmacy technician.

_____ 2. The pharmacy medication reconciliation technician is an essential part of patient safety.

_____ 3. The number of elderly patients has increased because of improved health care and discovery of more effective treatments for medical conditions and diseases.

_____ 4. The purpose of PBMs is to develop and manage broad and costly prescription drug benefits for a large group of patient populations.

_____ 5. A pharmacy technician trainer must have adequate experience in the practice area he or she is teaching.

_____ 6. It is unnecessary for a pharmacy technician trainee to complete a test proving the technician understands the tasks he or she needs to perform.

_____ 7. Pharmacy technician educators ideally should have retail and hospital pharmacy experience and an associate's or bachelor's degree.

_____ 8. A pharmaceutical sales representative must have a national pharmacy technician certification.

_____ 9. Specialized training is required for everyone handling radioactive material, including the pharmacist and pharmacy technician.

_____ 10. A pharmacy informatics technician must have additional pharmacy education, a bachelor's degree in computer science, and knowledge in pharmacology.

Complete each question by circling the best answer:

1. Between 2010 and 2020, the expected employment growth for pharmacy technicians is _____.
   A. 5%
   B. 24%
   C. 32%
   D. 50%

2. A pharmacy technician career ranks as the _____ fastest growing job overall in the United States.
   A. First
   B. Tenth
   C. Twenty-second
   D. Sixtieth

3. Performing medication reconciliation tasks can prevent _____.
   A. Drug omissions
   B. Duplications
   C. Drug-drug interactions
   D. All of the above

4. A _____ pharmacy technician requires experience in the pharmacy field and preferably call center experience.
   A. Medication reconciliation
   B. Managed care
   C. Purchasing
   D. Nuclear

5. A(n) _____ pharmacy technician is most commonly found working for an accredited college or university, either on campus or online.
   A. Educator
   B. Medication reconciliation
   C. Purchasing
   D. Nuclear

6. A pharmacy technician educator must possess a national certification, meet her or his state's regulations for practice, and have, at minimum, _____ of experience in the pharmacy setting.
   A. 6 months
   B. 1 year
   C. 2 years
   D. 3 years

7. A _____ will have important information on hand, including up-to-date knowledge on clinical studies and side effects, as well as the pharmacology knowledge of the medication she or he is trying to sell.
   A. Nuclear pharmacy technicians
   B. Managed care pharmacy technician
   C. Pharmaceutical sales representative
   D. Pharmacy technician trainer

8. The special class of drugs used in the nuclear pharmacy setting is known as _____.
   A. Radioactive prescriptions
   B. Radiopharmaceuticals
   C. Radiohazards
   D. Radiation

9. _____ is an example of radiopharmaceutical medication.
   A. Fluorodeoxyglucose
   B. Diethylenetriamine penta-acetic acid
   C. Pertechnetate
   D. All of the above

10. _____ focuses on the use of information technology and drug information to optimize medication use.
   A. Pharmacy informatics
   B. Nuclear pharmacy
   C. Telepharmacy
   D. Medication reconciliation

MATCHING

Match the following advanced level pharmacy technicians with their correct description

A. Managed care pharmacy technician
B. Medication reconciliation technician
C. Nuclear pharmacy technician
D. Pharmaceutical sales representative
E. Pharmacy informatics technician
F. Pharmacy purchasing agent
G. Pharmacy technician trainer
H. Telepharmacy technician

_____ 1. Provides support for pharmacy information in clinical systems

_____ 2. Provides benefit information to the patient/client; determines the proper usage of benefits

_____ 3. Performs on-the-job training for new employees or for technicians in new roles

_____ 4. Takes specific safety precautions when prepares radioactive products as ordered

_____ 5. Travels to clients' sites and promotes his or her company's assigned medications

_____ 6. Performs duties much like those of a technician at a community or hospital setting without a pharmacist physically on site

_____ 7. Interviews patients about their at-home medications including prescription and over-the-counter medications, vitamins, or herbal supplements to help the provider make informed decisions about a patient's medication regimen

_____ 8. Places daily orders to keep the department stocked to fulfill the orders/prescription requests to satisfy the patient in need and works closely with pharmacy management in implementing cost-saving opportunities

FILL IN THE BLANKS

Answer each question by completing the statement in the space provided.

1. Employers hiring pharmacy technicians in an _____ _____ pharmacy setting often seek those individuals who have had prior formal training and certification.

2. With the increased amount of medications being prescribed, pharmacies need at least one employee to do the _____ for the department.

3. The goal of the medication reconciliation position is to avoid _____ _____.

4. Most elderly patients take multiple medications, increasing the need for the management of prescription _____ _____.

5. An experienced pharmacy technician can take on a role as an _____ at an accredited school or _____ _____ for new pharmacy employees.

6. The requirements for a pharmaceutical sales representative include an associate's or bachelor's degree in fields such as, _____, _____, _____, _____, or a related field.

7. Because of the risks associated with the _____ _____ setting, the pay in this area of pharmacy is most often higher than that of a traditional pharmacy setting.

8. The _____ _____ technician assists in building new systems to be used by the pharmacy staff and must also be available to help troubleshoot if anything needs to be fixed.

9. A minimum of _____ _____ experience in a community or hospital setting is required to be a prospective candidate in pharmacy informatics.

10. _____ is the most important characteristic of any candidate seeking a position in any health care position.

SHORT ANSWER

Write a short response to each question in the space provided.

1. List three reasons for the increased need of a highly qualified pharmacy technician.

_____

_____

_____

2. List three responsibilities of the pharmacy purchasing agent.

_____

_____

_____

3. List three responsibilities of a managed care pharmacy technician.

_____

_____

_____

4. List three attributes a pharmaceutical sales representative must possess.

_____

_____

_____

5. List three important competencies required of the nuclear pharmacy technician.

_____

_____

_____

RESEARCH ACTIVITIES

Follow the instructions given in each exercise and provide a response.

1. Call or visit a local nuclear pharmacy. Ask the lead technician or the pharmacist in charge the following questions:

   A. What qualifications do you require for technicians in your pharmacy?

   B. What duties do your technicians perform?

   C. Do you require certification and/or additional training?

2. Access the website *https://www.pbmi.com/* and answer the following questions:

   A. What services do they provide?

   B. How many co-pay tiers do they offer?

   C. What opportunities are available for pharmacy technicians?

REFLECT CRITICALLY

CRITICAL THINKING

Reply to each question based on what you have learned in the chapter.

1. What opportunities are available to you in your area at an advanced level pharmacy? How could you prepare yourself for that opportunity?

2. Medication reconciliation is becoming more important in a hospital setting. What attributes do you possess that could help you become a medication reconciliation technician? What skills would be necessary?

RELATE TO PRACTICE

LAB SCENARIOS

Advanced Pharmacy Technician Positions

Objective: To prepare a pharmacy technician student for an advanced pharmacy technician position

> As the roles of a pharmacist and pharmacy technician change, it will become important to begin thinking about how well prepared you are to move into an advanced pharmacy technician position. As you work in a pharmacy as a pharmacy technician, you should begin to take stock of your strengths and work toward obtaining skills to highlight those strengths. This will help prepare you for an advanced pharmacy technician position in the future.

Lab Activity #10.1: Preparing for an advanced pharmacy technician position

Equipment needed:

- Computer with Internet access
- Paper
- Pencil/pen

Time needed to complete this activity: 90 minutes

You are a certified pharmacy technician who is looking for an advanced pharmacy technician position. Perform a web search to begin looking for available positions in your area. Based on your web search, answer the following questions:

1. What advanced pharmacy technician positions are available in your area?

_____

_____

2. Which advanced pharmacy technician position most interests you?

_____

_____

3. What pharmacy technician training can help prepare you for that position?

_____

_____

_____

_____

4. Will you need additional education for your interested position? If so, what education is required?

_____

_____

5. Does your interested position require certification? If so, which one(s)?

_____

_____

6. Why would you be successful as an advanced pharmacy technician?

_____

_____

7. Why do you want to work as an advanced pharmacy technician?

_____

_____

8. What in your background prepares you for this advanced pharmacy technician position?

_____

_____

9. How will this opportunity contribute to your overall goal of being a pharmacy technician?

_____

_____

10. What type of job duties is required for this advanced pharmacy technician position?

_____

_____

11. What skills do you need to improve or obtain for this advanced pharmacy technician position?

_____

_____

_____

12. What coursework, if any, would you need to obtain for this advanced pharmacy technician position?

_____

_____

13. What is your greatest strength that could help you with this advanced pharmacy technician position?

_____

_____

14. What is your greatest weakness that could hinder you with this advanced pharmacy technician position? How can you overcome this weakness?

_____

_____

_____

_____

Lab Activity #10.2: Read the following statement located at *http://www.ashp.org/doclibrary/bestpractices/ autoitstptrolepharminform.aspx* from ASHP concerning the role of the pharmacy technician in pharmacy informatics.

Equipment needed:
- Computer with Internet access
- Computer printer
- Paper
- Pencil/pen

Time needed to complete this activity: 30 minutes

After reading the statement, answer the following questions:

1. What are the roles and responsibilities of a pharmacy technician informaticist?

_____

_____

_____

_____

2. List three ways pharmacy technician informaticists integrate software applications for technological services.

_____

_____

_____

3. List three responsibilities associated with end-user training and education.

_____

_____

_____

4. List two responsibilities associated with reporting.

_____

_____

_____

5. List five skills a pharmacy technician informaticist must have.

_____

_____

_____

_____

_____

Maintaining Your Education

Objective: To keep up with advanced pharmacy technician information, roles, and education.

> To maintain your pharmacy technician certification, it will soon be required to complete pharmacy technician–specific continuing education. To keep ahead of the times and to help prepare for an advanced pharmacy technician position, it is in the best interest of pharmacy technicians to seek continuing education programs related to advanced pharmacy technician roles.

Lab Activity #10.3: Participate in pharmacy technician continuing education–related to an advanced pharmacy technician role.

Equipment needed:

- Computer with Internet access
- Computer printer
- Paper
- Pencil/pen

Time needed to complete this activity: 90 minutes

Using the Internet, select a pharmacy continuing education article related to an advanced pharmacy technician role from one of the following websites:

- *www.freece.com*
- *www.modernmedicine.com*
- *www.pharmacychoice.com*
- *www.pharmacytimes.com*
- *www.powerpak.com*
- *www.rxschool.com*
- *www.uspharmacist.com*

Read the article, take the examination, and print out the continuing education certificate. Provide the certificate to your instructor.

11 Bulk Repackaging and Non-Sterile Compounding

TERMS AND DEFINITIONS

Select the correct term from the following list and write the corresponding letter in the blank next to the statement.

A. Blister Pack
B. Bulk Repackaging
C. Calibration
D. Compounding
E. Compounding Record
F. Cream
G. Elixir
H. Emulsion
I. Excipient
J. Formulation Record
K. Good Manufacturing Practices
L. Hydrophilic
M. Hydrophobic
N. Non-Sterile Compounding
O. Ointment
P. Oleaginous Base
Q. Punch Method
R. Reconstitution
S. Solute
T. Solution
U. Solvent
V. Strip Pack
W. Suspension
X. Syrup
Y. Triturate
Z. Troche

_____ 1. Manual filling of capsules with powdered medication that has been premixed

_____ 2. The greater part of a solution that dissolves a solute

_____ 3. A mixture of two or more liquids that do not usually blend together, which are mixed using a stabilizing agent

_____ 4. Federal guidelines that must be followed by all entities that prepare and package medication or medical devices

_____ 5. The ingredient that is dissolved into a solution

_____ 6. The process by which the pharmacy transfers a medication manually, or by means of an automated system, from a manufacturer's original container to another type of container unrelated to dispensing a prescriber's order

_____ 7. A flat disk-like tablet that dissolves between the gum and cheek

_____ 8. Consists of compounding two or more medications in a non-sterile environment

_____ 9. A strip of heat-sealed packets each holding one tablet or capsule used in the bulk repackaging process

_____ 10. Document of non-sterile compounding

_____ 11. The act of mixing, reconstituting, and packaging a drug

_____ 12. Any substance that easily mixes in water

_____ 13. A water base in which the ingredient or ingredients are dissolved completely

_____ 14. A hydrophobic product such as petroleum jelly

_____ 15. A base solution that is a mixture of alcohol and water

_____ 16. A sugar-based liquid

_____ 17. The markings on a measuring device

_____ 18. Document similar to a recipe used in preparation of non-sterile compounds

_____ 19. A solution in which the powder does not dissolve into the base and must be shaken before use

_____ 20. Ingredient used in compounding that does not dissolve in water

_____ 21. A hydrophilic base

_____ 22. To grind or crush powder such as a tablet into fine particles

_____ 23. Inert substance added to a drug to form a suitable consistency for dosing

_____ 24. A preformed card with 28, 30, and 31 day depressions that can hold medications

_____ 25. To mix a liquid and a powder to form a suspension or solution

_____ 26. Any substance that does not mix or dissolve in water

TRUE OR FALSE

Write T or F next to each statement.

_____ 1. Repackaging of medication is a common process in a hospital pharmacy.

_____ 2. No expiration date is necessary for repackaged products.

_____ 3. The process of repackaging should be done in a horizontal flow hood.

_____ 4. If the expiration date includes the month and year; the drug expires on the first day of the month.

_____ 5. Part of the preparation for repackaging is accurate calculations.

_____ 6. Jars and syringes are the only packages that do not have childproof caps or lids.

_____ 7. All records are to be kept in the pharmacy for only 1 year from the time the medication was prepared.

_____ 8. The record-keeping part of compounding is extremely important.

_____ 9. Capsule size 000 is the smallest size.

_____ 10. Graduated cylinders are available in conical and cylindrical shapes.

MULTIPLE CHOICE

Complete each question by circling the best answer.

1. Which of the following is _not_ a reason the pharmacy repackages a bulk drug into unit dose?
   A. Unit dose is easier to count.
   B. Manufacturers do not package the drug in unit dose.
   C. Unit dose medications can be recycled and used on another patient.
   D. The cost is lower when this process is done by the hospital.

2. The dosage form normally repackaged in a pharmacy is the:
   A. Tablet form
   B. Capsule form
   C. Liquid form
   D. All of the above

3. The expiration date on a drug is 2/12; the drug expires on:
   A. The first day of February 2012
   B. The last day of February 2012
   C. The first day of December 2002
   D. The last day of December 2002

4. A factor that can affect the stability of a drug is:
   A. Light
   B. Air
   C. Temperature
   D. All of the above

5. The punch method is used to prepare:
   A. Solutions
   B. Tablets
   C. Capsules
   D. Ointments

6. Good manufacturing practices do not include which of the following?
   A. Equipment in good and clean condition
   B. Medications checked by a technician
   C. Appropriate packaging for the drugs
   D. Records logged for referencing

7. Which of the following could be used as a base when preparing a compounded ointment?
   A. Aquaphor
   B. Mannitol
   C. Bentonite
   D. Kaolin

8. Which of the following is commonly used as an additive when compounding tablets?
   A. Lanolin
   B. Dextrose
   C. PEG
   D. Plastibase

9. Simple syrup is made on March 15, 2014, from the following products:
   Sucrose 85 g   Expires: November 2016
   Purified water qs 100mL
   What would be the expiration date?
   A. March 29, 2014
   B. April 14, 2014
   C. September 15, 2014
   D. November 15, 2014

10. Using the punch method, you prepare 100 acetaminophen 500 mg capsules on May 30, 2014, from the following products:
    Acetaminophen 500 mg tablets   Expires: 10/14
    Size 0 gelatin capsules   Expires: 11/2015
    What beyond-use date would you assign this compounded product?
    A. June 14, 2014
    B. June 30, 2014
    C. October 31, 2014
    D. November 30, 2014

MATCHING

Matching I

Match the following additives with their correct description.

A. Gums
B. Coatings
C. Disintegrants
D. Lubricants
E. Suspending agents
F. Plasticizers
G. Emulsifying agents

_____ 1. Added to a tablet or capsule blend to help break up compacted mass when put into a fluid environment; especially important for rapid-release agents

_____ 2. Have a wide variety of functional properties (retarding drug release) and allow for flexibility in coating

_____ 3. Surrounding layer of polymeric material of a tablet, capsule, or pellet; is done to change color; protect active ingredient from moisture, light, pH of stomach; avoid bad taste or odor when taken by mouth

_____ 4. Maintains dispersion of finely divided liquid droplets in a liquid vehicle; made from two or more immiscible liquids, such as water and oil, and can be liquid or semisolid (creams and lotions)

_____ 5. Additive for powder blend to prevent compacted powder mass from sticking to equipment during process of making tablets or capsules

_____ 6. Naturally occurring plant derivatives that are water soluble; provide a variety of properties, including gelling, thickening, and film forming

_____ 7. Insoluble particles that are dispersed in a liquid; act by increasing the viscosity of the liquid vehicle; reduces rate of sedimentation of particles

Matching II

Match the following dosage forms with their auxiliary labels.

_____ 1. Ophthalmics

_____ 2. Otics

_____ 3. Ointments, creams, lotions

_____ 4. Suppositories

_____ 5. Suspensions

_____ 6. Patches

A. For topical use; external use
B. Apply to skin
C. For rectal use
D. For the eye
E. For the ear
F. Shake well

FILL IN THE BLANKS

Answer each question by completing the statement in the space provided.

1. All repackaging equipment should be kept _____ and in _____ condition at all times.

2. The process of repackaging should take place in a designated area of the pharmacy, away from _____ areas.

3. Once a bulk bottle is opened and the medication repackaged, the manufacturer's expiration date is no longer

   _____.

4. The FDA requires that compounded products adhere to the _____ standards, although they do not specifically regulate compounding.

5. A class III balance, also called a _____ balance, is a torsion balance and is required by most states' BOPs.

6. Flavorings are often added to medications to mask the _____ _____ of the ingredients.

7. When reading the calibrations of a beaker or graduated cylinder, you must have the liquid at _____ _____ and read the bottom of the _____.

8. For maximum accuracy in measuring liquids, use the _____ rule.

9. Every pharmacy has an _____ _____ with information regarding all chemical products and how to handle spillage or contact.

10. _____ _____ is the special use of finishing technique to give the final product a professional look.

SHORT ANSWER

Write a short response to each question in the space provided.

1. Why is it necessary to use tweezers to grasp metal weights?

_____

_____

2. Why is it necessary to clean counting trays?

_____

_____

RESEARCH ACTIVITIES

Follow the instructions given in each exercise and provide a response.

1. Access the following compounding websites:
   - *www.pccarx.com*
   - *www.pharmacytimes.com/compounding*

   A. What types of services do they provide?

   B. Find an interesting compounding recipe (if published). Print it and share it with the class.

   C. Is membership required to use these sites and to obtain their products?

2. Access the website *www.ehso.com/msds.php* and find the MSDS for polyethylene glycol.

A. What is the physical state and appearance of polyethylene glycol?

B. What is the boiling point for polyethylene glycol?

C. How should polyethylene glycol be stored?

D. What first aid measures should be taken if polyethylene glycol gets in your eyes?

REFLECT CRITICALLY

CRITICAL THINKING

Reply to each question based on what you have learned in the chapter.

1. Pediatric medications sometimes require special compounding. What are some ways the pharmacy staff can accommodate pediatric patients to foster their compliance in taking their medications?

2. Preparing capsules using the punch method can be messy. What techniques for preparing capsules can you develop to minimize the mess?

3. Mrs. Foster has been coming to your pharmacy for years. Lately, she has become hard of hearing and often misinterprets the pharmacist's directions about her medications.

A. How can you, as a technician, aid in this process?

B. What tools can you develop to help Mrs. Foster understand how to take her medications?

LAB SCENARIOS

Pharmacy Equipment Used in Compounding Nonsterile Preparations

Objective: To introduce the pharmacy technician to the equipment used in preparing non-sterile preparations.

Lab Activity #11.1: Correctly identify the following pharmacy equipment used in extemporaneous compounding and its purpose.

Equipment needed:

- Beaker
- Compounding record
- Conical graduate
- Counterbalance
- Cylindrical graduate
- Droppers
- Electronic scale
- Erlenmeyer flask
- Filter paper
- Forceps
- Funnel
- Glass funnel
- Glass mortar and pestle
- Glassine paper
- Hot plate
- Latex gloves
- Masks
- Metric weights
- Ointment slab
- Parchment paper
- Pipette
- Porcelain mortar and pestle
- Reconstitution tube
- Rubber spatula
- Safety glass
- Stainless steel spatula
- Stirring rod
- Suppository molds
- Tongs
- Torsion balance
- Wedgewood mortar and pestle
- Weighing boat

Time needed to complete this activity: 30 minutes

Equipment	Correctly Identified (Yes/No)	Purpose
Beaker		
Compounding record		
Conical graduate		
Cylindrical graduate		
Counterbalance		
Dropper		
Electronic scale		
Erlenmeyer flask		
Filter paper		
Forceps		
Funnel		
Glass funnel		
Glass mortar and pestle		
Glassine paper		
Hot plate		
Latex gloves		
Masks		
Metric weights		
Ointment slab		
Parchment papers		
Pipette		
Porcelain mortar and pestle		
Reconstitution tube		
Rubber spatula		
Safety glasses		
Stainless steel spatula		
Stirring rod		
Suppository molds		
Tongs		
Torsion balance		
Wedgewood mortar and pestle		
Weighing boat		

Lab Activity #11.2: Define the following terms used in non-sterile compounding.

Equipment needed:
- Medical dictionary
- Pencil/pen

Time needed to complete this activity: 15 minutes

1. Blending

_____

2. Comminution

_____

3. Diluent

_____

4. Geometric dilution

_____

5. Inert substance

_____

6. Levigation

_____

7. Pulverization

_____

8. Punch method

_____

9. Sifting

_____

10. Solvent

_____

11. Spatulation

_____

12. Trituration

_____

13. Tumbling

_____

The Class A Scale and Weighing Ingredients

Objective: Demonstrate proper procedures in weighing solids in the practice of pharmacy.

Weighing refers to the determination of a definite weight of a material to be used in the compounding of a prescription or the manufacturing of a dosage form. Weight is measured by means of a balance. Four types of balances are used in pharmacy practice: single beam (equal-arm or unequal), compound lever, torsion, and electronic. All pharmacies are required to have a Class A (III) balance, which can be a torsion balance. An unequal arm balance is used to measure weights greater than 60 g and is commonly used in manufacturing.

A torsion balance must have a maximum sensitivity of 6 mg with no load, and with full load to one pan must cause the indicator or the rest point to be shifted not less than one division on the index point. A torsion balance can weigh up to 120 g. An electronic balance has a sensitivity of less than 10 mg and can weigh quantities of a drug more accurately than a torsion balance.

If a pharmacy uses a torsion balance, it must have a set of metric weights that consists of one 50-g, two 20-g, one 10-g, one 5-g, two 2-g, one 1-g, one 500-mg, two 200-mg, one 100-mg, one 50-mg, two 20-mg, and one 10-mg weight. These weights are made of brass, and forceps must be used in placing the weight on the pan.

Lab Activity #11.3: Identify the following components of a Class A prescription balance.

Equipment needed:

■ Class A balance

Time needed to complete this activity: 5 minutes

Identifying the Parts of a Class A Balance Evaluation	Yes/No	Purpose
Calibrated dial		
Graduate dial		
Index plate		
Leveling screw feet		
Locking or arrest arm		
Weighing pans		

Lab Activity #11.4: Calibrate a Class A prescription balance.

Equipment needed:

■ Class A prescription balance

Time needed to complete this activity: 5 minutes

Procedure
1. Arrest the balance by turning the arrest arm.
2. Level the balance from front to back by turning the leveling screw feet. Move leveling screw feet until all four sides of the balance are at the same distance from the surface on which they are resting.
3. Turn the calibrated dial to zero.
4. Level balance from left to right by adjusting the leveling screw feet.

Calibrating a Class A Balance Evaluation	Yes/No
Arrested the balance	
Leveled the balance	
Calibrated the balance to zero	
Leveled the balance	

Lab Activity #11.5: Use a torsion or electronic balance to weigh the proper quantity of ingredient.

Equipment needed:

- Disinfecting agent/cleanser
- Forceps
- Latex gloves
- Lint-free paper towels
- Metal spatula
- Metric weights
- Sink with running hot and cold water
- Solid powder such as flour or sugar
- Torsion balance
- Weighing boats or glassine paper

Time needed to complete this activity: 30 minutes

Procedure

1. Wash hands thoroughly and put on latex gloves.
2. Organize materials on workbench.
3. Calibrate the Class A balance.
4. Lock balance.
5. Place a weighing boat or glassine paper on each pan.
6. Unlock the balance by releasing the arrest knob.
7. Make sure the pointer is resting at the center of the index.
8. Arrest the balance.
9. Place the correct weights on the right pan by using forceps.
10. Place the material to be weighed on the left pan using a spatula.
11. Release the balance.
12. If the pointer moves to the left, there is too much ingredient on the left pan. If the pointer moves to the right, there is not enough ingredient on the left pan.
13. Remove or add ingredient by using the spatula. Arrest the balance each time before material is added or released.
14. Double-check that the amount weighed on the left pan is correct.

Weight	Amount Weighed
20 mg	
65 mg	
83 mg	
554 mg	
858 mg	
1.25 g	
10 g	
21.25 g	
28.37 g	
45.3 g	

Procedure	Yes/No
Proper equipment and materials were selected.	
Ensured that equipment, supplies, and compounding area were clean/disinfected	
Materials organized.	
Washed hands and put on latex gloves.	
Calibrated the Class A balance.	
Locked balance.	
Placed a weighing boat or glassine weigh paper on each pan.	
Unlocked the balance by releasing the arrest knob.	
Made sure the pointer was resting at the center of the index.	
Arrested the balance.	
Placed the correct weights on the right pan by using forceps.	
Placed the material to be weighed on the left pan using a spatula.	
Released the balance.	
Used pointer as reference to determine if enough ingredient on the left pan.	
Removed or added ingredient by using the spatula. Arrested the balance each time before material was added or released.	
Double-checked that the amount weighed on the left pan was correct.	

Measuring Liquids

Objective: Demonstrate the proper procedures in measuring liquids in the practice of pharmacy.

> Measuring refers to the exact determination of a definite volume of liquid. Glass measures are preferred for measuring liquids because they can indicate volume more accurately by the transparency of the glass.
>
> When an aqueous or alcoholic liquid is poured into a graduate, surface forces cause its surface to become concave; the portion in contact with the liquid is drawn upward resulting in the formation of a meniscus. Two types of graduates are available: cylindrical and conical. The conical graduate is suitable for some measurements, but cylindrical graduates are more accurate because of their uniform and smaller average diameter. Pipettes are more accurate and convenient than very small graduates in measuring very small volumes. The very narrow bore permits greater distances between graduations on the apparatus, thus allowing greater accuracy in making the reading.

Lab Activity #11.6: Using a graduated cylinder of correct size, measure the following volumes and indicate the volume of the graduated cylinder that was used and why it was selected.

Equipment needed:

- Disinfecting agent/cleanser
- Latex gloves
- Lint-free paper towels
- Sink with running hot and cold water
- Various sizes of graduated cylinders from 5mL to 150 mL
- Water

Time needed to complete this activity: 30 minutes

Procedure

1. Collect the appropriate equipment and supplies for this procedure.
2. Ensure that equipment, supplies, and compounding area are clean and disinfected.

3. Organize materials on workbench.
4. Wash hands thoroughly and put on latex gloves.
5. Select a graduate of proper size; the selected graduate should not measure less than 20% of the capacity of the graduate.
6. Hold the graduate in the left hand and grasp the original container with the label in such a position that any excess of liquid will not soil the label if it should run down the container.
7. Raise the graduate and hold it at eye level, so that the graduation point to be read is level with the eye, and measure the liquid.
8. Pour the liquid slowly into the graduate.
9. Remove excess liquid or add additional liquid to measure the proper quantity of liquid.
10. Place the graduated cylinder on a stable surface. Read the graduation point of the meniscus at eye level.

Volume	Amount Measured	Size of Graduate Cylinder Used	Reason for Selection of Graduate
2.5 mL			
5 mL			
9 mL			
10 mL			
24 mL			
30 mL			
38 mL			
48 mL			
66 mL			
88 mL			

Procedure	Yes/No
Proper equipment and materials selected	
Ensured equipment, supplies, and compounding area were clean/disinfected	
Materials organized	
Washed hands and put on latex gloves	
Selected a graduate of proper size; the selected graduate did not measure less than 20% of the capacity of the graduate	
Did not soil the label of product being measured while pouring it into the graduated cylinder	
Raised the graduate and held it at eye level, so that the graduation point to be read was level with the eye, and measured the liquid	
Poured the liquid slowly into the graduate	
Removed excess liquid or added additional liquid to measure the proper quantity of liquid	
Placed the graduated cylinder on a stable surface to read the graduation point of the meniscus at eye level	

Lab Activity #11.7: Measuring a liquid using a pipette.

Equipment needed:

- Disinfecting agent/cleanser
- Empty containers (2)
- Latex gloves

- Lint-free paper towels
- Pipette
- Pipette filler
- Sink with running hot and cold water
- Water

Time needed to complete the activity: 15 minutes

Procedure

1. Collect the appropriate equipment and supplies for this procedure.
2. Ensure that equipment, supplies, and compounding area are clean/disinfected.
3. Organize materials on workbench.
4. Wash hands thoroughly and put on latex gloves.
5. Insert the pipette into the liquid to be withdrawn.
6. Squeeze the pipette bulb slowly.
7. Gently release your grip until the correct amount is withdrawn.
8. Remove the pipette from the liquid and hold above the container to which the liquid is being added.
9. Remove the bulb while holding your finger over the top of the pipette, slowly allowing the correct amount of liquid to flow into the empty container by releasing your finger from the top of the pipette.
10. Verify final measurement of liquid in the pipette.

Measuring a Liquid Using a Pipette Evaluation	Yes/No
¼ of a pipette	
½ of a pipette	
¾ of a pipette	
1 pipette	

Procedure	Yes/No
Proper equipment and materials selected	
Ensured equipment, supplies, and compounding area were clean/disinfected	
Materials organized	
Washed hands and put on latex gloves	
Inserted the pipette into the liquid to be withdrawn	
Squeezed the pipette bulb slowly	
Gently released grip until the correct amount was withdrawn	
Removed the pipette from the liquid and held above the container to which the liquid was being added	
Removed the bulb while holding a finger over the top of the pipette, slowly allowed the correct amount of liquid to flow into the empty container by releasing the finger from the top of the pipette	

Preparing Powders and Capsules

Objective: Demonstrate proper techniques in preparing capsules by using the punch method. Complete a compounding log, and assign the correct beyond-use date.

A powder is a solid dosage form that can be taken orally and externally, depending on the drug being used. Powders are used in compounding tablets, capsules, and suspensions. A capsule is a solid dosage form in which the drug substance is enclosed in a hard or soft, soluble container or shell of a suitable form of gelatin. A hard gelatin capsule, also known as a dry-filled capsule, consists of two sections. These capsules range in size from 000 to 5, measuring from 600 to 30 mg. A soft elastic capsule is a soft, globular gelatin shell somewhat thicker than that of a hard gelatin capsule. A capsule dissolves in the stomach after 10 to 30 minutes, and the drug is released. A capsule eliminates objectionable tastes and odors of certain drugs.

A compounding log or mixing record is an official detailed record of the processes and materials used in the compounding process. A compounding log contains the name of the final product; the quantity prepared; a copy of the patient label; the recipe; the names, lot numbers, and quantities of all products and ingredients used; a record of the steps followed to prepare the prescription; the lot number assigned to the final product; and a beyond-use date.

Manufactured drug products are assigned an expiration date for the drug product. USP 795 (non-sterile preparations) requires that all compounded products have beyond-use dating. Under USP 795, a refrigerated aqueous solution has a beyond-use date of 14 days, and for a nonaqueous formulation the sooner of 6 months or the expiration date of any of the ingredients. For all other formulations, the beyond-use date is not later than the intended duration of therapy, or 30 days, whichever is earlier.

Lab Activity #11.8: Preparing powders.

Equipment needed:

- Electronic or torsion balance
- Disinfecting agent/cleanser
- Label
- Latex gloves
- Lint-free paper towels
- Mortar and pestle
- Powder papers
- Sieve
- Sink with running hot and cold water
- Spatula
- Ointment slab
- Powder A
- Powder B
- Powder C
- Powder papers
- Weighing boats

Time to needed complete this activity: 30 minutes

Procedure
1. Collect the appropriate equipment and supplies for this procedure.
2. Ensure that equipment, supplies, and compounding area are clean and disinfected.
3. Organize materials on workbench.
4. Wash hands properly and place gloves on hands.
5. Triturate (grind) each powder using geometric dilution in the correct mortar and pestle; triturate in a circular motion to reduce the particle size of each powder.
6. Blend (mix) all three powders until the particle size is uniform and the powders are mixed thoroughly.
7. Stir the powder thoroughly using the appropriate spatula.
8. Pour the mixed powders through a sieve to an ointment slab.
9. Place weighing boats or glassine weigh paper on the balance pan(s), and then tare the balance.
10. Weigh the correct quantity of powder.
11. Empty the ingredients from the weighing boat into a powder paper.
12. Fold powder paper.
13. Complete compounding log.
14. Label product.
15. Clean equipment and compounding area.

Pharmacy Compounding Log							
Product Compounded:							
Patient Name:				**Date Prepared:**			
				Date Dispensed:			
MRN or Rx #:				**Pharmacy Lot #:**			
Storage Requirements:				**Beyond-Use Date:**			
Drug Products/Ingredients Used							
Drug Name	**Mfg. Name and NDC**	**Mfg. Lot #**	**Mfg. Exp Date**	**Quantity Measured**	**Measured By**	**Verified By**	

Compounding Powder Evaluation	Yes/No
Proper equipment and materials selected	
Ensured equipment, supplies, and compounding area were clean/disinfected	
Materials organized	
Washed hands properly and put on latex gloves	
Properly triturated powders using geometric dilution	
Powders added in correct order	
Powder blended properly	
Stirred powders properly with a spatula	
Sifted powders properly	
Weighed the proper quantity of powder for each powder paper	
Poured powder into papers and folded properly to avoid spillage	
Observed the finished preparation to ensure it appeared as expected. Investigated any discrepancies and took appropriate actions to rectify before dispensing.	
Correct beyond-use date assigned	
Properly completed compounding record	
Properly labeled compounded product	
Cleaned equipment and compounding area	

Lab Activity #11.9: Preparing capsules using the punch method.

Equipment needed:

- 10 Acetaminophen 500 mg tablets
- 10 Empty size 0 gelatin capsules
- Clean gauze
- Counting tray
- Disinfecting agent/cleanser
- Electronic or torsion balance
- Label
- Latex gloves
- Lint-free paper towels
- Metal spatula
- Mortar card
- Ointment slab
- Sink with running hot and cold water
- Soap
- Wedgewood or porcelain mortar and pestle
- Weighing boat or glassine weigh paper

Time to needed complete this activity: 30 minutes

Procedure

1. Gather supplies necessary for this exercise.
2. Ensure that equipment, supplies, and compounding area are clean and disinfected.
3. Organize materials on workbench.
4. Wash hands thoroughly and put on latex gloves.
5. Count out 10 acetaminophen 500 mg tablets on a counting tray.
6. Pour tablets into a Wedgewood mortar. Triturate with Wedgewood pestle.
7. Pour acetaminophen powder from mortar onto ointment slab.
8. Scrape remaining acetaminophen from mortar with spatula or mortar card onto ointment slab.
9. Using the spatula, form the powder into a "cake."
10. Place weighing boats or glassine weigh paper on the balance pan(s), and then tare the balance.
11. Place an empty capsule in weighing boat or on glassine weigh paper, and obtain reading.
12. Tare the balance again to reset the scale to zero.
13. Remove empty capsule from weighing boat or glassine weigh paper.
14. Remove the capsule cap from the capsule body.
15. Take the body of the capsule, open side down with thumb and first finger.
16. Punch capsule into acetaminophen powder. After reaching the bottom of the powder on the ointment slab, turn the capsule lightly and pinch the open end of the capsule.
17. Repeat the process with the same capsule until body of capsule is filled.
18. Place the capsule cap on the body of the capsule.
19. Place the filled capsule on the weighing boat or glassine weigh paper and weigh the capsule.
20. If the capsule weighs more than 500 mg, gently remove the cap from the body of the capsule and take out some of the powder from the capsule; reweigh the capsule. If the capsule weighs less than 500 mg, remove the cap from the body of the capsule, add powder from the ointment slab, and reweigh the filled capsule.
21. Wipe off powder from exterior of capsule with a dry piece of gauze.
22. Repeat this process four additional times and record the weight of each capsule in the table below.
23. Complete the compounding record.
24. Label product.
25. Clean equipment and compounding area.

Capsule #	Desired Weight	Actual Weight	Difference
1	500 mg		
2	500 mg		
3	500 mg		
4	500 mg		
5	500 mg		
6	500 mg		
7	500 mg		
8	500 mg		
9	500 mg		

Pharmacy Compounding Log

Product Compounded:

Patient Name:	Date Prepared:
	Date Dispensed:
MRN or Rx #:	Pharmacy Lot #:
Storage Requirements:	Beyond-Use Date:

Drug Products/Ingredients Used

Drug Name	Mfg. Name and NDC	Mfg. Lot #	Mfg. Exp Date	Quantity Measured	Measured By	Verified By

Evaluation of Capsule Preparation	Yes/No
Proper equipment and materials selected	
Ensured equipment, supplies, and compounding area were clean/disinfected	
Materials organized	
Washed hands properly and put on latex gloves	
Counted out proper quantity of acetaminophen tablets	
Used Wedgewood or porcelain mortar and pestle	
Triturated tablets to a fine powder	
Tared balance before and after punching capsule; did not include capsule weight in the final capsule weight	

Continued

Evaluation of Capsule Preparation	Yes/No
Filled capsules properly using punch method	
Final weight of capsules within 2 mg of desired weight	
Excess powder removed from exterior of capsule	
Observed the finished preparation to ensure it appeared as expected. Investigated any discrepancies and took appropriate actions to rectify before dispensing.	
Correct beyond-use date assigned	
Properly completed compounding log	
Properly labeled compounded product	
Cleaned equipment and compounding area	

Reconstituting a Solid

Objective: Demonstrate the proper steps in reconstituting a powder into a solution.

> Reconstitution is the process by which a predetermined quantity of liquid is added to a powder to form a solution or a suspension. The drug manufacturer provides on the drug label the quantity and type of liquid to be added to the powder.

Lab Activity #11.10: Reconstituting a solid.

Equipment needed:

- 6 fl oz amber bottle
- Disinfecting agent/cleanser
- Distilled water
- Electronic or torsion balance
- Label
- Lint-free paper towels
- Reconstitution tube
- "Shake well" label
- Sink with running hot and cold water
- Steel spatula
- Sugar
- Weighing boat/glassine weigh paper

Time needed to complete this activity: 15 minutes

Procedure

1. Gather supplies necessary for this exercise.
2. Ensure that equipment, supplies, and compounding area are clean and disinfected.
3. Organize materials on workbench.
4. Wash hands thoroughly and put on latex gloves.
5. Measure 2 g of sugar and pour into 6 fl oz amber bottle.
6. Bring amber bottle with sugar to reconstitution area.
7. Make sure the lower clamp on the reconstitution tube is clamped closed by pinching the clamp until it clicks shut.
8. Open the upper clamp on the reconstitution tube by clicking the clamp open.
9. Allow 88 mL of distilled water to flow into the reconstitution tube. When the tube is filled to 88 mL, close the upper clamp by pinching it shut.
10. Shake the amber bottle to loosen the sugar, and remove the bottle top.
11. Place the tip of the lower tube of reconstitution tube into mouth of amber bottle.

12. Open the lower clamp to allow approximately two thirds of the water (60 mL) to enter the amber bottle slowly. Close the lower clamp.
13. Place bottle top back on amber bottle and shake amber bottle with distilled water-sugar solution until solution is evenly dissolved.
14. Remove bottle top and place the reconstitution tube into the mouth of the amber bottle; add remaining water from reconstitution tube into amber bottle and shake well.
15. Tightly recap the amber bottle and shake thoroughly.
16. Complete the compounding log.
17. Label product.
18. Clean equipment and compounding area.

Pharmacy Compounding Log						
Product Compounded:						
Patient Name:			**Date Prepared:**			
			Date Dispensed:			
MRN or Rx #:			**Pharmacy Lot #:**			
Storage Requirements:			**Beyond-Use Date:**			
Drug Products/Ingredients Used						
Drug Name	**Mfg. Name and NDC**	**Mfg. Lot #**	**Mfg. Exp Date**	**Quantity Measured**	**Measured By**	**Verified By**

Reconstituting a Solid Powder Evaluation	Yes/No
Proper equipment and materials selected	
Ensured equipment, supplies, and compounding area were clean/disinfected	
Materials organized	
Washed hands properly and put on latex gloves	
Electronic or torsion balance tared	
2 g of sugar weighed properly	
Sugar transferred to amber bottle	
88 mL of distilled water measured properly in reconstitution tube	
Loosened sugar then added 2/3 of water from reconstitution tube into amber bottle with sugar	

Continued

Reconstituting a Solid Powder Evaluation	Yes/No
Shook amber bottle with distilled water-sugar solution until solution was evenly dissolved	
Remaining water from reconstitution tube emptied into amber bottle with sugar solution; shook solution thoroughly	
Observed the finished preparation to ensure it appeared as expected. Investigated any discrepancies and took appropriate actions to rectify before dispensing.	
Affixed "Shake well" label to amber bottle	
Correct beyond-use date assigned	
Properly completed compounding log	
Properly labeled compounded product	
Cleaned equipment and compounding area	

Non-Sterile Compounding of Syrups and Elixirs

Objective: Demonstrate the proper technique for preparing oral syrup.

A syrup is a concentrated, viscous, aqueous solution of sugar or sugar substitute with or without flavors and medical substances. When purified water alone is used in making the solution of sucrose, the preparation is known as a syrup or simple syrup if the sucrose concentration is 85%. Sometimes alcohol is included in the preparation of syrup as a preservative and a solvent for flavors. A medicated syrup is one that contains a medicinal syrup. A flavored syrup is not usually medicated and is intended as a vehicle or flavor for prescriptions.

Syrups possess the ability to mask the taste of bitter or saline drugs. Disadvantages of syrups include the possibility of producing cavities and gingivitis in individuals. Another concern regarding syrups is the calorie content resulting from sugar.

Syrups can be compounded by using one of the following four techniques: solution with heat, solution by agitation, addition of sucrose to a liquid medication or flavored vehicle, and percolation. Solution with heat can be used if the ingredients are not volatile or can be broken down by heat. Purified water is heated to 80 to 85° C; it is removed from its source of heat and sucrose is added. Other ingredients can be added at this time, and the solution is able to cool down. Agitation without heat is used when heat would cause the ingredients to break down. During this process, sugar is dissolved in purified water in a container that is larger than the volume being prepared and is shaken vigorously. Addition of sucrose to a liquid medication or a flavored extract is often used with fluid extracts and tinctures. A disadvantage of this process is that a precipitate may develop. Percolation is the process by which purified water is passed slowly over a bed of crystalline sugar, resulting in a syrup.

An elixir is a clear, pleasantly flavored, sweetened hydroalcoholic liquid for oral use. The primary ingredients in an elixir are ethanol and water, but glycerin, sorbitol, propylene glycol flavoring agents, preservatives, and syrups are also used. An elixir is more fluid than syrup because it contains less sucrose than syrup. An elixir can be used as a vehicle for flavors and medications. An elixir does not mask the taste of saline ingredients. A major disadvantage of elixirs is their many incompatibilities with medications.

Lab Activity #11.11: Compounding Simple Syrup-NF.

Equipment needed:

- 4-Ounce prescription bottle
- Beaker
- Disinfecting agent/cleanser
- Graduated cylinder
- Label
- Latex gloves
- Lint-free paper towels
- Metric weights

- Purified water
- Sink with running hot and cold water
- Sucrose
- Torsion or electronic balance

Time needed to complete this activity: 30 minutes

Procedure

1. Gather supplies necessary for this exercise.
2. Ensure that equipment, supplies, and compounding area are clean and disinfected.
3. Organize materials on workbench.
4. Wash hands thoroughly and put on latex gloves.
5. Place weighing boat on balance.
6. Tare torsion or electronic balance.
7. Weigh 85 g of sucrose and place in a beaker that has a capacity greater than 100 mL.
8. Measure 100 mL of purified water in graduate cylinder.
9. Add purified water to sucrose.
10. Agitate (shake) sucrose solution slowly.
11. Pour sucrose solution into a 4-ounce bottle and qs up to 120 mL.
12. Complete the compounding log.
13. Label product.
14. Clean equipment and compounding area.

Pharmacy Compounding Log						
Product Compounded:						
Patient Name:			**Date Prepared:** **Date Dispensed:**			
MRN or Rx #:			**Pharmacy Lot #:**			
Storage Requirements:			**Beyond-Use Date:**			
Drug Products/Ingredients Used						
Drug Name	**Mfg. Name and NDC**	**Mfg. Lot #**	**Mfg. Exp Date**	**Quantity Measured**	**Measured By**	**Verified By**

Compounding a Syrup Evaluation	Yes/No
Proper equipment and materials selected	
Ensured equipment, supplies, and compounding area were clean/disinfected	
Materials organized	
Washed hands properly and put on latex gloves	
Electronic or torsion balance tared	

Continued

Compounding a Syrup Evaluation		Yes/No
Sucrose weighed properly		
Purified water measured properly		
Ingredients added properly		
Sucrose solution thoroughly shaken		
Sucrose solution poured into prescription bottle of proper size		
Syrup qs to 120 mL with purified water		
Observed the finished preparation to ensure it appeared as expected. Investigated any discrepancies and took appropriate actions to rectify before dispensing.		
Compounding log completed		
Properly labeled compounded product		
Cleaned equipment and compounding area		

Lab Activity #11.12: Compounding an elixir.

Prepare 4 fluid ounces of acetaminophen elixir using the following formula:

Acetaminophen	4 g
Propylene glycol	50 mL
Ethanol	200 mL
Sorbitol solution	600 mL
Saccharin sodium	5 g
Flavor	qs
Purified water	qsad 1000 mL

Equipment needed:

- 4-Ounce prescription bottle
- Acetaminophen tablets
- Calculator
- Disinfecting agent/cleanser
- Ethanol
- Filter paper
- Flavoring
- Funnel
- Graduated cylinders
- Label
- Latex gloves
- Lint-free paper towels
- Propylene glycol
- Purified water
- Saccharin sodium
- Sink with running hot and cold water
- Sorbitol solution
- Spatula
- Torsion or electronic balance
- Wedgewood or porcelain mortar and pestle
- Weighing boat

Time needed to complete this activity: 30 minutes

Procedure

1. Perform the necessary calculations using a calculator to reduce the formula to 4 fluid ounces.
2. Gather supplies necessary for this exercise.
3. Ensure that equipment, supplies, and compounding area are clean and disinfected.
4. Organize materials on workbench.
5. Wash hands thoroughly and put on latex gloves.
6. Count out the correct number of acetaminophen tablets; weigh them on the balance.
7. Triturate acetaminophen tablets.
8. Weigh the triturated acetaminophen in weighing boat on balance.
9. Count out the correct quantity of saccharin sodium tablets.
10. Triturate the saccharin sodium tablets.
11. Weigh the triturated saccharin sodium in weighing boat on balance.
12. Measure the proper volumes of sorbitol solution, ethanol, and purified water in graduated cylinders.
13. Dissolve water-soluble ingredients in part of water.
14. Add and solubilize the sucrose in the aqueous solution.
15. Prepare an alcoholic solution containing the other ingredients.
16. Add the aqueous phase to the alcoholic solution.
17. Fold filter paper and place in funnel on top of graduated cylinder.
18. Filter the elixir.
19. Qs the elixir to 120 mL with purified water.
20. Transfer elixir to 4-ounce prescription bottle.
21. Complete compounding log.
22. Label product.
23. Clean equipment and compounding area.

Pharmacy Compounding Log						
Product Compounded:						
Patient Name:			**Date Prepared:**			
			Date Dispensed:			
MRN or Rx #:			**Pharmacy Lot #:**			
Storage Requirements:			**Beyond-Use Date:**			
Drug Products/Ingredients Used						
Drug Name	**Mfg. Name and NDC**	**Mfg. Lot #**	**Mfg. Exp Date**	**Quantity Measured**	**Measured By**	**Verified By**

Compounding an Elixir Evaluation	Yes/No
Reduced formula to 120 mL	
Proper equipment and materials selected	
Ensured equipment, supplies, and compounding area were clean/disinfected	
Materials organized	
Washed hands properly and put on latex gloves	
Correct quantities of acetaminophen and saccharin tablets	
Acetaminophen triturated and weighed	
Saccharin triturated and weighed	
Liquids measured properly in correct graduates	
Water-soluble ingredients dissolved in water	
Sucrose mixed in aqueous phase	
Alcoholic solution prepared	
Aqueous solution added to alcoholic solution	
Elixir filtered	
Transferred elixir to prescription bottle of proper size	
Observed the finished preparation to ensure it appeared as expected. Investigated any discrepancies and took appropriate actions to rectify before dispensing.	
Compounding log completed	
Properly labeled compounded product	
Cleaned equipment and compounding area	

Non-Sterile Compounding of Suspensions

Objective: Demonstrate the proper technique in preparing a suspension.

A suspension is a coarse dispersion containing finely divided insoluble material suspended in a liquid. All suspensions require that a suspending agent be used in their preparation. Examples of suspending agents include Avicel, Methocel, Metocel, Tylopur, Culminol, Celocel, Ethicel, Natrasol, Cellocize, Bermacol, Tylose, Carbopol, Povidone, and Kollidon. Sometimes a product can be prepared in dry form and is placed in the form of a suspension, with water added at the time of dispensing. A suspension may be taken orally, injected intramuscularly or subcutaneously, instilled intranasally, inhaled into the lungs, applied as a topical preparation, or used as an ophthalmic or otic agent.

Suspensions offer the following advantages over other dosage forms:

- They offer an alternative oral dosage form for patients who are unable to swallow a tablet or capsule, especially pediatric and geriatric patients.
- Some medications are poorly water soluble and cannot be formulated as solutions.
- Some drugs have an unpleasant taste, and a suspension allows for less interaction with the taste receptors in the mouth.
- Suspensions offer a method to provide sustained release of a drug by parenteral, topical, and oral routes of administration.

It is important to remember the size of the dispersed particles so they do not settle rapidly in their container. However, if the particles do settle in the container, they should be able to be redispersed with minimum effort by the patient. In addition, the suspension should be easy to pour, should have a pleasant taste, and should be resistant to microbial attack.

Lab Activity #11.13: Compounding a suspension.

Equipment needed:

- 120 mL of Syrpalta (or other wetting agent)
- Acetaminophen 500 mg tablets or caplets, 24 tablets
- Class A balance
- Disinfecting agent/cleanser
- Glass mortar and pestle
- Graduate
- Label
- Latex gloves
- Light-resistant bottle
- Lint-free paper towels
- "Shake well" label
- Sink with running hot and cold water
- Size 100 sieve
- Spatula
- Stirring rod
- Wedgewood or porcelain mortar and pestle

Time to needed complete this activity: 30 minutes

Procedure

1. Gather supplies necessary for this exercise.
2. Ensure that equipment, supplies, and compounding area are clean and disinfected.
3. Organize materials on workbench.
4. Wash hands thoroughly and put on latex gloves.
5. Weigh the dry ingredients.
6. Triturate all dry ingredients with Wedgewood or porcelain mortar and pestle.
7. Filter a pulverized powder through a size 100 mesh sieve.
8. Measure 120 mL of Syrpalta into a graduate cylinder.
9. Transfer pulverized powder to glass mortar.
10. In the glass mortar, wet the powder with Syrpalta in the mortar.
11. Using the glass pestle, levigate pulverized powder with Syrpalta until it forms a thick paste.
12. Pour the mixture into a graduate.
13. Add the remaining Syrpalta until the desired volume is obtained.
14. Stir mixture until it is mixed thoroughly.
15. Pour suspension into a container of appropriate size.
16. Complete compounding log.
17. Label product.
18. Clean equipment and compounding area.

Pharmacy Compounding Log

Product Compounded:

Patient Name:	**Date Prepared:**
	Date Dispensed:
MRN or Rx #:	**Pharmacy Lot #:**
Storage Requirements:	**Beyond-Use Date:**

Drug Products/Ingredients Used

Drug Name	Mfg. Name and NDC	Mfg. Lot #	Mfg. Exp Date	Quantity Measured	Measured By	Verified By

Compounding a Suspension Evaluation	Yes/No
Proper equipment and materials selected	
Ensured equipment, supplies, and compounding area were clean/disinfected	
Washed hands properly and put on latex gloves	
Materials organized	
Counted out the correct quantity of tablets or caplets of acetaminophen	
Measured Syrpalta correctly	
Triturated ingredients properly	
Filtered powder with sieve	
Levigated pulverized powder properly	
Paste qs'd to proper volume	
Suspension properly mixed	
Poured suspension into container of proper size	
Observed the finished preparation to ensure it appeared as expected. Investigated any discrepancies and took appropriate actions to rectify before dispensing.	
Compounding log completed	
Properly labeled compounded product	
Cleaned equipment and compounding area	

Non-Sterile Compounding of Emulsions

Objective: Demonstrate the proper technique for preparing an emulsion.

An emulsion is a dispersed system containing at least two immiscible liquid phases. An emulsion consists of at least three components: the dispersed phase, the dispersion medium, and an emulsifying agent. One of the two immiscible liquids is aqueous, and the second is oil. The emulsifying agent used and the quantities of aqueous and oil phases will determine whether the emulsion is oil-in-water (O/W) or water-in-oil (W/O). An oil-in-water emulsion finds oil dispersed as droplets in the aqueous phase. Conversely, when water is dispersed in the oil phase, it is known as a water-in-oil emulsion. Oral emulsions are normally oil-in-water; emulsified lotions may be O/W or W/O, depending on their usage.

Two distinct processes occur in the preparation of an emulsion. Flocculation is the process of clumping together particles or drops. Meanwhile, coalescence occurs when two immiscible liquids are shaken together. An emulsifying agent reduces the possibility that coalescence may occur. An emulsifying agent should:

- Be able to reduce surface tension
- Absorb quickly around the dispersed drops, which will prevent the drops from coalescing
- Provide an electrical potential, so drops repel each other
- Increase the viscosity of the emulsion
- Be effective in low concentration

Emulsifying agents may be classified as synthetic, natural, or finely divided. Examples of emulsifying agents include potassium laureate, triethanolamine stearate, sodium lauryl sulfate, dioctyl sodium sulfosuccinate, acacia, gelatin, lecithin, cholesterol, and Bentonite. In some situations, multiple emulsifying agents may be used in the preparation of an emulsion.

Lab Activity #11.14: Compounding an emulsion using the dry gum method.

Equipment needed:

- Active ingredients
- Class A balance
- Disinfecting agent/cleanser
- Glass mortar and pestle
- Graduate
- Gum acacia
- Label
- Latex gloves
- Light-resistant container
- Lint-free paper towels
- Oil
- Sink with running hot and cold water
- Spatula
- Water
- Weighing boats

Time to needed complete this activity: 30 minutes

Procedure

1. Gather supplies necessary for this exercise.
2. Ensure that equipment, supplies, and compounding area are clean and disinfected.
3. Organize materials on workbench.
4. Wash hands thoroughly and put on latex gloves.
5. Measure oil in graduated cylinder and pour the oil into the glass mortar.
6. Place the desired amount of gum acacia into the mortar.
7. Levigate until the acacia is thoroughly wet and smooth.
8. Measure the appropriate amount of water desired for the aqueous phase in a clean graduate.
9. Levigate the mixture with a firm motion and quick movement until the primary emulsion is formed. The emulsion will change from a transparent liquid to a white liquid. The sound associated with the trituration process will change.
10. Add the remaining ingredients until the final volume is reached.

201

11. Homogenize the emulsion.
12. Pour into a container of appropriate size.
13. Complete compounding log.
14. Label product.
15. Clean equipment and compounding area.

Pharmacy Compounding Log						
Product Compounded:						
Patient Name:			**Date Prepared:**			
			Date Dispensed:			
MRN or Rx #:			**Pharmacy Lot #:**			
Storage Requirements:			**Beyond-Use Date:**			
Drug Products/Ingredients Used						
Drug Name	**Mfg. Name and NDC**	**Mfg. Lot #**	**Mfg. Exp Date**	**Quantity Measured**	**Measured By**	**Verified By**

Compounding an Emulsion (Dry Gum Method) Evaluation	Yes/No
Proper equipment and materials selected	
Ensured equipment, supplies, and compounding area were clean/disinfected	
Washed hands properly and put on latex gloves	
Materials organized	
Oil measured properly and poured into the proper mortar	
Weighed the correct amount of acacia and poured into mortar	
Levigated acacia properly	
Measured water properly in the correct graduate	
Levigated oil-acacia-water mixture properly	
Mixture qs to proper volume	
Poured emulsion into bottle of proper size	
Observed the finished preparation to ensure it appeared as expected. Investigated any discrepancies and took appropriate actions to rectify before dispensing.	
Compounding log completed	
Properly labeled compounded product	
Cleaned equipment and compounding area	

Lab Activity #11.15: Compounding an emulsion using the wet gum method.

Equipment needed:

- Active ingredients
- Disinfecting agent/cleanser
- Glass mortar and pestle
- Graduate
- Gum acacia
- Label
- Latex gloves
- Light-resistant container
- Lint-free paper towels
- Oil
- Sink with running hot and cold water
- Syrup
- Water

Time needed to complete this activity: 30 minutes

Procedure

1. Gather supplies necessary for this exercise.
2. Ensure that equipment, supplies, and compounding area are clean and disinfected.
3. Organize materials on workbench.
4. Wash hands thoroughly and put on latex gloves.
5. Place the desired amount of gum acacia into a glass mortar.
6. Slowly add the desired amount of water while levigating the mixture.
7. Gradually add the correct volume of oil while levigating the mixture.
8. Measure syrup and weigh active ingredient.
9. Add remaining ingredients to mixture and qs to proper volume.
10. Pour mixture into container of proper size.
11. Complete compounding log.
12. Label product.
13. Clean equipment and compounding area.

Pharmacy Compounding Log						
Product Compounded:						
Patient Name:			**Date Prepared:**			
			Date Dispensed:			
MRN or Rx #:			**Pharmacy Lot #:**			
Storage Requirements:			**Beyond-Use Date:**			
Drug Products/Ingredients Used						
Drug Name	**Mfg. Name and NDC**	**Mfg. Lot #**	**Mfg. Exp Date**	**Quantity Measured**	**Measured By**	**Verified By**

Continued

Compounding an Emulsion (Wet Gum Method) Evaluation	Yes/No
Proper equipment and materials selected	
Ensured equipment, supplies, and compounding area were clean/disinfected	
Washed hands properly and put on latex gloves	
Materials organized	
Acacia weighed correctly and poured into correct mortar and pestle	
Water measured in correct graduate	
Water poured into mixture and levigated	
Oil measured, poured into mixture, and levigated	
Syrup measured correctly	
Active ingredient weighed properly and incorporated in mixture	
Emulsion poured into container of proper size	
Observed the finished preparation to ensure it appeared as expected. Investigated any discrepancies and took appropriate actions to rectify before dispensing.	
Compounding log completed	
Properly labeled compounded product	
Cleaned equipment and compounding area	

Non-Sterile Compounding of Creams and Ointments

Objective: Demonstrate the proper technique in preparing an ointment.

An ointment is a semisolid preparation intended for external application to the skin or mucous membranes. Normally, it contains a medication. Four different types of bases are used in the preparation of an ointment: hydrocarbon (oleaginous), absorption, water-removable (water washable), and water-soluble bases.

A hydrocarbon base is selected when the ointment will maintain prolonged contact with the skin and produces an emollient effect. An advantage of a hydrocarbon ointment base is that it will retain moisture in the skin. Examples of hydrocarbon bases include White Petrolatum USP and White Ointment USP.

Absorption bases have the ability to absorb water and are often W/O emulsions. They have the ability to allow aqueous solutions to be incorporated into them and provide an emollient effect. Examples of absorption bases include Hydrophilic Petrolatum USP and Lanolin USP.

Water removable (water washable) bases are O/W emulsions and are the most commonly used type of ointment base. These ointment bases are easily removed from the skin, can be diluted with water, and allow the absorption of discharges from the skin (Hydrophilic Ointment USP).

A water-soluble ointment base consists of soluble components or may include jelled aqueous solutions. These ointment bases are water washable and leave no water-insoluble residue. Polyethylene Glycol Ointment NF is an example of a water-soluble base.

An ointment is prepared by dispersing the drug uniformly throughout the vehicle base. The drug material is a fine powder or is present in a solution before it is incorporated into the vehicle base.

A cream is another topical dosage form that may be a viscous liquid or a semisolid emulsion (O/W or W/O). A pharmaceutical cream is classified by the USP as a water removable base. Often creams are used for cosmetic purposes. O/W creams are used as hand and foundation cream; W/O creams include cold and emollient creams.

Lab Activity #11.16: Compounding an ointment.

Prepare 4 ounces of the following formula:

Salicylic acid		2%
White petrolatum	qs	4 ounces

Equipment needed:

- Calculator
- Disinfecting agent/cleanser
- Label
- Latex gloves
- Lint-free paper towels
- Ointment jar
- Ointment slab or parchment paper
- Salicylic acid
- Sink with running hot and cold water
- Spatula
- Torsion or electronic balance
- Wedgewood or porcelain mortar and pestle
- Weighing boats
- White petrolatum

Time needed to complete this activity: 30 minutes

Procedure
1. Perform the necessary calculations for the prescription.
2. Gather supplies necessary for this exercise.
3. Ensure that equipment, supplies, and compounding area are clean and disinfected.
4. Organize materials on workbench.
5. Wash hands thoroughly and put on latex gloves.
6. Weigh proper quantity of salicylic acid in weighing boat on torsion or electronic balance.
7. Transfer salicylic acid to Wedgewood or porcelain mortar and pestle, and triturate.
8. Weigh proper quantity of white petrolatum in a weighing boat on torsion or electronic balance.
9. Transfer white petrolatum to corner of ointment slab or parchment paper.
10. Add salicylic acid to other corner of ointment slab or parchment paper.
11. Add a small amount of the white petrolatum to the salicylic acid, and mix thoroughly using an S pattern with the spatula.
12. Continue adding white petrolatum to white petrolatum–salicylic acid compound, and mix thoroughly.
13. Ointment should not appear to have a gritty appearance; if it does, continue to mix it until the ointment has a uniform consistency.
14. Transfer ointment to an ointment jar of proper size. The top of the ointment in the ointment jar should be smooth and level.
15. Complete compounding log.
16. Label product.
17. Clean equipment and compounding area.

Pharmacy Compounding Log

Product Compounded:

Patient Name:	Date Prepared:
	Date Dispensed:
MRN or Rx #:	Pharmacy Lot #:
Storage Requirements:	Beyond-Use Date:

Drug Products/Ingredients Used

Drug Name	Mfg. Name and NDC	Mfg. Lot #	Mfg. Exp Date	Quantity Measured	Measured By	Verified By

Compounding an Ointment Evaluation	Yes/No
Calculations correct	
Proper equipment and materials selected	
Ensured equipment, supplies, and compounding area were clean/disinfected	
Washed hands properly and put on latex gloves	
Materials organized	
Correct quantity of salicylic acid weighed	
Salicylic acid triturated to a fine powder in Wedgewood or porcelain mortar and pestle	
Correct quantity of white petrolatum weighed	
Salicylic acid and white petrolatum transferred to ointment slab or parchment paper	
Used S motion to incorporate salicylic acid into white petrolatum	
Texture of salicylic acid-white petrolatum compound is evenly mixed. No visible signs of salicylic acid powder. Ointment is not gritty.	
Salicylic acid-white petrolatum ointment transferred to ointment jar of proper size	
Final product has a pharmaceutically elegant appearance	
Observed the finished preparation to ensure it appeared as expected. Investigated any discrepancies and took appropriate actions to rectify before dispensing.	
Compounding log completed	
Properly labeled compounded product	
Cleaned equipment and compounding area	

Non-Sterile Compounding of Molded Tablets

Objective: To be able to calibrate the mold before making molded tablets and accurately compound pharmaceutically elegant tablets with a mold.

Molded tablets, also known as tablet triturates, have a limited use because they disintegrate quickly when exposed to moisture and are limited to substances that require a smaller dose. This dosage form also requires a base and additional additives to the active drug ingredient. Common additives include dextrose, lactose, and sucrose. A wetting agent, typically a hydroalcoholic solution (50% to 80% alcohol), is used to bind the tablet ingredients; alcohol is used to dry the triturate while the water causes sugar to dissolve and bind the tablet. The ingredients are pressed into a tablet mold and allowed to completely dry. Because each tablet mold varies in size, calibrating the mold to the specific strength of each molded tablet compounded is necessary. Therefore, it takes great skill and experience to make molded tablets. For more information about molded tablets and to view a video of calibrating a molded tablet and preparing molded tablets, visit *http://pharmlabs.unc.edu/labs/tablets/molded.htm.*

Lab Activity #11.17: Calibrating the tablet mold.

Equipment needed:

- 80- to 100-Mesh sieve
- Active drug ingredient
- Calculator
- Disinfecting agent/cleaner
- Glass mortar and pestle
- Glassine weigh paper
- Latex gloves
- Tablet mold
- Ointment slab
- Powder base
- Sink with running hot and cold water
- Spatula
- Torsion or electronic balance
- Wetting agent (alcohol and water)

Time needed to complete this activity: 30 minutes

Procedure

1. Gather supplies necessary for this exercise.
2. Ensure that equipment, supplies, and compounding area are clean and disinfected.
3. Organize materials on workbench.
4. Wash hands thoroughly and put on latex gloves.
5. Make tablets that contain only a powder base first. Weigh the entire batch and then average the weight per tablet.
6. Determine the average weight of only the active drug; fill a few cavities in the mold and determine the average weight per tablet.
7. Divide the quantity of drug required per tablet in the prescription by the average weight per tablet of the active drug to get the percentage of the cavity that will be active drug.
8. Subtract the percentage in step 7 from 100%; this equals the percentage of the cavity that will be inactive powder base.
9. Use percentages of both the active drug in the cavity and the base in the cavity to calculate the amount of base and drug to weigh.
   For example, if the mold holds 10 cavities, each holding 100 mg, then 1000 mg of mixture is needed to fill the entire mold. From this calculation, calculate the base and drug to weigh; multiply 1000 mg by the two different percentages from steps 7 and 8.
10. Prepare 5% to 10% excess mixture.
11. Clean equipment and compounding area.

Calibrating the Tablet Mold Evaluation	Yes/No
Proper equipment and materials selected	
Ensured equipment, supplies, and compounding area were clean/disinfected	
Organized materials on workbench	
Washed hands thoroughly and put on latex gloves	
Made tablets that contained only a powder base first. Weighed the entire batch and then averaged the weight per tablet	
Determined the average weight of only the active drug; filled a few cavities in the mold and averaged the weight per tablet	
Divided the quantity of the total prescription by the average weight of each tablet's active ingredient	
Subtracted the percentage in step 7 from 100% and determined the volume (%) available for the base	
Used percentages of both the active drug in the cavity and the base in the cavity to calculate the amount of base and drug to weigh	
Prepared 5% and 10% excess mixture	
Cleaned equipment and compounding area	

Lab Activity #11.18: Using the calculations determined in Lab Activity #11.17, compounding molded tablets.

Equipment needed:

- 80- to 100-Mesh sieve
- Active drug ingredient
- Disinfecting agent/cleaner
- Glass mortar and pestle
- Glassine weigh paper
- Latex gloves
- Ointment slab
- Powder base
- Sink with running hot and cold water
- Spatula
- Tablet mold
- Torsion or electronic balance
- Wetting agent (alcohol and water)

Time needed to complete this activity: 30 minutes

Procedure

1. Gather supplies necessary for this exercise.
2. Ensure that equipment, supplies, and compounding area are clean and disinfected.
3. Organize materials on workbench.
4. Wash hands thoroughly and put on latex gloves.
5. Prepare the power mixture using proper techniques for that specific recipe; sift the mixture through an 80- to 100-mesh sieve.
6. Moisten the powder mixture with the wetting agent (alcohol/water) until it adheres to the pestle.
7. Place the cavity plate on the ointment slab.
8. Take the molded form and press mixture into the cavity plate using a hard rubber spatula.
9. Apply sufficient pressure onto each cavity to make sure all cavities are filled entirely and fully.
10. Inspect the cavity plate to ensure all cavities are filled to capacity; very little mixture should be left unused.
11. Align the cavity plate onto the peg plate and then slowly press down evenly onto the peg plate.
12. The cavity plate will fall, having pushed out the tablets onto the pegs.
13. Allow the tablets to dry in the pegs, approximately 1 to 2 hours.
14. Invert the plate and press the tablets off.

15. Complete compounding log.
16. Package and label product.
17. Clean equipment and compounding area.

Pharmacy Compounding Log						
Product Compounded:						
Patient Name:			**Date Prepared:**			
			Date Dispensed:			
MRN or Rx #:			**Pharmacy Lot #:**			
Storage Requirements:			**Beyond-Use Date:**			
Drug Products/Ingredients Used						
Drug Name	**Mfg. Name and NDC**	**Mfg. Lot #**	**Mfg. Exp Date**	**Quantity Measured**	**Measured By**	**Verified By**

Compounding Molded Tablets Evaluation	Yes/No
Proper equipment and materials selected	
Ensured equipment, supplies, and compounding area were clean/disinfected	
Organized materials on workbench	
Washed hands thoroughly and put on latex gloves	
Prepared the power mixture using proper techniques for the specific recipe; sifted the mixture through an 80- to 100-mesh sieve	
Moistened the powder mixture with the wetting agent (alcohol/water) until it adhered to the pestle	
Placed the cavity plate on the ointment slab	
Used the molded form and press mixture into the cavity plate using a spatula. Chose correct spatula for the tablets being prepared.	
Applied sufficient pressure onto each cavity to make sure all cavities were filled entirely and fully	
Inspected the cavity plate to ensure all cavities are filled to capacity; very little mixture was left unused	
Aligned the cavity plate onto the peg plate and slowly pressed down evenly onto the peg plate	
Pushed out the tablets onto the pegs	
Allowed the tablets to dry in the pegs	

Continued

Chapter **11** **Bulk Repackaging and Non-Sterile Compounding**

Compounding Molded Tablets Evaluation	Yes/No
Inverted the plate and pressed the tablets off	
Observed the finished preparation to ensure it appeared as expected. Investigated any discrepancies and took appropriate actions to rectify before dispensing	
Completed compounding log	
Packaged and labeled product	
Cleaned equipment and compounding area	

Repackaging Bulk Medications

Objective: To be able to use good manufacturing practices when packaging a unit dose or single dose container, properly label each unit dose, and properly document repackaging.

Pharmacies will often repackage bulk medications into single (unit) doses. This is done to help lower pharmacy cost and to help decrease dosing errors. When repackaging, good manufacturing practices must be followed, each unit dose must be labeled appropriately, and the procedure must be documented.

Lab Activity #11.19: Repacking bulk medications.

Equipment needed:

- Alcohol prep pads
- Counting tray and spatula
- Latex gloves
- Sink with running hot and cold water
- Unit dose packing of choice—plastic cups/oral syringes, blister packs/ADS supplies
- Various medications as assigned

Time needed to complete this activity: 60 minutes

Procedure

1. Gather supplies necessary for this exercise.
2. Ensure that equipment, supplies, and compounding area are clean and disinfected.
3. Organize materials on workbench.
4. Wash hands thoroughly and put on latex gloves.
5. Repackage the medications as listed by your instructor using good manufacturing practices and proper labeling.
6. Document each medication repackaged in the Unit Dose Log.
7. Have pharmacist verify unit doses/single doses and Unit Dose Log.
8. Clean equipment and work area.
9. Store unit doses in proper place in the pharmacy.

	Date	Drug	Strength	Dosage Form	Amount	Mfg.	Mfg. Lot #	Mfg. Exp. Date	Pharmacy Exp. Date	Pharmacy Lot #	Tech	RPh
1												
2												
3												
4												
5												
6												
7												
8												
9												
10												
11												
12												
13												
14												
15												
16												
17												
18												
19												
20												
21												
22												
23												
24												
25												

Procedure	Yes/No
Proper equipment and materials selected	
Ensured equipment, supplies, and compounding area were clean/disinfected	
Organized materials on workbench	
Washed hands thoroughly and put on latex gloves	
Repackaged the medications as listed in the table using good manufacturing practices	
Properly labeled each unit/single dose	
Documented each medication repackaged in the Unit Dose Log	
Had pharmacist verify unit doses/single doses and verify the Unit Dose Log	
Cleaned equipment and work area	
Placed unit doses in proper storage area in the pharmacy	

Chapter **11** Bulk Repackaging and Non-Sterile Compounding

12 Aseptic Technique and Sterile Compounding

TERMS AND DEFINITIONS

Select the correct term from the following list and write the corresponding letter in the blank next to the statement.

A. Aseptic Technique
B. Beyond-Use Date
C. Biological Safety Cabinet
D. Clean Room
E. Compounded Sterile Preparations (CSPs)
F. Gauge
G. Hazardous Drug
H. Hazardous Waste
I. Healthcare-Associated Infection (HAI)
J. Horizontal Laminar Flow Hood
K. Hyperalimentation
L. Infection Control
M. Laminar Flow Hood
N. Parenteral Medication
O. Peripheral Parenteral
P. Peripheral Parenteral Nutrition (PPN)
Q. Precipitate
R. Reconstitute
S. Standard Operating Procedures (SOPs)
T. Standard Precautions
U. Sterile Preparation
V. Total Parenteral Nutrition
W. USP <797>
X. Vertical Laminar Flow Hood

_____ 1. Any drug that has been proved to have dangerous effects during animal or human testing; it may cause cancer or harm to certain organs or pregnant women

_____ 2. Intravenous nutrition administered through the veins located on the periphery of the body, instead of a central vein or artery

_____ 3. Parenteral nutrition for persons who are unable to eat solids or liquids

_____ 4. A contained and controlled environment within the pharmacy that has a low level of environmental pollutants such as dust, airborne microbes, aerosol particles, and chemical vapors

_____ 5. To add a diluent such as saline or sterile water to a powder

_____ 6. The date or time after which a CSP shall not be administered, stored, or transported, determined from the date the preparation is compounded

_____ 7. Large-volume intravenous nutrition administered through a central vein which allows for a higher concentration of solutions

_____ 8. Medication that bypasses the digestive system but is intended for systemic action

_____ 9. To separate from solution or suspension; a solid that emerges from a liquid solution

_____ 10. Environment for the preparation of compounded sterile preparations where air originating from the back of the hood moves forward across the hood and into the room

_____ 11. Environment for the preparation of chemotherapeutic and hazardous agents in which air originating from the roof of the hood moves downward and is captured in a vent located on the floor of the hood

_____ 12. The procedures used to eliminate the possibility of a drug becoming contaminated with microbes or particles

_____ 13. Environment for the preparation of sterile products

_____ 14. Any waste that meets the RCRA characteristic of ignitability, corrosivity, reactivity, or toxicity

_____ 15. A set of standards that lowers the possibility of contamination and lowers the risk of transmission of infectious disease

_____ 16. Preparations prepared in a sterile environment using nonsterile ingredients or devices that must be sterilized before administration

_____ 17. An infection that patients acquire during the course of receiving treatments for other conditions within an institutional setting

_____ 18. A preparation that contains no living microorganisms

_____ 19. Injection of a medication into the veins located on the periphery of the body, instead of a central vein or artery

_____ 20. The size of the needle opening

_____ 21. Written guidelines and criteria that list specific steps for various competencies

_____ 22. A set of enforceable sterile compounding standards which describes the guidelines, procedures and compliance requirements for compounding sterile preparations and sets the standards that apply to all settings in which sterile preparations are compounded

_____ 23. Policies and procedures put in place to minimize the risk of spreading infections in hospitals or other health care facilities

_____ 24. A hood that should be used for hazardous sterile preparations within the clean room

TRUE OR FALSE

Write T or F next to each statement.

_____ 1. One of the most trivial responsibilities that a hospital pharmacy technician can have is the proper preparation of parenteral medications.

_____ 2. All parenteral and ophthalmic medications should be prepared within a laminar flow hood.

_____ 3. Cost can be a determining factor in the choice of some pharmacy equipment.

_____ 4. All syringes must have a transfer needle if transported out of the pharmacy.

_____ 5. Flexible bags and bottles are the main types of piggyback containers.

_____ 6. Most syringes are made of glass and are meant to be sterilized and reused.

_____ 7. Low-risk CSPs can be stored in the refrigerator for 14 days after compounding.

_____ 8. Medium-risk CSPs can be stored at room temperature for 48 hours after compounding.

_____ 9. All chemotherapeutic agents can be prepared in a vertical flow hood.

_____ 10. All IV rooms have references that can be used to find special instructions for all types of parenteral medications.

MULTIPLE CHOICE

Complete each question by circling the best answer.

1. Amiodarone should go in _____.
   A. 1/2NS
   B. D5W
   C. Metered dose ventilator
   D. None of the above

2. Which of the following is not a parenteral route of administration?
   A. IV
   B. IM
   C. SL
   D. SubQ/Subcut

3. Nitroglycerin must be put only into _____.
   A. Glass containers
   B. Small-volume drips
   C. Syringe pumps
   D. Viaflex bags

4. Which of the following is not an example of a medication administration system?
   A. Cassette pump
   B. CRIS
   C. CADD pump
   D. None of the above

5. A chunk of rubber from the vial stopper is dislodged and falls into the vial, which is known as _____.
   A. Filtering
   B. Beveling
   C. Coring
   D. Piggybacking

6. To ensure sterility, which part of the needle should not be touched?
   A. Hub
   B. Shaft
   C. Bevel
   D. All of the above

7. When aseptic technique is used, what should *not* be worn?
   A. Gloves
   B. Artificial nails
   C. Hair ties
   D. All of the above

8. For proper hand washing technique, you should wash which areas for 30 to 90 seconds?
   A. Hands, nails, face, and forearms
   B. Hands, nails, wrists, and forearms
   C. Fingernails, wrists, and underarms
   D. Fingernails, hands, and face

9. To clean the hood, you should use _____.
   A. Soap and water
   B. Antimicrobial soap and hot water
   C. 70% isopropyl alcohol
   D. Hydrogen peroxide

10. The horizontal and vertical flow hoods must be turned on at least _____ before use.
    A. 30 minutes
    B. 60 minutes
    C. 2 hours
    D. 8 hours

11. The laminar flow hood should be cleaned and disinfected _____.
    A. Monthly
    B. Weekly
    C. Daily
    D. At the start of each shift

12. Walls, ceilings, and storage shelves in the clean room should be disinfected _____.
    A. Monthly
    B. Weekly
    C. Daily
    D. At the start of each shift

13. Counters and work surfaces in the clean room should be cleaned and disinfected _____.
    A. Monthly
    B. Weekly
    C. Daily
    D. At the start of each shift

14. Ciprofloxacin must be put in a _____.
    A. Glass container
    B. Amber bag to protect from light
    C. Multiple dose vial
    D. CADD pump

15. While continuous compounding is taking place, the biological safety hood should be cleaned every _____.
    A. Day
    B. Shift
    C. 12 hours
    D. 30 minutes

FILL IN THE BLANKS

Answer each question by completing the statement in the space provided.

1. All parenteral medications should be prepared in a manner that reduces the possibility of _____.

2. Large-volume drips include Viaflex bags in _____ and _____, _____, and _____ volumes.

3. _____-_____ _____ is a method of administration that allows the patient to control the rate at which the drug is delivered for the relief of pain.

4. A _____ dose of a PCA regimen is a preset amount of drug that can be administered by the patient when pain intensifies.

5. Two types of syringes that are commercially available are _____ and _____.

6. The rule to remember when sizing needles is that the gauge number of the needle is _____ _____ to the bore size of the needle.

7. The smallest filter is _____ _____, which removes all unwanted particles from the solution.

8. A BSC must be turned on at least _____ _____ before use.

9. All work done in the hood is to be done _____ within the hood.

10. The _____ _____ is a special filter is that traps all particles larger than 0.2 micrometers.

MATCHING

Match the following terms with their meanings.

A. Ante area
B. Buffer area
C. Compounding aseptic isolator (CAI)
D. Critical site
E. Direct compounding area (DCA)
F. First air
G. Media-fill test
H. Multidose vial (MDV)
I. Negative pressure room
J. Positive pressure room
K. Primary engineering control (PEC)
L. Single dose vial (SDV)

_____ 1. An area exposed to air or touch, such as vial, needle, or ampule

_____ 2. A practice in which an ISO Class 5 system is in place that provides safety for admixtures

_____ 3. An isolator cabinet designed to contain all contaminants; prevents contaminants from escaping IVs and being transferred to surrounding area

_____ 4. A room that has a lower pressure than the adjacent rooms; net airflow is into the room.

_____ 5. A test performed on compounded products to ensure no contamination has taken place during preparation phase

_____ 6. An area in which all preparations for IV admixture are gathered, including labels, gowning, and drug materials

_____ 7. The air from the HEPA filter that passes over materials; this air is contaminant free

_____ 8. A vial or container that can only be used once

_____ 9. A room that has a higher pressure than the adjacent rooms; net airflow is out of the room.

_____ 10. An area in which hoods are kept and IV preparation takes place

_____ 11. A vial or container that can be used for more than one admixture; normally contains preservatives

_____ 12. A critical area within the hood (ISO Class 5) where areas are exposed to filtered air; also known as "first air"

SHORT ANSWER

Write a short response to each question in the space provided.

1. Name two types of hyperalimentation.

_____

_____

2. List two substances that are used to make needles.

_____

_____

3. What two items can be used to draw up medications from an ampule?

_____

_____

4. Describe the process for breaking an ampule.

_____

_____

_____

5. How are chemotherapy wastes disposed?

_____

_____

_____

6. Why are dextrose, amino acids, and lipids used in TPNs?

_____

_____

7. Why are syringes not reused when a change is made from one drug to another?

_____

_____

8. Why is the placement of the hands so important when sterile products are prepared?

_____

_____

RESEARCH ACTIVITIES

Follow the instructions given in each exercise and provide a response.

Access the website *https://www.ashp.org/s_ashp/docs/files/DiscGuide797-2008.pdf*. Read the *Summary of Revisions to the USP Chapter <797> for Compounding Sterile Preparations* developed by the ASHP, then answer the following questions.

1. What nine steps should be taken toward USP <797> compliance?

2. What is the new risk level that is exempt from USP <797> guidelines?

3. What are the requirements for the immediate-use category classification?

4. What is the beyond-use date for single-dose containers?

5. What is the beyond-use date for multiple-dose containers?

CRITICAL THINKING

Reply to each question based on what you have learned in the chapter.

1. You have been preparing injections in the IV room and suddenly stick your finger with a needle. What went wrong? What mistake did you make that caused you to stick your finger?

2. If you stick your finger with a sterile needle, is it necessary to go to the emergency department for treatment?

3. You have been assigned to work in the IV preparation room for your shift. What are the first items you need to take care of when you walk into the IV room? What aseptic technique requirements need to be followed before you begin preparation of IVs?

4. What should you do at the end of your shift to ensure a smooth workflow when your replacement technician comes to relieve you?

RELATE TO PRACTICE

LAB SCENARIOS

Pharmacy Equipment Used in Preparation of Sterile Compounds
Objective: To familiarize the pharmacy technician with equipment used in the preparation of sterile compounds.

> Parenteral dosage forms differ from all other drug dosage forms because they are injected directly into body tissues through the skin and mucous membranes. Some of the many routes by which parenteral medications are injected into the body include intravenous, intramuscular, subcutaneous, and intradermal. Parenteral dosage forms differ from other pharmaceutical dosage forms for the following reasons:
>
> - All products must be sterile.
> - All products must be free from pyrogenic contamination.
> - Injectable solutions must be free from visible particulate matter.
> - Parenteral products should be isotonic; however, the degree of isotonicity will vary according to the route of administration of the medication.
> - All parenteral products must be stable chemically, physically, and microbiologically.
> - These products must be compatible with IV diluents, delivery systems, and other drug products that are co-administered.
>
> Pharmacy technicians need to be familiar with various solutions that serve as vehicles for parenteral drugs. In addition, the technician must be familiar with equipment used in sterile compounding and its purpose.

Lab Activity #12.1: Identify the meaning of the following abbreviations used as infusion liquids.

Equipment needed:

- Pencil/pen
- Medical dictionary

Time needed to complete this activity: 15 minutes

1. BWFI _____

2. SWFI _____

3. D5W _____

4. D10W _____

5. D20W _____

6. D5LR _____

7. D5 1/4 S _____

8. D5 1/2 S _____

9. D5NS _____

10. D5R _____

11. D10NS _____

12. LR _____

13. R _____

14. NS _____

Lab Activity #12.2: Correctly identify equipment used in the preparation of sterile compounds and its purpose.

Equipment needed:

- Administration set
- Alcohol pads
- Ampule
- Depth filter
- Disinfecting cleaning solution
- Filter needle
- Filter straw
- Gloves (powder free)
- Gown
- Hair cover
- Hypodermic needle
- Hypodermic syringe
- In-line filter
- Insulin syringe
- Intravenous piggyback
- Large-volume parenteral
- Mask
- Membrane filter
- Multidose vial
- Nonsterile gauze swabs
- Nonvented administration set
- Port adapters
- Scrubs
- Sharps container
- Shoe covers

- Single-dose vial
- Small-volume parenteral
- Sterile gauze swabs
- Syringe caps
- Transfer needle
- Tuberculin syringe
- Vented administration set

Time needed to complete this activity: 30 minutes

Equipment	Correctly Identified (Yes/No)	Purpose
Administration set		
Alcohol pads		
Ampule		
Depth filter		
Disinfecting cleaning solutions		
Filter needle		
Filter straw		
Gloves		
Gown		
Hair cover		
Hypodermic needle		
Hypodermic syringe		
In-line filter		
Insulin syringe		
Intravenous piggyback		
Large-volume parenteral (LVP)		
Mask		
Membrane filter		
Multiple dose vial		
Nonsterile gauze swabs		
Nonvented administration set		
Port adapters		
Scrubs		
Sharps container		
Shoe covers		
Single-dose vial		
Small-volume parenteral (SVP)		
Sterile gauze swabs		
Syringe caps		
Transfer needle		
Tuberculin syringe		
Vented administration set		

Lab Activity #12.3: Correctly identify parts of a needle.

Equipment needed:

■ Needle

Time needed to complete this activity: 5 minutes

Parts of a Needle	Correctly Identified (Yes/No)
Bevel	
Hilt	
Hub	
Lumen	
Point	
Shaft	

Lab Activity #12.4: Correctly identify parts of a syringe.

Equipment needed:

■ Tuberculin syringe

Time needed to complete this activity: 5 minutes

Parts of a Syringe	Correctly Identified (Yes/No)
Barrel	
Plunger	
Needle	
Cap	

Calculations, Compatibility, and Storage for Sterile Compounds

Objective: To become familiar with calculations, compatible solutions, and storage when preparing CSPs.
Lab Activity #12.5: Answer the following questions to prepare the following CSPs.

Equipment needed:

■ Calculator
■ *Handbook on Injectable Drugs*
■ Pencil/pen
■ Paper

Time to complete this activity: 45 minutes

1. Cefepime HCl is available as a 1-g vial for reconstitution.

   A. How many milliliters of diluent would need to be added to reconstitute to a concentration of 100 mg/mL?

   _____

   B. For intravenous injection, which diluents would be compatible for reconstitution?

   _____

   C. After reconstitution, how long will this reconstitution be stable at room temperature? In the refrigerator?

   _____

2. You receive an order to prepare an IV bag for ampicillin 1000 mg in 50 mL NS q6h. Ampicillin sodium is available in 125-mg, 250-mg, 500-mg, 1-g, or 2-g vials for reconstitution.

   A. Which vial would you choose to make this IV bag?

   _____

   B. Which diluents would be compatible for reconstitution? How many milliliters would you need to draw up to reconstitute this product?

   _____

   C. If you prepare the IV bag at 11:30 on a Monday, what expiration date and time would you need to put on the IV bag label?

   _____

3. You receive an order to prepare an IV bag of furosemide 100 mg in 100 mL D$_5$W. Furosemide is available in 2-mL, 4-mL, and 10-mL vials with a concentration of 10 mg/mL.

   A. How many milliliters of furosemide will you need to make this IV bag?

   _____

   B. Which vial should you choose? How many vials would you need?

   _____

   C. How long would this IV bag be stable at room temperature? How long would this IV bag be stable if refrigerated?

   _____

4. You need to prepare cefazolin IV bags for 5 different patients as follows:
   - Patient 1—cefazolin 1500 mg in 250 mL NS q6h
   - Patient 2—cefazolin 1000 mg in 100 mL NS q8h
   - Patient 3—cefazolin 750 mg in 100 mL NS q8h
   - Patient 4—cefazolin 500 mg in 100 mL NS q8h
   - Patient 5—cefazolin 1000 mg in 100 mL NS q6h

Cefazolin is available in 500-mg, 1-g, and 10-g vials for reconstitution.

   A. How many IV bags will you need to make for a 24-hour period for each patient?

   _____

   B. Which vial would you choose to make these IV bags? How many vials would you need?

   _____

   C. Which diluents would be compatible for reconstitution? How many milliliters would you need to draw up to reconstitute this product?

   _____

   D. After reconstitution, how many milliliters of cefazolin would you need to draw up to make each IV bag?

   _____

   E. How long would each IV bag be stable at room temperature? How long would each IV bag be stable if refrigerated?

   _____

5. You receive an order to prepare an IV bag for Ranitidine 50 mg in 50 mL D_5W. Ranitidine is available in 2-mL, 6-mL, and 40-mL vials with a concentration of 25 mg/mL.

   A. How many milliliters of Ranitidine will you need to make this IV bag?

   _____

   B. Which vial should you choose? How many vials would you need?

   _____

   C. How long would this IV bag be stable at room temperature? How long would this IV bag be stable if refrigerated?

   _____

6. You need to prepare 4 vancomycin IV bags—750 mg, 1250 mg, and 2 bags with 1500 mg each. Vancomycin is available in 500-mg, 1-g, 5-g, and 10-g vials for reconstitution.

   A. Which vial would you choose to make these IV bags? How many vials would you need?

   _____

   B. Which diluents would be compatible for reconstitution?

   _____

   C. How many milliliters of diluent would you need to draw up to reconstitute this product to a concentration of 100 mg/mL?

   _____

   D. After reconstitution, how many milliliters of vancomycin would you need to draw up to make each IV bag?

   _____

   E. How long would each IV bag be stable at room temperature? How long would each IV bag be stable if refrigerated?

   _____

7. You receive an order to prepare an IV bag for tobramycin 110 mg in 100 mL NS. Tobramycin is available in 2-mL and 30-mL vials with a concentration of 40 mg/mL.

   A. How many milliliters of tobramycin will you need to make this IV bag?

   _____

   B. Which vial should you choose? How many vials will you need?

   _____

   C. How long would this IV bag be stable at room temperature? How long would this IV bag be stable if refrigerated?

   _____

8. You receive an order to prepare an IV bag for pantoprazole sodium 40 mg in 100 mL NS. Pantoprazole sodium is available as a 40-mg vial for reconstitution.

   A. Which diluents would be compatible for reconstitution?

   _____

   B. How many milliliters of diluent would you need to draw up to reconstitute this product to a concentration of 4 mg/mL?

   _____

223

C. After reconstitution, how many milliliters of pantoprazole sodium would you need to draw up to make the IV bag?

_____

D. How long would the IV bag be stable at room temperature? How long would the IV bag be stable if refrigerated?

_____

9. You need to prepare 10 PCA syringes with a concentration of 0.1% hydromorphone, 30 mL each for an opioid tolerant patient. Hydromorphone is available in a 20-mL multidose vial with a concentration of 2 mg/mL.

A. How many milliliters of hydromorphone 2 mg/mL will you need to make one 30-mL PCA syringe with a concentration of 0.1% hydromorphone?

_____

B. The syringes are to be qs'd with NS to 30 mL. How much NS will you need to add to each syringe?

_____

C. How many milliliters of hydromorphone 2 mg/mL will you need to make 10 PCA syringes with a concentration of 0.1% hydromorphone? How many vials will you need?

_____

D. How long can these PCA syringes be stored at room temperature?

_____

10. You receive an order to prepare an IV bag for acyclovir 340 mg in 50 mL NS q8h. Acyclovir sodium is available in 500-mg or 1-g vials for reconstitution.

A. Which vial would you choose to make this IV bag? How many vials would you need?

_____

B. Which diluents would be compatible for reconstitution? How many milliliters would you need to draw up to reconstitute this product?

_____

C. After reconstitution, how many milliliters of acyclovir sodium would you need to draw up to make this IV bag?

_____

D. How long would the IV bag be stable at room temperature? How long would the IV bag be stable if refrigerated?

_____

Proper Hand Washing in Aseptic Compounding

Objective: To perform a complete hand washing procedure as necessary before sterile compounding.

The United States Pharmacopeia (USP) is a nongovernmental, official public standards–setting authority for prescription and over-the-counter medicines and other health care products manufactured in the United States. The USP establishes standards for the quality, purity, strength, and consistency of these products. The United States Pharmacopeia publishes the USP-NF, which is the official compendium for the United States. Chapter 797 of the USP addresses sterile compounding and is designed to cut down on infections transmitted to patients through pharmaceutical products. USP 797 addresses appropriate hand washing before preparation of compounded sterile products.

224

Lab Activity #12.6: Aseptic hand washing.

Equipment needed:

- Biohazard waste container
- Disinfecting agent/cleanser
- Lint-free paper towels
- Nailbrush
- Sink with hot and cold running water

Procedure

1. Remove all cosmetics, visible jewelry, watches, and objects up to the elbow.
2. Turn on water faucets with a paper towel if not foot operated.
3. Make sure water temperature is lukewarm.
4. Avoid unnecessary splashing during washing process.
5. Use a nailbrush to clean under every fingertip.
6. Apply sufficient disinfecting/cleansing agent to hands in a circular motion, holding the fingertips downward.
7. Clean all four surfaces of each finger, and rub well between the fingers.
8. Clean all surfaces of hands, wrists, and arms up to the elbows in a circular motion.
9. Rinse well.
10. Repeat the scrubbing process a second time and rinse.
11. Dry hands with paper towels.
12. Do not touch the sink, faucet, or other objects that could contaminate hands.
13. Turn off the water using a paper towel.
14. Discard paper towels in biohazard waste container.

Time needed to complete this activity: 15 minutes

Evaluation of Hand Washing	Procedural Steps	Yes/No
Removed all cosmetics, visible jewelry, watches, and objects up to the elbow		
Was not wearing acrylic nails or nail polish		
Started water and adjusted to the correct temperature		
Avoided unnecessary splashing during process		
Used a nailbrush to clean under every fingertip		
Used sufficient disinfecting agent/cleanser		
Cleaned all four surfaces of each finger		
Cleaned all surfaces of hands, wrists, and arms up to the elbows in a circular motion		
Did not touch the sink, faucet, or other objects that could contaminate the hands		
Rinsed off all soap residue		
Rinsed hands, holding them upright and allowing water to drip to the elbow		
Repeated the scrubbing process a second time and rinsed hands, holding them upright and allowing water to drip to the elbow		
Did not turn off water until hands were completely dry		
Turned water off with a clean, dry, lint-free paper towel		
Did not touch the faucet while turning off the water		

225

Personal Protective Equipment (PPEs)

Objective: Identify personal protective equipment, explain its purpose in sterile compounding, and demonstrate proper techniques in donning personal protective equipment in the correct sequence.

The Occupational Safety and Health Administration requires the use of personal protective equipment (PPE) to reduce the exposure of employees to hazards. In the practice of pharmacy, PPEs are worn in the compounding of sterile products. These PPEs include foot and hair covers, face masks, gowns, and latex (or latex-free) gloves.

Gowns are worn to protect the skin and to prevent soiling of clothing during procedures that are likely to generate splashes. Masks, eye protection, and face shields are worn to protect the mucous membranes of the eyes, nose, and mouth during procedures that are likely to produce splashes. In addition, masks prevent moisture from being forced out from the mouth and nose during normal activities such as breathing or talking. Gloves are worn to prevent the spread of disease and to avoid possible contamination. However, the individual who wears gloves must still wash his/her hands before gloving. A pharmacy technician should never wash his/her hands with gloves on, because hand washing may damage the glove's pores, allowing microorganisms to enter the glove.

Lab Activity #12.7: Identify the following personal protective equipment worn in the practice of sterile compounding, and state its purpose.

Equipment needed:

- Face mask
- Foot coverings
- Goggles
- Hair covering
- Facial hair covering
- Sterile gown
- Sterile latex or latex-free gloves

Time needed to complete this activity: 5 minutes

Personal Protective Equipment	Purpose
Face mask	
Foot coverings	
Goggles	
Hair covering, facial hair covering	
Sterile gown	
Sterile latex (or latex-free) gloves	

Lab Activity #12.8: Donning personal protective equipment.

Equipment needed:

- Disinfecting agent/cleanser
- Face mask
- Foam alcohol
- Foot covering
- Hair covering, facial hair covering
- Lint-free paper towels
- Nailbrush
- Sink with hot and cold running water
- Sterile gown
- Sterile latex (or latex-free) gloves

Procedure

1. Remove all cosmetics, jewelry up to the elbows, and remove necklaces and earrings.
2. Remove all outer garments such as coats and hats.
3. Wash hands thoroughly with soap and water.
4. Pull shoe cover over the toe of the shoe first, around the bottom of the shoe, and finally over the heel of the shoe. Please note that shoe covers are not designated as left and right but are interchangeable.
5. Apply foam alcohol to the palm of one hand, and rub hands thoroughly. Allow hands to air dry.
6. Put on hair cover by gathering loose hair and placing it into the back of the hair cover. Pull front of hair cover over forehead. No hair should be outside of the hair cover.
7. Apply foam alcohol to the palm of one hand, and rub hands thoroughly. Allow hands to air dry.
8. Slip on face mask by situating the top of the mask at the bridge of the nose. Pull the two top ties of the face mask and attach them together. Attach the two lower ties behind the neck. The mask should cover the nose, mouth, and chin.
9. Wash hands using aseptic technique.
10. Open the package of the sterile gown. The gown should never make contact with any surface.
11. Slip one arm into the sleeve of the sterile gown, and pull it up to the shoulder. Repeat this procedure with the other arm. Tie the neck strings behind the neck, and repeat with the waist strings.
12. Apply foam alcohol to the palm of one hand, and rub hands thoroughly. Allow hands to air dry.
13. Open package containing sterile latex (or latex-free) gloves. Remove glove from package and maintain fingers within the cup of the gown. Place glove on palm of hand with the thumb side of the glove toward the palm. Pull the glove's cuff so that it covers the gown's cuff. Unfold the glove's cuff so that it covers the cuff of the gown. Take hold of the glove and gown at waist level. Pull glove onto the hand and work fingers into the glove. Repeat procedure for the other glove.

Time needed to complete this activity: 15 minutes

Evaluation of Donning Personal Protective Equipment	Yes/No
Cosmetics and jewelry removed; was not wearing acrylic nails or nail polish	
Hands washed properly before donning PPE	
Shoe covers put on	
Applied foam alcohol to hands and allowed to air dry	
Hair cover(s) put on properly	
Applied foam alcohol to hands and allowed to air dry	
Face mask put on properly	
Proper aseptic hand washing performed	
Sterile gown put on properly	
Foam alcohol applied	
Sterile gloves put on properly	

Lab Activity #12.9: Removal of personal protective equipment.

Equipment needed:

- Hair covering
- Sterile gown
- Sterile latex (or latex-free) gloves
- Face mask
- Foot covering
- Biohazard container

Procedure

1. Use your dominant hand to grasp the glove of the opposite hand near the palm.
2. Pull glove inside out until you reach your fingers.
3. Place your thumb of the non-gloved hand inside the cuff of the other glove. Pull glove inside out until you reach your fingers and pull over the first removed glove.

227

4. Dispose of gloves in biohazard container.
5. Remove gown.
6. Remove face mask.
7. Remove hair cover.
8. Remove shoe covers
9. Dispose of gown, face mask, hair cover, and shoe covers in biohazard container.

Time needed to complete this activity: 5 minutes

Evaluation of Personal Protective Equipment Removal	Yes/No
Glove removed and disposed of properly	
Gown removed correctly	
Face mask removed properly	
Hair cover removed correctly	
Shoe covers removed properly	
Personal protective equipment disposed of appropriately	

Laminar Airflow Workbench

Objective: Demonstrate the proper cleaning of a horizontal laminar airflow workbench.

A laminar airflow workbench is used in the compounding of sterile products. Laminar airflow workbenches are used to filter bacteria and other particulate matter from the air and to maintain constant airflow to prevent contamination. Several types of laminar airflow workbenches are available, including vertical (biological safety cabinet) and horizontal laminar airflow cabinets. Both types of flow hoods are built to allow the flow of sterile air across a work surface. Air particles are removed through the use of a high-efficiency particulate air (HEPA) filter. HEPA filters should be tested every 6 months.

The vertical or biological safety cabinet (BSC) is used in the preparation of chemotherapeutic agents and antineoplastic agents. The vertical airflow workbench filters air from the top down to the workbench and can remove particles 0.3 microns and larger. Horizontal laminar flow workbenches are the most common type used in the preparation of sterile products; they are capable of filtering particulate matter of 0.2 microns or larger. They blow air from the back of the hood to the front of the hood. Horizontal laminar flow workbenches are less likely to wash organisms into the sterility test media. Unfortunately, any airborne particulate matter generated in the unit is blown toward the pharmacy personnel and into the room. Regardless of the type of laminar flow workbench used, the pharmacist or pharmacy technician must be trained properly on its uses and proper maintenance. A laminar airflow workbench must be turned on for at least 30 minutes before it is used.

Lab Activity #12.10: Cleaning a horizontal laminar airflow hood.

Equipment needed:

- Disinfecting agent/cleanser
- Horizontal laminar airflow hood
- Isopropyl alcohol 70%
- Lint-free paper towels
- PPEs (foot covers, head cover, mask, gown, and sterile latex or latex-free gloves)
- Sink with running hot and cold water
- Sterile water
- Sterile gauze pad

Procedure

1. Turn horizontal laminar airflow workbench on for at least 30 minutes.
2. Wash hands using aseptic technique.
3. Don PPEs in proper sequence.
4. Remove any items from within the hood.
5. Deposit sterile, lint-free cleaning pads 6 inches inside laminar workflow.
6. Lightly moisten sterile gauze pads with sterile water.

7. Take moist gauze pads and begin to clean the back inside corner of laminar workbench, beginning with the ceiling. Cleaning should be performed using overlapping side-to-side motions, from left to right working from back to front. After ceiling has been cleaned, discard gauze pads.
8. Use moist gauze pads to wipe the horizontal IV poles and any hooks or brackets using a smooth motion from left to right. After IV pole, hooks and brackets have been cleaned, discard gauze pads.
9. Use moist gauze pads to clean the right-side section with overlapping up-down motion beginning in the back corner, and move forward to front of laminar airflow workbench; discard used gauze pads.
10. Repeat process on the left-side section of laminar airflow workbench, beginning in the back corner, with overlapping up-down motion; move forward; discard used gauze pads.
11. Repeat process on the work surface of the workbench. Begin in the back right-hand corner, going side-to-side with overlapping motion. Clean to the outer edge of the laminar airflow workbench.
12. Inspect all surfaces for any crystallized solutions. Clean those with sterile water before continuing.
13. Repeat steps 7 through 12 in the same order, using 70% isopropyl alcohol instead of sterile water.
14. Allow 70% alcohol to remain on surfaces to be disinfected for at least 30 seconds before CSPs are prepared in the hood.
15. Record initials, date, and time on the cleaning log.

Time needed to complete this activity: 20 minutes

Evaluation of Cleaning a Horizontal Laminar Airflow Hood	Yes/No
Cosmetics and jewelry removed; was not wearing acrylic nails or nail polish	
Proper aseptic hand washing procedure followed	
Personal protective equipment donned in proper sequence	
Laminar airflow workbench was on for at least 30 minutes	
Removed items from within the hood	
Clean, sterile gauze/sponge and disinfectant used to clean the hood	
Cleaned ceiling using sterile water and proper techniques	
Cleaned IV pole, hooks, and brackets using sterile water and proper techniques	
Cleaned the right side of the hood using sterile water with the appropriate motions. Started at the top and worked from side to side with overlapping strokes	
Cleaned left side of hood using sterile water with correct motions. Started at the top and worked from side to side with overlapping strokes	
Cleaned the rear wall of the hood using sterile water with appropriate motions. Started at the top and worked down to the bottom	
Cleaned the work surface last using sterile water and appropriate strokes. Started at the back and worked from side to side with overlapping strokes	
Inspected all surfaces for any crystallized solutions. Cleaned with sterile water before moving on	
Cleaned ceiling with 70% isopropyl alcohol and proper technique	
Cleaned IV pole, hooks, and brackets with 70% isopropyl alcohol and proper techniques	
Cleaned right side with 70% isopropyl alcohol with appropriate motions. Started at the top and worked from side to side with overlapping strokes	
Cleaned left side of hood using 70% isopropyl alcohol with correct motions. Started at the top and worked from side to side with overlapping strokes	
Cleaned the work surface last using 70% isopropyl alcohol and water with appropriate strokes. Started at the back and worked from side to side with overlapping strokes	
Did not contaminate the laminar airflow hood	
Did not at any time block airflow from HEPA filter or air intake grills	
Completed cleaning log	

Cleaning Log		
Date of Laminar Airflow Cleaning	Time of Cleaning	Initials of Person Completing the Cleaning

1. What is the difference between a vertical and a horizontal laminar airflow hood? When should they be used?

_____

_____

_____

_____

_____

_____

2. In what direction does air flow in a horizontal airflow workbench?

_____

3. In what direction does air flow in a vertical airflow workbench?

_____

4. How often should the HEPA filter be checked?

_____

Sterile Compounding

Objective: Demonstrate the proper sterile compounding techniques in performing a straight draw, reconstituting a powdered vial, and withdrawing a medication from an ampule.

Lab Activity #12.11: Performing a straight draw.

Equipment needed:

- Alcohol swabs
- Biohazard container
- Disinfecting agent/cleanser
- Horizontal laminar airflow hood
- Isopropyl alcohol 70%
- Lint-free paper towels
- Personal protective equipment (foot covers, head cover, mask, gown, and sterile latex or latex-free gloves)
- Sharps container
- Single or multidose vial
- Sink with running hot and cold water
- Sterile gauze pad
- Sterile water
- Syringe with needle

Procedure

1. Gather all materials needed for manipulation.
2. Wash hands using proper aseptic technique.

3. Don PPEs in the proper sequence.
4. Properly clean laminar airflow workbench.
5. Check the expiration of the single or multidose vial.
6. Select syringe of proper size. (Note: The syringe should not exceed five times the volume of the drug to be withdrawn into the syringe.)
7. Place all necessary materials in the laminar flow hood.
8. Swab the rubber top with alcohol. Allow the alcohol to dry.
9. Make sure the needle is firmly attached to the syringe.
10. Pull the plunger back on the syringe to slightly less than the amount needed to be withdrawn.
11. Hold the syringe with the thumb and the index and middle fingers.
12. Remove cap from needle. Place cap onto the alcohol swab with the opening pointing toward the HEPA filter of the hood.
13. Insert the needle at a 45-degree angle into the rubber stopper of the vial with beveled part of the needle facing upward.
14. Hold the vial with the hand that is opposite the hand holding the syringe.
15. Push the plunger, forcing the air in the syringe into the vial, and release, gently allowing the fluid to be drawn into the syringe.
16. Withdraw the correct amount.
17. Tap the syringe to force air bubbles out of it.
18. Withdraw the needle and carefully recap.
19. Discard syringe in sharps container

Time needed to complete this activity: 30 minutes

Evaluation of a Straight Draw	Yes/No
Gathered all materials needed	
Cosmetics and jewelry removed; was not wearing acrylic nails or nail polish	
Washed hands using proper aseptic technique	
Properly donned PPEs in correct sequence	
Laminar airflow workbench was on for at least 30 minutes	
Properly cleaned laminar airflow workbench	
Checked expiration dates of medications	
Performed all necessary calculations correctly prior to drug preparation	
Brought the correct drugs and concentrations into the hood for preparation	
Inspected all products for particulate matter/contamination prior to use	
Brought the correct supplies into the hood prior to preparation	
Cleaned rubber top of vial with alcohol swab	
Selected syringe of proper size	
Pulled plunger back to slightly half of amount to be withdrawn	
Removed needle cap	
Inserted needle into rubber stopper of vial	
Pushed air from plunger into vial	
Withdrew correct volume of medication	
Tapped air bubbles out of syringe	
Withdrew needle and recapped	
Discarded syringe/needle in sharps container	
Did not contaminate the needle or syringe during preparation	

Continued

Evaluation of a Straight Draw	Yes/No
Did not contaminate the laminar airflow hood	
Did not at any time block airflow from HEPA filter or air intake grills	
Did not utilize the outer 6 inches of the hood opening	
Did not core or puncture rubber stopper on vial	
Properly discarded waste, including sharps	
Removed PPEs in proper sequence	
Discarded PPEs in appropriate container	
Completed the cleaning log	

Cleaning Log		
Date of Laminar Airflow Cleaning	Time of Cleaning	Initials of Person Completing the Cleaning

Lab Activity #12.12: Using a syringe and needle of proper size, remove the following volumes from a multidose vial within a laminar flow workbench.

Equipment needed:

■ Alcohol swabs
■ Horizontal laminar airflow workbench
■ Multidose vial
■ Syringes of multiple sizes with needle
■ PPEs (foot covers, head cover, mask, gown, and sterile latex or latex-free gloves)
■ Sharps container

Prescribed Volume	Measured Volume
0.25 mL	
0.5 mL	
0.75 mL	
1.2 mL	
1.5 mL	

Lab Activity #12.13: Reconstituting a powdered vial.

Equipment needed:

■ Alcohol swabs
■ Laminar airflow hood
■ PPEs (foot covers, head cover, mask, gown, and sterile latex or latex-free gloves)
■ Sharps container
■ Single or multidose vial
■ Diluent for reconstitution
■ Sink with running hot and cold water
■ Syringe with needle
■ Vented needle

Procedure

1. Gather all materials needed for manipulation.
2. All compounding calculations should be performed and checked by instructor.
3. Wash hands using proper aseptic technique.
4. Don PPEs in the proper sequence.
5. Properly clean laminar airflow workbench.
6. Check the expiration date on the powdered vial and diluent.
7. Select syringe of proper size. (Note: The syringe should not exceed five times the volume of the drug to be withdrawn into the syringe.)
8. Place all necessary materials in the laminar flow hood.
9. Swab the rubber top with alcohol. Allow the alcohol to dry.
10. Make sure the needle is firmly attached to the syringe.
11. Prepare the syringe by adding the amount of air that will be equal to the amount of diluent to be withdrawn into the syringe.
12. Hold the syringe with the thumb and the index and middle fingers.
13. Remove cap from needle. Place cap onto the alcohol swab with the opening pointing toward the HEPA filter of the hood.
14. Insert the needle at a 45-degree angle into the rubber stopper of the vial with beveled part of the needle facing upward.
15. Hold the vial with the hand that is opposite the hand holding the syringe.
16. Push the plunger, forcing the air in the syringe into the vial, and release, gently allowing the fluid to be drawn into the syringe.
17. Tap the syringe to force air bubbles out of it.
18. Draw up the correct amount of diluent needed for reconstitution.
19. Pull the back on the plunger to clear the neck of the syringe. Remove the needle and replace with a vented needle.
20. Remove all excess air from syringe.
21. Swab the top of the powdered vial with an alcohol swab.
22. Insert vented needle of the syringe at a 45-degree angle into the rubber top of the powdered vial and push the diluent into the vial.
23. Gently shake or swirl to dissolve. The powder must dissolve completely.
24. Place needle and syringe into the sharps container.

Time needed to complete this activity: 30 minutes

Evaluation of Reconstituting a Powdered Vial	Yes/No
Gathered all materials needed	
Cosmetics and jewelry removed; was not wearing acrylic nails or nail polish	
Hands washed using proper aseptic technique	
PPEs donned in proper sequence	
Laminar airflow workbench on for at least 30 minutes	
Laminar airflow workbench properly cleaned	
Checked expiration dates of medications	
Performed all necessary calculations correctly prior to drug preparation	
Brought the correct drugs and concentrations into the hood for preparation	
Inspected all products for particulate matter/contamination prior to use	
Brought the correct supplies into the hood prior to preparation	
Vial top cleaned with alcohol	
Correct needles used during reconstitution	
Air bubbles removed from syringe	
Correct amount and type of diluent added to vial per directions on the vial	
Powder dissolved	

Continued

Evaluation of Reconstituting a Powdered Vial	Yes/No
Syringe and needle disposed into sharps container	
Did not contaminate the needle or syringe during preparation	
Did not contaminate the laminar airflow hood	
Did not at any time block airflow from HEPA filter or air intake grills	
Did not utilize the outer 6 inches of the hood opening	
Did not core or puncture rubber stopper on vials	
Properly discarded waste, including sharps	
Removed PPEs in proper sequence	
Discarded PPEs in appropriate container	
Completed the cleaning log	

Cleaning Log		
Date of Laminar Airflow Cleaning	Time of Cleaning	Initials of Person Completing the Cleaning

Lab Activity #12.14: Ampule preparation.

Equipment needed:

- Alcohol swabs
- Ampule
- Filter needle
- Laminar airflow hood
- PPEs (foot covers, head cover, mask, gown, and sterile latex or latex-free gloves)
- Sharps container
- Sink with running hot and cold water
- Syringe with needle
- IV bag

Procedure

1. Gather all materials needed for manipulation.
2. All compounding calculations should be performed and checked by instructor.
3. Wash hands using proper aseptic technique.
4. Don PPEs in the proper sequence.
5. Properly clean laminar airflow workbench.
6. Check the expiration date of the ampule.
7. Select syringe of proper size. (Note: The syringe should not exceed five times the volume of the drug to be withdrawn into the syringe.)
8. Place all necessary materials in the laminar flow hood.
9. Tap the top of the ampule, forcing all liquid at the top and neck of the ampule to fall into the body of the ampule.
10. Clean the neck of the ampule with an alcohol swab.
11. Hold the body of the ampule with your thumb and index finger.
12. Using your stronger hand, place the thumb and forefinger over the top of the ampule.
13. Apply pressure to the neck of the ampule with a sudden motion of the wrist.
14. Place the head of the ampule into the sharps container, and place the ampule on the work surface of the laminar flow workbench.
15. Attach filter needle to syringe.

16. Hold the barrel of the syringe with the hand and remove the cap of the needle.
17. Place cap onto the alcohol swab with the opening pointing toward the HEPA filter of the hood.
18. Hold barrel of syringe so the needle is pointing downward.
19. Cautiously insert the needle into the ampule so the needle is entered into the fluid of the ampule.
20. Pull the plunger of the syringe until the syringe contains more than the desired volume.
21. Hold ampule with your other hand as the first hand holds the barrel of the syringe and releases the plunger.
22. Remove the syringe from the ampule, invert the syringe upward, and recap.
23. Remove air bubbles from the syringe by tapping it.
24. Pull plunger downward, causing fluid from the ampule to enter into the syringe.
25. Push remaining air from the syringe by releasing the plunger.
26. Remove the filter needle and attach a new needle to the syringe.
27. Remove excess air and cap syringe.
28. Clean port of IV bag with alcohol swab.
29. Inject drug into IV bag.
30. Properly seal additive port of IV bag.
31. Discard syringe into sharps container.

Time needed to complete this activity: 30 minutes

Evaluation of Ampule Preparation	Yes/No
Gathered all materials needed	
Cosmetics and jewelry removed; was not wearing acrylic nails or nail polish	
Hands washed using aseptic technique	
PPEs donned in proper sequence	
Laminar airflow workbench on for at least 30 minutes	
Laminar airflow workbench cleaned	
Checked expiration dates of medications	
Performed all necessary calculations correctly prior to drug preparation	
Brought the correct drugs and concentrations into the hood for preparation	
Inspected all products for particulate matter/contamination prior to use	
Brought the correct supplies into the hood prior to preparation	
Cleaned ampule neck correctly before breaking	
Wrapped ampule neck correctly before breaking	
Broke ampule correctly	
Attached filter device to syringe correctly	
Drew up ampule correctly without spilling contents	
Removed filter needle and replaced it with new needle before injecting into final container	
Drew up correct amount of drug and checked measurement before injecting into container	
Cleaned additive port on final container before injecting drug	
Did not core or puncture side of additive port when adding drug to the final container	
Properly mixed contents of container and inspected for incompatibilities or particulate matter	
Properly sealed additive port of container	
Did not contaminate the needle or syringe during preparation	
Did not contaminate the laminar airflow hood	

Continued

Evaluation of Ampule Preparation	Yes/No
Did not at any time block airflow from HEPA filter or air intake grills	
Did not utilize the outer 6 inches of the hood opening	
Properly discarded waste, including sharps	
Removed PPEs in proper sequence	
Discarded PPEs in appropriate container	
Completed the cleaning log	

Cleaning Log		
Date of Laminar Airflow Cleaning	Time of Cleaning	Initials of Person Completing the Cleaning

Preparing Small- and Large-Volume Parenterals

Objective: To introduce the pharmacy technician to the preparation of small- and large-volume parenterals.

The most common type of sterile product prepared by a pharmacy technician is an intravenous (IV) bag that contains a medication. Intravenous bags are classified as small volume or large volume. Small-volume IV bags are considered to be 250 milliliters or less, including 50, 100, 150, and 250 mL sizes. Large-volume IV bags include 500 mL, 1 L, 2 L, and 3 L sizes. Some of the medications found in IV bags include antibiotics, antiviral agents, antineoplastics, and analgesics. During the preparation of IV bags, it is extremely important that aseptic techniques are followed.

Lab Activity #12.15: Prepare an intravenous compound.

Equipment needed:

- Alcohol swabs
- Diluent
- Laminar airflow hood
- Large-volume parenteral (LVP) or small-volume parenteral (SVP)
- PPEs
- Sharps container
- Single-dose vial (SDV) or multidose vial
- Sink with running hot and cold water
- Syringe with needle
- IV bag

Procedure

1. Gather all materials needed for activity.
2. All compounding calculations should be performed and checked by instructor.
3. Wash hands properly using aseptic technique.
4. Don PPEs in the proper sequence.
5. Clean laminar flow workbench in the proper manner, using the correct supplies and techniques.
6. Collect the medication to be compounded.
7. Check expiration dates on both the vial and the parenteral IV bag.
8. Place all necessary materials in the laminar flow hood.
9. Swab the rubber top with alcohol. Allow the alcohol to dry.
10. Make sure the needle is firmly attached to the syringe.
11. Prepare the syringe by adding the amount of air that will be equal to the amount of medication to be withdrawn into the syringe.

12. Hold the syringe with the thumb and the index and middle fingers.
13. Remove cap from needle. Place cap onto the alcohol swab with the opening pointing toward the HEPA filter of the hood.
14. Insert the needle at a 45-degree angle into the rubber stopper of the vial with beveled part of the needle facing upward.
15. Hold the vial with the hand opposite the hand that is holding the syringe.
16. Invert the vial and pull back on the plunger.
17. Push the plunger, forcing the air in the syringe into the vial, and release gently, allowing the fluid to be drawn into the syringe.
18. Tap the syringe to force air bubbles out of it.
19. Withdraw the correct amount of medication.
20. Remove excess air and cap syringe.
21. Clean port of IV bag with alcohol swab.
22. Inject drug into IV bag.
23. Properly seal additive port of IV bag.
24. Discard syringe into sharps container.
25. Remove PPEs in the proper sequence, and discard.
26. Record initials, date, and time on the cleaning log.

Time needed to complete this activity: 30 minutes

Evaluation of Intravenous Bag Preparation	Yes/No
Gathered all materials needed	
Cosmetics and jewelry removed; was not wearing acrylic nails or nail polish	
Hands washed using aseptic technique	
PPEs donned in proper sequence	
Laminar airflow workbench was on for at least 30 minutes	
Followed proper procedure and technique in cleaning the hood	
Performed all necessary calculations correctly prior to drug preparation	
Brought the correct drugs and concentrations into the hood for preparation	
Checked expiration dates of medications	
Brought the correct supplies into the hood prior to preparation	
Inspected all products for particulate matter/contamination prior to use	
Withdrew correct amount of drug and checked measurement before injecting into container	
Cleaned additive port on final container before injecting drug	
Did not core or puncture side of additive port when adding drug to the final container	
Properly mixed contents of container and inspected for incompatibilities or particulate matter	
Properly sealed additive port of container	
Did not contaminate the needle or syringe during preparation	
Did not contaminate the laminar airflow hood	
Did not at any time block airflow from HEPA filter or air intake grills	
Did not utilize the outer 6 inches of the hood opening	
Properly discarded waste, including sharps	
Removed PPEs in proper sequence	
Discarded PPEs in appropriate container	
Completed cleaning log	

Cleaning Log		
Date of Laminar Airflow Cleaning	**Time of Cleaning**	**Initials of Person Completing the Cleaning**

Preparing Cytotoxic Parenterals

Objective: To introduce the pharmacy technician to proper techniques in compounding cytotoxic parenteral medications and disposing of hazardous waste.

A pharmacy technician may be required to prepare an antineoplastic or cytotoxic medication for a patient diagnosed with a form of cancer. These agents are used to kill a specific type or form of cancer cell found in a patient. Although these agents have many benefits for the patient, they are unable to distinguish a cancer cell from a healthy cell. Therefore special measures must be taken to protect the pharmacist or pharmacy technician from being exposed to these agents accidentally.

Compounding cytotoxic medications is very similar to compounding sterile medications, with a few exceptions. First, cytotoxic compounds are prepared in biological safety cabinets (vertical laminar airflow workbenches), which are similar to horizontal laminar airflow workbenches except the air is blown from the top of the hood vertically to prevent fumes inside the hood. Also, biological safety cabinets (BSCs) may take the form of a glove box isolator, wherein the pharmacist or pharmacy technician slips his/her hands into a glove-like component contained in the cabinet.

Many of the policies and procedures used in preparing a sterile compound are applied when cytotoxic agents are prepared.

Lab Activity #12.16: Cleaning a biological safety cabinet (BSC).

Equipment needed:

- 70% isopropyl alcohol
- Biological safety cabinet (a laminar airflow workbench in the absence of a biological safety cabinet)
- Biological safety cabinet cleaner
- Deionized water
- Sterile water
- Germicidal cleanser
- Goggles
- Lint-free cloth
- Personal protective equipment
- Sink with running hot and cold water
- Hazardous waste container

Procedure

1. Gather all materials needed for activity.
2. Wash hands properly using aseptic technique.
3. Don PPEs in the proper sequence.
4. **MAKE SURE THE BLOWER IS ON!**
5. Remove any items from within the hood.
6. Using the lint-free cloth and sterile water, begin cleaning the bar at the top of the hood and any hooks or brackets using a smooth motion from left to right.
7. Using the lint-free cloth and sterile water, clean each side panel next going from the top of the panel to the bottom of the panel using overlapping strokes.
8. Using the lint-free cloth and sterile water, clean the back panel of the hood; clean the top of the panel in a side-to-side motion, moving toward the bottom.
9. Using the lint-free cloth and sterile water, wipe the inside of the front shield using a side-to-side motion from left to right, beginning at the top and working down to the bottom.

10. Using the lint-free cloth and sterile water, clean the base of the workbench, moving from the rear forward using a sideward motion.
11. Scrub from top to bottom of the workbench, using the cleaner.
12. Inspect all surfaces for any crystallized solutions. Clean with sterile water before continuing.
13. Rinse cabinet with deionized water.
14. Repeat process with 70% isopropyl alcohol.
15. Allow the 70% alcohol to remain on surfaces for 30 seconds to be disinfected before preparing CSPs.
16. Discard cleaning cloths in a hazardous waste container.
17. Record initials, date, and time on the cleaning log.

Time needed to complete this activity: 15 minutes

Evaluation of Cleaning a Biological Safety Cabinet	Yes/No
Gathered all materials needed	
Cosmetics and jewelry removed; was not wearing acrylic nails or nail polish	
Hands washed using aseptic technique	
PPEs donned in proper sequence; goggles worn	
Made sure biological safety cabinet blower was on	
Removed items from the hood	
Lint-free cloth used	
Inside of biological safety cabinet cleaned in proper sequence	
Biological safety cabinet cleaner used inside of cabinet	
Biological cabinet rinsed inside with deionized water	
70% isopropyl alcohol used to clean inside of biological safety cabinet	
Did not contaminate the BSC	
Did not at any time block airflow from HEPA filter or air intake grills	
Discarded cleaning cloths in hazardous waste container	
Completed the cleaning log	

Cleaning Log		
Date of Laminar Airflow Cleaning	Time of Cleaning	Initials of Person Completing the Cleaning

If a laminar airflow workbench is used, remember that in a hospital pharmacy, cytotoxic compounds are prepared in a biological safety cabinet.

Lab Activity #12.17: Vial preparation—hazardous drugs.

Equipment needed:

- 70% isopropyl alcohol
- Biohazardous waste bag
- Biological safety cabinet (a laminar airflow workbench in the absence of a biological safety cabinet)
- Biological safety cabinet cleaner
- Calculator

- Chemo mat
- Chemo spill kit
- Deionized water
- Eyewash station
- Foil
- Gauze
- Germicidal cleanser
- Goggles
- Hazardous waste container
- Large-volume or small-volume parenteral IV bag
- Luer-Lock syringe with needle
- 0.2 micron filter
- Lint-free cloth
- Personal protective equipment
- Sharps container
- Sink with running hot and cold water
- Vial
- Zip seal bag

Procedure

1. Gather all materials needed for activity.
2. All compounding calculations should be performed and checked by instructor.
3. Wash hands properly.
4. Don PPEs in the proper sequence.
5. **MAKE SURE THE BLOWER IS ON!**
6. Clean biological safety cabinet.
7. Place chemo mat inside of biological safety cabinet.
8. Check all ingredients for particulate matter and possible contamination.
9. Clean the top of the vial with alcohol swab.
10. Pull the plunger of the Luer-Lock syringe halfway back for the amount of drug to be drawn into the syringe.
11. Take off the cap from the needle.
12. Insert the needle into the center of the vial with the beveled tip of the needle up.
13. Hold vial so that air is being blown onto the syringe and the stopper of the vial.
14. Holding the syringe from the bottom, gradually push the air from the syringe into the vial.
15. Withdraw the correct amount of medication from the vial by slowly pulling the syringe's plunger back.
16. Remove the needle from the vial once the correct amount of drug has been measured.
17. Remove air bubbles from syringe.
18. Recap the syringe.
19. Clean medication port with alcohol swab.
20. Inject medication into IV bag.
21. Thoroughly mix the medication that has been injected into the IV bag.
22. Check for any particulate matter.
23. Clean the outside of the IV bag with moist gauze, as well as all IV ports.
24. Properly seal additive port of IV bag.
25. Label final product, and place inside zip seal bag.
26. Place used syringe and needle into sharps container.
27. Remove PPEs in proper sequence, and place in a hazardous waste container.
28. Record initials, date, and time on the cleaning log.

Time needed to complete this activity: 20 minutes

Evaluation of Preparing a Hazardous Drug from a Vial	Yes/No
Gathered all materials needed	
Made sure biological safety cabinet blower was on	
Eyewash station in compounding area	
Chemo spill kit in compounding area	
Compounding calculations checked by instructor	
Cosmetics and jewelry removed; was not wearing acrylic nails or nail polish	
Hands washed using proper aseptic technique	
PPEs donned in proper sequence	
Biological safety cabinet cleaned properly using correct tools and in proper sequence	
Chemo mat in biological safety cabinet	
Performed all necessary calculations correctly prior to drug preparation	
Brought the correct drugs and concentrations into the hood for preparation	
Checked expiration dates of medications	
Brought the correct supplies into the hood prior to preparation	
Inspected all products for particulate matter/contamination prior to use	
Vial top cleaned with alcohol	
Needle inserted into vial properly to prevent possible coring	
Used a venting device that had a 0.2 micron hydrophobic filter	
Air bubbles removed from syringe before removal of the syringe from the vial	
Needle removed from syringe, resulting in no spillage	
Drew up correct amount of drug and checked measurement before injecting into container	
Medication port of IV bag cleaned before injecting medication into IV bag	
IV bag mixed thoroughly with no visible signs of particulate matter	
Final product labeled and placed in zip seal bag	
Placed syringe in sharps container	
Removed PPEs and goggles in proper sequence	
Discarded PPEs in hazardous waste container	
Completed the cleaning log	

Cleaning Log		
Date of Laminar Airflow Cleaning	Time of Cleaning	Initials of Person Completing the Cleaning

13 Pharmacy Billing and Inventory Management

TERMS AND DEFINITIONS

Select the correct term from the following list and write the corresponding letter in the blank next to the statement.

A. Adjudication
B. Closed Formulary
C. Coinsurance
D. Copayment
E. Deductible
F. Direct Manufacturer Ordering
G. Inventory
H. Just-in-Time Ordering
I. Medicare Modernization Act (MMA)
J. National Provider Identifier (NPI)
K. Open Formulary
L. PAR
M. P&T Committee
N. POS
O. Prime Vendors
P. Prior Authorization
Q. Safety Data Sheets (SDS)
R. Treatment Authorization Request (TAR)
S. Wholesalers

_____ 1. The enactment of prescription drug coverage provided for persons covered under Medicare

_____ 2. Companies that stock a variety of drug manufacturers' medications and normally have a "just-in-time" turnaround for ordered drugs

_____ 3. The amount paid by a policyholder out-of-pocket before the insurance company will pay a claim

_____ 4. Medical staff composed of physicians, pharmacists, pharmacy technicians, nurses, and dieticians who provide necessary information and advice to the institution or insurer on whether a drug should be added to a formulary

_____ 5. Information sheets supplied to the pharmacy from the manufacturer of chemical products; lists hazards of the product and procedures to follow if exposed to that product

_____ 6. Refers to the amount of product a pharmacy has for sale

_____ 7. A type of insurance in which the policyholder pays a share of the payment made against a claim

_____ 8. Number assigned to any health care provider that is used for the purpose of standardizing health data transmissions

_____ 9. A system that orders a product just before it is used

_____ 10. A tightly restricted list of medications that are preapproved by the health plan provider or pharmacy benefits manager for reimbursement

_____ 11. The process used for Medicare and Medicaid preapproval for assistive technology devices with a cost of more than $100

_____ 12. Insurance-required approval for a restricted, non-formulary, or noncovered medication before a prescription medication can be filled

_____ 13. System that allows inventory to be tracked as it is used

_____ 14. Directly contracting with and ordering from the manufacturer to obtain better pricing; may join a GPO

_____ 15. Electronic insurance billing for medication payment

_____ 16. Periodic automatic replenishment of stock levels to a certain number of allowed units

_____ 17. Large distributors of medications and retail products that contract with the pharmacy to deliver the bulk of their medications in exchange for lower prices

_____ 18. The portion of the prescription bill that the patient is responsible for paying

_____ 19. A list that is essentially unrestricted in the types of drug choices offered or that can be prescribed and reimbursed under the health provider plan or pharmacy benefit plan

TRUE OR FALSE

Write T or F next to each statement.

_____ 1. A pharmacy technician often is put in charge of billing.

_____ 2. A formulary is a book that contains compounding recipes.

_____ 3. Many formulary drugs are generic versions of proprietary products.

_____ 4. Generic drugs are less expensive because they are less effective than brand name drugs.

_____ 5. In a PPO, the patient must select a physician from the insurance plan's list.

_____ 6. A PPO plan usually has a higher copayment than an HMO.

_____ 7. Each insurance plan has specific guidelines that must be followed for reimbursement.

_____ 8. The cost of prescriptions is the same from pharmacy to pharmacy.

_____ 9. If the cardholder's information does not match the processor's information, the patient does not have coverage.

_____ 10. When the shipment arrives, all included medications and supplies must be verified against the inventory list.

_____ 11. One of the best ways to learn drug names and to become familiar with their locations in your pharmacy is to put away new stock.

_____ 12. Recall notices arrive by voice mail.

_____ 13. Storing medications in the proper location is the responsibility of everyone working in the pharmacy.

_____ 14. Cytotoxic drugs require special packaging when they are returned to the manufacturer.

_____ 15. Medications taken out of the pharmacy by a patient can be returned to stock.

MULTIPLE CHOICE

Complete the question by circling the best answer.

1. Who is responsible for maintaining the inventory stock in the pharmacy?
   A. Pharmacist
   B. Technician
   C. Inventory technician
   D. All of the above

2. The types of drugs typically included in a formulary are:
   A. New drugs
   B. Generic drugs and common branded drugs for which no generic is available in the drug class
   C. Uncommon drugs
   D. Extremely expensive drugs

3. In third-party billing, the third party is the:
   A. Pharmacy
   B. Patient
   C. Insurance company
   D. All of the above

4. Which of the following is not a type of health insurance plan in use today?
   A. POS
   B. HMO
   C. PPO
   D. Medicare

5. Which of the following is not a special feature of an HMO?
   A. Primary care physician
   B. Independent physicians' association
   C. Copayment
   D. Workers' compensation

6. Which of the following is not a difference between HMOs and PPOs?
   A. A PPO plan has no requirements for a PCP
   B. PPO plans have a copayment
   C. PPO plans have a deductible
   D. All of the above are differences

7. The amount a patient must pay before the copay starts is called the:
   A. Share of cost
   B. Penalty period
   C. Deductible
   D. Grace period

8. Which of the following is not a government-run insurance program?
   A. Medicare
   B. Medicaid
   C. Long-term disability
   D. Workers' compensation

9. Which group is not covered by Medicare?
   A. Healthy infants
   B. Disabled patients
   C. Seniors
   D. Dialysis patients

10. The insurance company decides the amount of coverage per medication based on:
    A. AWP
    B. Copay
    C. DAW
    D. A and B

11. Which of the following is not a reason for the insurance company to reject a claim?
    A. Coverage has expired
    B. Use of a generic drug
    C. Refill too soon
    D. NDC not covered

12. Sometimes insurance companies refill medications early because:
    A. The patient lost the medication
    B. The patient is going on a vacation
    C. The physician told the patient to increase the dosage
    D. All of the above

13. Which of the following is *not* an example of an inventory system that can keep a running inventory of medications, as well as order them?
    A. SOC system
    B. POS system
    C. Order card system
    D. Handheld computer inventory system

14. Which of the following is *not* a reason to return medications to the warehouse or manufacturer?
    A. Drug recalled
    B. Drug damaged during delivery
    C. Drug incorrectly reconstituted
    D. Drug expired

15. Manufacturers are required by law to recall any product that has been found to have which of the following guideline violations?
    A. Labeling is wrong
    B. Product was not packaged or produced properly
    C. Drug batch was contaminated
    D. All of the above

16. Drug utilization evaluation (DUE) is an important process used to screen the medication order for:
    A. Duplicate therapy
    B. Possible errors
    C. Drug-drug interactions
    D. All of the above

17. A zero for a DAW code means _____.
    A. No refills
    B. Dispense order as written
    C. Generic substitution authorized
    D. Patient would like brand name only

18. A one for DAW code means _____.
    A. No refills
    B. Dispense order as written
    C. Generic substitution authorized
    D. Patient would like brand name only

19. Point-of-sale billing allows the insurance company to _____.
    A. Price a claim
    B. Verify eligibility
    C. Identify covered drugs
    D. All of the above

20. Reasons for obtaining a prior authorization may include _____ .
    A. Patient is demanding the drug
    B. Drug of choice not formulary
    C. Physician is requesting
    D. None of the above

FILL IN THE BLANKS

Answer each question by completing the statement in the space provided.

1. Everyone working in the pharmacy is responsible for maintaining the _____ _____.

2. For medications to become part of a formulary, they must meet certain requirements such as _____ and _____.

3. _____ is a method of payment in which the doctor receives a fixed amount for each member patient regardless of how many times the patient visits the physician.

4. If the patient must self-bill the insurance company for reimbursement, then the patient will need the _____ to submit to the insurance company.

5. A percentage of each _____ _____ is applied toward Medicaid.

6. Regardless of the patient's type of insurance, you should always treat people with _____.

7. The term _____-_____ _____ refers to the portion of payment reimbursed by insurance companies.

8. Falsely billing charges for medication that was not dispensed is a _____.

9. _____ _____ focuses on ordering stock, proper storage of medication and supplies, repackaging, disposal of used and unused pharmaceutical products, and distribution systems.

10. A _____ _____ can identify the drug, strength, dosage form, quantity, cost, package size, and any other information necessary about a drug.

MATCHING

Match the types of insurance with its corresponding description.

A. CHAMPVA
B. HMO
C. Medicaid
D. Medicare
E. Medigap plans
F. PPO
G. TRICARE
H. Workers' compensation

_____ 1. Supplemental insurance policies provided through private insurance companies to help cover costs not reimbursed by the Medicare plan, such as co-insurance, co-pays, and deductibles

_____ 2. Allows coverage for in-network only physicians and services

_____ 3. A health benefit program for active-duty and retired personnel in all seven uniformed services; also covers dependents of military personnel who were killed while on active duty

_____ 4. Government-managed insurance program that provides health care services to low-income children, the elderly, blind, and those with disabilities

_____ 5. Government-managed insurance program composed of several coverage plans for health care services and supplies for individuals 65 years or older, younger than 65 with long-term disabilities, or those suffering from end-stage renal disease

_____ 6. Government-required and government-enforced medical coverage for workers injured on the job, paid for by the employer

_____ 7. A program for veterans with permanent service-related disabilities and their dependents, and spouses and children of veterans who died from service-connected disability

_____ 8. Allows patients to choose a physician with reduced costs for medical services

SHORT ANSWER

Write a short response to each question in the space provided.

1. When a pharmacy is billing for medication, what is the minimum information the insurance company requires?

   _____

   _____

   _____

2. List four common reasons a prescription may not be covered.

   _____

   _____

   _____

   _____

3. One of the most common problems resulting in a claim rejection is a non-ID match. What patient information should be double-checked in these cases?

   _____

   _____

   _____

4. Why do many pharmacies have a policy of pulling any medication off the shelves that will expire in 3 months or sooner?

   _____

   _____

   _____

5. What are the three main responsibilities of automated return companies?

   A. _____

   B. _____

   C. _____

6. What are the four Medicare levels available?

   A. Medicare Part A

   _____

   B. Medicare Part B

   _____

C. Medicare Part C

_____

D. Medicare Part D

_____

7. List and describe the three classes of drug recalls.

_____

_____

_____

8. List the medication storage temperature requirements for each of the following:

A. Freezer _____

B. Refrigerator _____

C. Room temperature _____

RESEARCH ACTIVITIES

Follow the instructions given in each exercise and provide a response.

1. Access the website *www.fda.gov* for FDA news, recalls, and product safety.

   A. Find and list three drugs that have been recalled within the last 30 days.

   B. What were the reasons for the recalls?

2. Access the website *http://www.deadiversion.usdoj.gov/drug_disposal/takeback/* for the DEA National Take-Back Initiative.

   A. What is the goal of the Take-Back Initiative?

   B. When is the next scheduled National Take-Back Initiative day scheduled?

CRITICAL THINKING

Reply to each question based on what you have learned in the chapter.

1. Should Medicare cover all medical and prescription costs for elderly patients? Give three pros and three cons for this issue.

2. Many Canadian pharmacies are offering prescription drugs at vastly reduced prices compared with U.S. prices. Is there any reason not to "go across the border" for your medications?

3. Choosing an insurance health plan can be overwhelming. What type of coverage would best meet your needs? Outline all items you would need to have total health coverage.

LAB SCENARIOS

Purchase of Pharmaceuticals

Objective: To follow the legal requirements of ordering and receiving Schedule II medications and to become familiar with various types of medication recalls.

Lab Activity #13.1: Completion of a DEA Form 222.

Equipment needed:

- Sample DEA Form 222
- Internet access
- *Physicians' Desk Reference* or *Drug Facts and Comparisons*
- *Drug Topics Red Book* or *FDA National Drug Code Directory*
- Black ink pen

See Reverse of PURCHASER'S Copy for Instructions	No order form may be issued for Schedule 1 and II substances unless a completed application form has been received. (21 CFR 1305.04).			**OMB APPROVAL No. 1117-0010**	
TO: *(Name of Supplier)*		STREET ADDRESS			
CITY and STATE	DATE		**TO BE FILLED IN BY SUPPLIER**		
			SUPPLIERS DEA REGISTRATION No.		

LINE No.	No. of Packages	Size of Package	Name of Item	National Drug Code	Packages Shipped	Date Shipped
			TO BE FILLED IN BY PURCHASER			
1						
2						
3						
4						
5						
6						
7						
8						
9						
10						

◄ **LAST LINE COMPLETED**	*(MUST BE 10 OR LESS)*	SIGNATURE OF PURCHASER OR ATTORNEY OR AGENT	
Date Issued	DEA Registration No.	Name and Address of Registrant	
20010101	DEAREGNO	VOID VOID VOID VOID VOID VOID VOID VOID VOID	
Schedules			
XXXXXXXXXXXX		VOID VOID VOID	
Registered as a	No. of this Order Form	VOID VOID VOID VOID VOID VOID	
XXXXXXXXXXXX	000000005		

DEA Form -222 (Oct. 2004)	**U.S. OFFICIAL ORDER FORMS - SCHEDULES I & II** DRUG ENFORCEMENT ADMINISTRATION SUPPLIER'S Copy 1	107051797

Time needed to complete this activity: 15 minutes

Procedure

1. Using a black ink pen, enter the name of the supplier; the supplier's street address, city, and state; and the date the DEA Form 222 is being completed.
2. Enter the number of packages, the bottle size, and the name of the medication on the DEA Form 222.
3. Using the *Drug Topics Red Book* or *FDA National Drug Code Directory*, enter on the DEA Form 222 the NDC number of medications being ordered.
4. Sign the document.

You have been asked to order the following quantities of Schedule II substances for the pharmacy:

- 5 bottles of 100 tablets of Roxicet-5 (oxycodone 5 mg/APAP 325 mg)
- 1 bottle of 100 tablets of Percodan (oxycodone 5 mg/ASA 325 mg)
- 2 boxes of Fentanyl-50
- 4 bottles of 100 tablets of methylphenidate 10 mg
- 5 bottles of 100 tablets of methylphenidate 5 mg
- 1 bottle of 100 tablets of methylphenidate 20 mg
- 2 bottles of 100 capsules Adderall XR 10 mg
- 3 bottles of 100 tablets of Oxycontin 10 mg
- 1 bottle of 100 tablets of hydromorphone 2 mg

1. The DEA Form 222 is a three-part form; what is done with the three parts of the form?

_____

_____

2. What would you do with a DEA Form 222 if you made an error filling it out?

_____

_____

3. How long must the pharmacy retain a completed DEA Form 222?

_____

_____

Lab Activity #13.2: Receiving a Schedule II order from a wholesaler.

Equipment needed:

- Sample DEA Form 222
- Blue ink pen

Time needed to complete this activity: 5 minutes

Procedure

The pharmacy has received its order of Schedule II medications that were ordered during the previous activity. The pharmacy has received all of the medications ordered, but received only 3 bottles of Methylphenidate 10 mg. Using the DEA Form 222 from the previous activity and a blue pen, complete the remainder of the DEA form.

1. How would you handle the shortage of Methylphenidate 10 mg?

_____

_____

2. Where does a pharmacy keep its Schedule II medications?

_____

_____

3. Describe how you would place the medication into stock.

_____

_____

_____

_____

Procedure	Yes/No
Had the appropriate invoice to accurately check in the order.	
Accounted for all boxes/items.	
Inspected all boxes/items for storage requirements; stored items needing refrigeration or freezing ASAP.	
Checked all information against the invoice including drug name, strength, dosage form, quantity, and that the expiration date is not too soon.	
Compared the invoice with the order form to ensure that only the items requested were received.	
Signed and dated the invoice and forwarded it for processing per pharmacy protocol.	
Placed the stock in the correct location per pharmacy protocol, placing new stock behind existing stock with the most current expiration dates in the front.	
Returned inventory cards to the medication box for future use.	
Filed invoice per pharmacy protocol.	

Lab Activity #13.3: Medication recall.

Equipment needed:

- Computer with Internet connection
- Paper
- Pen

Time needed to complete this activity: 30 minutes

Procedure

1. Using the Internet, go to *www.fda.gov*.
2. Click on Recalls.
3. Answer questions regarding specific medications.

January 10, 2013

1. What strength of Mitosol was recalled?

_____

2. Why was it recalled?

_____

3. What should the patient do if he/she has medication being recalled?

_____

May 10, 2013
1. Which company recalled piperacillin and tazobactam for injection?

_____

2. What is the indication for piperacillin and tazobactam for injection?

_____

3. Why were these lots recalled?

_____

4. What lot numbers and expiration dates were indicated in this drug recall?

_____

_____

_____

_____

_____

_____

November 1, 2013
1. What OTC medication did Perrigo recall?

_____

_____

_____

2. Why was the medication recalled?

_____

_____

3. What telephone number or e-mail address should an individual use to contact The Perrigo Company?

_____

_____

February 19, 2014

1. What strength of etomidate injection was recalled?

_____

2. Why was it recalled?

_____

3. What NDC numbers, lot numbers and expiration dates were indicated in this recall?

_____

_____

_____

_____

_____

_____

March 6, 2014

4. What three products did Pfizer recall?

_____

5. Why were they recalled?

_____

6. What should the patient do if he/she has medication being recalled?

_____

Lab Activity #13.4: Access the website *www.fda*.gov to define the various types of medication recalls and determine the type of recalls from the previous activity.

Equipment needed:

- Computer with Internet access
- Pencil/pen
- Paper

Time needed to complete this activity: 30 minutes

1. Define the following terms:

A. Class I Recall

_____

_____

_____

B. Class II Recall

_____

_____

_____

C. Class III Recall

_____

_____

_____

2. What type of Class Recall was involved with Mitosol 2 mg/vial? Why?

_____

_____

_____

3. What type of Class Recall was involved with piperacillin and tazobactam for injection? Why?

_____

_____

_____

4. What type of Class Recall was involved with Perrigo? Why?

_____

_____

_____

5. What type of Class Recall was involved with etomidate 2 mg/mL? Why?

_____

_____

_____

6. What type of Class Recall was involved with Pfizer? Why?

_____

_____

_____

Third-Party Formulary and Requirements

Objective: To become familiar with various third-party formularies and requirements.

Lab Activity #13.5: Third-party formulary and requirements.

Equipment needed:

- Internet access
- Pencil/pen

Time needed to complete this activity: 30 minutes

1. Access the website *www.caremark.com*. Click on the link named *For Pharmacists and Medical Professionals* and look up the *Performance Drug List* to answer the following questions:

   A. What are the therapeutic categories of the formulary?

   B. Which calcium channel blockers are covered?

   C. Which SNRIs are covered?

   D. What are the preferred alternatives to Lipitor?

   E. What are the preferred alternatives to Prevacid?

2. Access the website *www.bcbstx.com*. Click on the link named *Already a Member* and look up *Prescription Drug Information* for *Prescription Plans for Metallic Individual Plans* to answer the following questions under the 5-tier plan:

   A. What are the therapeutic categories of the formulary for the current year?

   B. Is Gabitril 12 mg tablet a preferred or non-preferred drug on the formulary?

C. Is divalproex sodium delayed release 500 mg tablet a preferred or non-preferred drug on the formulary?

D. Is Plavix 75 mg tablet a preferred or non-preferred drug on the formulary?

E. List three drugs that require step therapy.

F. List three drugs that require prior authorization.

3. Access the website *www.cigna.com* to answer the following questions:

A. Click on the link named *Find a Doctor*. Name three pharmacies within 5 miles of your zip code that accept Cigna prescription insurance.

B. Click on the link named *View Drug Lists* on the Cigna home page then view a *List of All Drugs*. Name three drugs on the Three Tier Plan Drug List that would require prior authorization.

14 Medication Safety and Error Prevention

TERMS AND DEFINITIONS

Select the correct term from the following list and write the corresponding letter in the blank next to the statement.

A. American Society of Health-System Pharmacists (ASHP)
B. Automated Dispensing Systems (ADS)
C. Institute for Healthcare Improvement (IHI)
D. Institute for Safe Medication Practices (ISMP)
E. Institute of Medicine (IOM)
F. Medication Error
G. Medication Error Prevention
H. MEDMARX
I. MedWatch
J. National Coordinating Council for Medication Error Reporting and Prevention (NCC MERP)
K. Pharmacy Technician Certification Board (PTCB)
L. Risk Evaluation and Mitigation Strategy (REMS)
M. Pharmacy Technician Educators Council (PTEC)
N. Society for the Education of Pharmacy Technicians (SEPhT)
O. United States Pharmacopeia (USP)

_____ 1. National pharmacy technician organization promoting the education and training of pharmacy technicians

_____ 2. Any preventable event that may cause or lead to inappropriate medication use or patient harm

_____ 3. Strategy to manage a known or potential serious risk associated with a drug or biological product

_____ 4. Program established by the FDA for reporting drug and medical product safety alerts and label changes; the program also provides a voluntary adverse event reporting system for medications, medical products, and devices

_____ 5. A nonprofit organization committed to the improvement of health care by promoting promising concepts through safety, efficiency, and other patient-centered goals

_____ 6. Founded by the USP, this is an independent council of more than 25 organizations gathered to address interdisciplinary causes of medication errors and strategies for prevention

_____ 7. A nonprofit organization devoted entirely to promoting safe medication use and preventing medication errors; gathers information on drug errors and suggests new safer standards to avoid such errors

_____ 8. U.S. organization that promotes teachers' strategies and instructions for pharmacy technician education

_____ 9. Methods used by pharmacy, nursing, and other allied health professionals to prevent medication errors

_____ 10. Association of pharmacists, pharmacy students, and technicians practicing in hospitals and health care systems, including home health care; has a long history of advocating patient safety and establishing best practices to improve medication use

_____ 11. Offers national certification for pharmacy technicians in the United States

_____ 12. Electronic systems used to dispense medications

_____ 13. National Internet-accessible database that hospitals and health care systems use to track adverse drug reactions and medication errors

_____ 14. This nonprofit organization provides scientifically informed analysis and guidance regarding health and health policy

_____ 15. Independent organization that strives to ensure the quality, safety, and benefit of medicines and dietary supplements by setting standards and certification processes

TRUE OR FALSE

Write T or F next to each statement.

_____ 1. Errors are always caught before they can possibly hurt someone.

_____ 2. Pharmacy technicians are on the front line when it comes to being able to prevent drug errors.

_____ 3. Combined sources suggest that more than 400,000 people per year suffer some type of preventable adverse event while in the hospital that contributes to their death.

_____ 4. All drug errors cause harm to the patient.

_____ 5. One common cause of medication error is illegible handwriting.

_____ 6. Medication errors only occur in hospital settings.

_____ 7. Even the most highly skilled person will make errors at one time or another.

_____ 8. One of the most serious types of errors is with parenteral medications.

_____ 9. A delayed-release drug may be substituted for an extended-release drug.

_____ 10. Many new systems are in place and are working toward decreasing errors.

_____ 11. The most important aspect of dealing with errors is the reporting process.

_____ 12. A drug error cannot be reported anonymously.

_____ 13. Misinterpreted abbreviations have resulted in drug errors and are an area of concern.

_____ 14. One of the best ways that errors are decreased is through trial and error.

_____ 15. It is imperative that every health care worker view drug error prevention as a priority.

MULTIPLE CHOICE

Complete each question by circling the best answer.

1. According to a Health and Human Services report, bad hospital care contributes to the deaths of _____ patients on Medicare in a given year.
   A. 440,000
   B. 210,000
   C. 180,000
   D. 7000

2. The Institute for Safe Medication Practices (ISMP) estimates that around _____ deaths per year are linked to actual medication errors.
   A. 440,000
   B. 210,000
   C. 180,000
   D. 7000

3. Which drug is *not* an example of an ISMP high-alert medication?
   A. Amoxicillin
   B. Warfarin
   C. Metformin
   D. Carbamazepine

4. Most reported medication errors are made in what type of setting?
   A. Hospital pharmacies
   B. Mail order pharmacies
   C. Retail pharmacies
   D. Both A and C

5. Which of the following is *not* an example of the barriers that pharmacy workers face to avoid errors?
   A. Stress
   B. When their lunch hour is
   C. Hard to read labels because of small print
   D. Medication names that sound alike

6. Anticoagulants such as warfarin have the potential for many interactions with:
   A. Dietary/herbal supplements
   B. Food
   C. Other drugs
   D. All of the above

7. Which of the following drugs is of great concern as a cause of error because it is commonly used to flush IV lines?
   A. Heparin
   B. Saline
   C. Potassium
   D. Dextrose

8. Which of the following abbreviations is not a suffix on a drug label?
   A. LA
   B. DA
   C. ER
   D. SR

9. Receiving care in the home also carries the risk of:
   A. Improper dosing
   B. Contamination of IV sets
   C. High costs
   D. Only A and B

10. Life expectancy in the United States has risen in the last century as a result of:
    A. Improved health care
    B. Increased activity
    C. Better dietary intake
    D. All of the above

11. Pharmacy technicians should always check each prescription _____ throughout the filling process.
    A. Once
    B. Twice
    C. Three times
    D. None of the above

12. Many pharmacies fill upwards of:
    A. 200 to 300 prescriptions per day
    B. 300 to 400 prescriptions per day
    C. 400 to 500 prescriptions per day
    D. 500 to 600 prescriptions per day

13. The Institute for Healthcare Improvement has reported that more than _____ of all errors in hospitals are caused by poor communication of medication orders.
    A. 50%
    B. 45%
    C. 60%
    D. 75%

14. What three steps are involved in medication reconciliation?
    A. Clarification
    B. Verification
    C. Reconciliation
    D. All of the above

15. The ability to prevent mistakes from happening will always fall on people involved in the prescribing, _____, and dosing of medications.
    A. Reading
    B. Writing
    C. Filling
    D. Filing

FILL IN THE BLANKS

Answer each question by completing the statement in the space provided.

1. Drug errors are unacceptable in any situation involving _____ _____ or _____.

2. It takes a _____ working together to prevent medication errors.

3. According to the ISMP, some medications that are considered _____ _____ in connection with errors are insulin, narcotics and opiates, methotrexate, warfarin, and potassium chloride injections.

4. Physicians' _____ has long been known for its illegibility.

5. The first response to an error is normally to _____ rather than to _____ the reasons behind such an occurrence.

6. Errors often occur when one task is _____ by an electronic device.

7. No one wants to make an error, but when it does happen, _____ feelings and _____ may emerge.

8. Medication _____ is the responsibility of all pharmacy personnel.

9. One of the best ways to decrease errors is through _____ and _____.

10. Accurate interpretation of _____ _____ can mean the difference between life and death to a patient.

MATCHING

Match the type of medication error with its correct description.

A. Prescribing error
B. Omission error
C. Wrong time error
D. Unauthorized drug error
E. Improper dose error
F. Wrong dosage form error
G. Wrong drug preparation error
H. Wrong administration
I. Deteriorated drug
J. Monitoring error
K. Compliance error

_____ 1. Failure to administer an ordered dose to a patient before the next dose is due, without an apparent reason or appropriate documentation

_____ 2. Medication administered in a dosage form other than what was ordered

_____ 3. Failure to review a prescribed medication for proper regimen, appropriateness, and dosage, or failure in using laboratory results to correctly adjust dose

_____ 4. Patient administered a dose that is greater or less than prescribed amount

_____ 5. Drug is given using wrong procedure or technique

_____ 6. Medication administered outside scheduled time frame

_____ 7. Drug is incorrectly formulated or manipulated, and medication is administered to patient

_____ 8. Prescriber orders a medication that is incorrect or is selected incorrectly based on indications or contraindications and medication reaches patient

_____ 9. Medication is administered that has expired or integrity of ingredients has been compromised

_____ 10. Patient does not adhere to prescribed medication regimen

_____ 11. Medication administered to a patient from an unauthorized prescriber; physician not licensed in that state or not an authorized prescriber

261

SHORT ANSWER

Write a short response to each question in the space provided.

1. List the five basic rights involving medication safety.

_____

_____

_____

_____

2. Why would a patient try to use medical supplies, intended for single use, more than once, and what risks are associated with this practice?

_____

_____

_____

_____

3. The FDA has recommended new labeling on over-the-counter (OTC) cough and cold medications for children. What does the new label say?

_____

_____

_____

_____

4. List the five guidelines used to share information with health care professionals about potentially dangerous events.

_____

_____

_____

_____

5. List five safety standards outlined by The Joint Commission to improve patient quality and safety.

_____

_____

_____

_____

_____

6. List four strategies a pharmacy technician can use to help reduce errors.

_____

_____

_____

_____

_____

RESEARCH ACTIVITIES

Follow the instructions given in each exercise and provide a response.

1. Access the website *http://www.accessdata.fda.gov/cdrh_docs/psn/video/mpeg/FDA-SHOW104-SEG6.MPG* and watch the video to answer the following questions:

   A. Fifty percent of letter-number errors come from what four basic mix-ups?

   B. What does ISMP recommend to avoid these mix-ups?

2. Access the website *http://www.ismp.org/NAN/default.asp*. List two special error alerts from ISMP. How could you help your pharmacy not make the mistakes listed in the alert?

3. Access the website at *www.ashp.org*.

   A. List the nine goal categories for the *Model Curriculum* for a pharmacy technician education and training program.

   B. Where is the nearest ASHP-accredited pharmacy technician training program you could attend located?

CRITICAL THINKING

Reply to each question based on what you have learned in the chapter.

1. An elderly patient has been diagnosed with rheumatoid arthritis. When she is admitted to the hospital, she tells the nurse she takes OTC NSAIDs but cannot remember the names of the medications. Because polypharmacy is a problem with many elderly adults, what steps should be taken by the hospital pharmacy?

2. Mark is an IV specialist working in a home infusion pharmacy. When he gets an order to prepare a TPN for a 7-year-old girl, he accidentally draws up the strength of the ingredients listed instead of the calculated volumes needed. What will be the consequences if this error is not caught?

3. Each individual reacts differently to medications. Metabolism changes occur over time. A technician should pay special attention to the preparation and administration of drugs for the older adult. List three factors that could lead to serious cumulative effects with medications in the elderly. Briefly explain the results of each.

4. Meticulous care should be taken in the preparation and administration of medications to reduce the chance of error. However, if a mistake is made, how should the technician handle the situation?

5. James is a pharmacy technician working in a large hospital pharmacy. The critical care nurse calls and asks for the evening dose of daptomycin. She states that the patient is taking the drug q8h. How should James handle this situation?

6. Brittany is working as an IV technician in a local hospital. She receives a medication order for dopamine for a seriously ill baby on the pediatric floor. The nurse states that it is needed stat. What are the most important factors that Brittany should keep in mind as she prepares the order?

LAB SCENARIOS

Pharmacy Abbreviations

Objective: To introduce the pharmacy technician to the many abbreviations encountered in the practice of pharmacy, regardless of the pharmacy setting.

> The pharmacy technician encounters abbreviations when reviewing a prescription/medication order and in pharmacy-related literature. Some of these abbreviations may indicate dosage forms, routes of administration, quantities to be taken, frequency of administration, compounding instructions, and even disease states.
>
> If a pharmacy technician is not familiar with a particular abbreviation, he or she should always ask the pharmacist for clarification of the abbreviations. The technician should never guess the meaning of an abbreviation. Guessing incorrectly will lead to a medication error and will possibly affect the patient's outcome.
>
> Throughout the years, numerous errors have been associated with misinterpreting abbreviations. As a result of these errors, The Institute of Safe Medication Practices formulated a list of error-prone abbreviations, symbols, and dose designations. Many health care organizations have adopted this list, and practitioners within the organization are not to use these abbreviations. However, pharmacy technicians may continue to see them in the community pharmacy setting.

Lab Activity #14.1: Write the meaning of the following pharmaceutical abbreviations.

Equipment needed

- Pencil/pen

Time needed to complete this activity: 20 minutes

Part 1

1. aa _____

2. dtd _____

3. pm _____

4. L _____

5. mcg _____

6. PO _____

7. qh _____

8. supp _____

9. tbsp _____

10. mOsmol _____

11. inj _____

12. gr _____

Part 2

1. ac _____

2. cc _____

3. elix _____

4. kg _____

5. non rep _____

6. noct _____

7. postop _____

8. sol _____

9. top _____

10. ATC _____

11. s _____

12. syr _____

Part 3

1. ad _____

2. caps _____

3. g _____

4. ID _____

5. mEq _____

6. NR _____

7. pr _____

8. susp _____

9. tid _____

10. amp _____

11. bid _____

12. qd _____

Part 4

1. ad lib _____

2. n/v _____

3. ft _____

4. IM _____

5. mg _____

6. prn _____

7. qs _____

8. prn p _____

9. WH/SOB _____

10. gtt _____

11. ml _____

12. disp _____

Part 5

1. AM _____

2. BSA _____

3. hs _____

4. IV _____

5. mg/kg _____

6. pulv _____

7. q _____

8. qs ad _____

9. tsp _____

10. aq _____

11. stat _____

12. ung _____

Part 6

1. Ca _____

2. EtOH _____

3. KCl _____

4. MVI _____

5. NS _____

6. DW _____

7. O_2 _____

8. H_2O _____

9. LR _____

10. ½ NS _____

11. D_5W _____

12. $D_{10}W$ _____

Lab Activity #14.2: Write the organization for each of the following acronyms.

Equipment needed:

■ Pencil/pen

Time needed to complete this activity: 5 minutes

1. AAPT _____

2. ACPE _____

3. ASHP _____

Chapter **14 Medication Safety and Error Prevention**

4. CDC _____

5. CMS _____

6. CPhT _____

7. DEA _____

8. ExCPT _____

9. FDA _____

10. ISMP _____

11. NABP _____

12. P&T _____

13. PTCB _____

14. PTEC _____

15. TJC _____

Medication Safety

Objective: To make the pharmacy technician aware that the names of many medications are similar to the names of other medications.

Lab Activity #14.3: Using the ISMP List of Confused Drug Names located at *www.ismp.org*, identify those medications that are commonly mistaken for the following drug listed in the table.

Equipment needed:

- Computer with Internet access
- Pencil/pen

Time needed to complete this activity: 30 minutes

Medication	Mistaken for
Aciphex	
Actos	
Alkeran	
Amaryl	
aMILoride	
Anacin	
Antivert	
Aricept	
Asacol	
Avandia	
Benicar	
CeleBREX	
Celexa	
Cerebyx	
Clonazepam	
Coumadin	

Medication	Mistaken for
Cozaar	
DAUNOrubicin	
Diovan	
Effexor	
FLUoxetine	
HumaLOG	
HumuLIN	
Jantoven	
Janumet	
Januvia	
Lasix	
Leukeran	
Levothyroxine	
Lipitor	
Lodine	
LORazepam	
Methadone	
Neumega	
Neurontin	
NovoLIN	
Ortho Tri-Cyclen	
Paxil	
Plendil	
Prednisone	
Procanbid	
Tobrex	
Topamax	
Wellbutrin SR	
Yasmin	
Zantac	
Zestril	
Zetia	
Zovirax	
ZyPREXA	

Lab Activity #14.4: Medication errors in the hospital have increased because specific drug classifications and medications are now used. You have been asked to highlight the labels of those medications with a fluorescent pink marker. Indicate whether the following medications should be highlighted using the ISMP List of High-Alert Medications located at *www.ismp.org*.

Equipment needed:

- Computer with Internet access
- Drug reference book of choice
- Pencil/pen

Time needed to complete this activity: 15 minutes

Medication	Yes	No
Actoplus Met		
Actos		
Alteplase		
Amoxicillin		
Avalide		
Avandia		
Cephalexin		
Ciprofloxacin		
Digoxin		
Humalog		
Lipitor		
Lovenox		
Magnesium sulfate injection		
Metformin		
Novolog Mix 70/30		
Oxytocin (IV)		
Plavix		
Promethazine (IV)		
Sodium chloride for injection (hypertonic)		
Total parenteral solutions		
Tricor		
Truvada		
Vytorin		
Warfarin		
Zetia		

Lab Activity #14.5: You are working in a hospital and you have been asked to serve on the Pharmacy and Therapeutics (P&T) Committee. Recently, medication errors caused by misinterpretation of pharmacy abbreviations have increased. The P&T committee has been asked to develop a list of approved abbreviations to be used in the hospital. Using the ISMP List of Error-Prone Abbreviations, Symbols, and Dose Designations located at *www.ismp*.org, indicate whether or not the following abbreviation can be used. If it should not be used, indicate why.

Equipment needed:

■ Computer with Internet access
■ Pencil/pen

Time needed to complete this activity: 15 minutes

Abbreviation	Yes, it may be used	No, it should not be used	If no, why?
AD			
Bid			
BT			
Cap			
D/C			
IN			
IU			
OD			
OS			
OU			
Qd			
Qod			
Qhs			
Ss			
Stat			
Susp			
Tab			
Tid			
TIW			
U			

Lab Activity #14.6: A patient comes to the pharmacy and states that she had difficulty taking the medication and would like to know if she can crush her medication and place it in some applesauce. Using the ISMP List of Oral Dosage Forms that Should Not Be Crushed located at *www.ismp.*org, indicate if the following medications can be crushed.

Equipment needed:

- Computer with Internet access
- Pencil/pen

Time needed to complete this activity: 20 minutes

Medication	Can it be crushed?	If no, explain
Aciphex		
Actonel		
Amoxicillin tablets		
Bactrim DS		
Boniva		
Cymbalta		
Depakote		
Dyazide		
Erythromycin stearate		
Fosamax		
Hydrea		
Imdur		
Inderal		
Keppra		
Motrin		
Naprosyn		
Nexium		
Oracea		
Paxil		
Ritalin		
Tegretol XR		
Topamax		
Toprol XL		
Xanax		
Zyban		

Medication Reconciliation

Objective: To understand the steps required to complete a medication reconciliation form. The goal is to ensure the patient is give then the correct medication at all points as he or she moves through the health care system.

Lab Activity #14.7: With a partner, role-play the patient interview process using the patient profiles provided by your instructor. Interview your partner to complete the medication reconciliation form.

Equipment needed:

- Medication reconciliation form
- Pen

Time needed to complete this activity: 20 minutes

Patient Name

MRN

MEDICATION RECONCILIATION FORM

ADMISSION / POINT OF ENTRY RECONCILIATION
▪ The first nurse to interview the patient should initiate completion of this form. Additional nurses and clinicians may continue to use the same form for the same patient.
▪ **Circle all sources of information:**   Patient   Caregiver   Rx bottle   EMS   Primary provider   Other:_____

ALLERGIES AND ADVERSE DRUG REACTIONS : _____

ACTIVE MEDICATION LIST			Date of Admission / Point of Entry:				RECONCILIATION
List below all medications patient was taking at time of admission. *(Dosing information REQUIRED, if available.)*							Continue on Admission?
Medication Name	Dose	Route	Frequency	Last Dose (Date/Time)	Date	Initials	Circle **Y** (yes) *or* **N** (no)*
1.							Y N
2.							Y N
3.							Y N
4.							Y N
5.							Y N
6.							Y N
7.							Y N
8.							Y N
9.							Y N
10.							Y N
11.							Y N
12.							Y N
13.							Y N
14.							Y N
15.							Y N
OTC Medications, Herbals, etc.							
							Y N
							Y N
							Y N
							Y N

*If order to be discontinued, see Admitting Note for comments.

Medication list recorded by RN/MD/PA/NP/LPN/RPh							
Initials	Print Name/Stamp	Signature	Date	Initials	Print Name/Stamp	Signature	Date

Reconciling Prescriber (MD/PA/NP/CNM)			
Print Name/Stamp	Signature	Title	Date

TRANSFER RECONCILIATION	DISCHARGE RECONCILIATION
▪ See Physician Orders for active medication orders upon transfer. ▪ See Medication Administration Record for last dose given.	▪ See Patient Discharge Plan for list of medications patient should continue after discharge. ▪ Discharge plan should include stopped medications.
Reconciling Prescriber (**Provide name, date, signature.**)	Reconciling Prescriber (**Provide name, date, signature.**)

☐   Check here if multiple pages needed. Please indicate: Page ____ of ____

Pilot Number 2/06

Procedure:

1. Verification—Attain the patient's medication history and other medical information. This includes all medications, OTC drugs, and herbal remedies.
2. Clarification—Make sure the medication and dosages are appropriate for the patient. *The current physician's orders are compared with the patient's medication list.
3. Reconciliation—Clinical decisions are made based on the comparison between the two drug lists. Resolving any observed discrepancies or errors through documentation and direct communication is the final step.

Procedure	Yes/No
Attained the patient's medication history and other medical information. This includes all medications, OTC drugs, and herbal remedies.	
Ensured medication and dosages are appropriate for the patient. *The current physician's orders are compared with the patient's medication list.	
*Clinical decisions were made based on the comparison between the two drug lists. Resolved any observed discrepancies or errors through documentation and direct communication as the final step.	

*These steps are usually completed by a nurse and may be viewed by the physician, nurse, pharmacist, or trained pharmacy technician.

15 Therapeutic Agents for the Nervous System

REINFORCE KEY CONCEPTS

TERMS AND DEFINITIONS

Select the correct term from the following list and write the corresponding letter in the blank next to the statement.

A. Afferent
B. Autonomic
C. Axon
D. Blood-Brain Barrier
E. Bradykinesia
F. Cell Body
G. Dendrites
H. Efferent
I. Myasthenia Gravis
J. Neuron
K. Neurotransmitters
L. Nerve Terminal
M. Parasympathetic
Nervous System
N. Peripheral Nervous
System
O. Polyneuropathy
P. Somatic
Q. Sympathetic Nervous
System
R. Tardive Dyskinesia

_____ 1. The motor neurons that control voluntary actions of the skeletal muscles

_____ 2. The main part of a neuron from which axons and dendrites extend

_____ 3. Unwanted, involuntary rhythmic movements

_____ 4. The segment of a neuron that branches out to bring impulses to the cell body

_____ 5. The conduction of electrical impulses away from the central nervous system (CNS) of the body

_____ 6. The part of a nerve cell that conducts impulses away from the cell body

_____ 7. Rare autoimmune disorder that affects the transmission of electrical impulses from the CNS to muscles throughout the body

_____ 8. Division of the autonomic nervous system (ANS) that functions during restful situations

_____ 9. Chemicals that are transmitted from one neuron to another as electrical nerve impulses

_____ 10. Slowed movements

_____ 11. Characterized by distal loss of sensation, burning, or weakness

_____ 12. The functional unit of the nervous system that includes the cell body, dendrites, axons, and terminals

_____ 13. The end portion of the neuron in which nerve impulses cause chemicals to be released; these cross a small space called a synaptic cleft to carry the impulse to another neuron

_____ 14. Division of the ANS that functions during stressful situations; the "flight or fight" part of the ANS

_____ 15. Self-controlling or involuntary

_____ 16. Division of the nervous system outside the brain and spinal cord

_____ 17. A barrier formed by special characteristics of capillaries that prevents certain chemicals from moving into the brain

_____ 18. The direction of neuronal impulses from the body toward the CNS

275

TRUE OR FALSE

Write T or F next to each statement.

_____ 1. The human nervous system is a simple body system.

_____ 2. The CNS consists of the brain and spinal cord.

_____ 3. The nerve impulses are transmitted by various chemicals called neurotransmitters.

_____ 4. Most drugs that can pass through the blood-brain barrier are water soluble.

_____ 5. The somatic nervous system is part of the CNS.

_____ 6. Sympathetic and parasympathetic systems are part of the ANS.

_____ 7. Individuals with Parkinson's disease have low levels of dopamine.

_____ 8. Few differences can be found between the sympathetic and parasympathetic systems.

_____ 9. Beta-blockers can be used for people who experience frequent migraines.

_____ 10. People with epilepsy are very in tune with their medication needs and may be allowed to dose their medications according to their symptoms on any given day with their physician's permission.

SYSTEM IDENTIFIER

Identify each component in this system and enter the term next to the corresponding number.

1. _____

2. _____

3. _____

4. _____

5. _____

6. _____

7. _____

8. _____

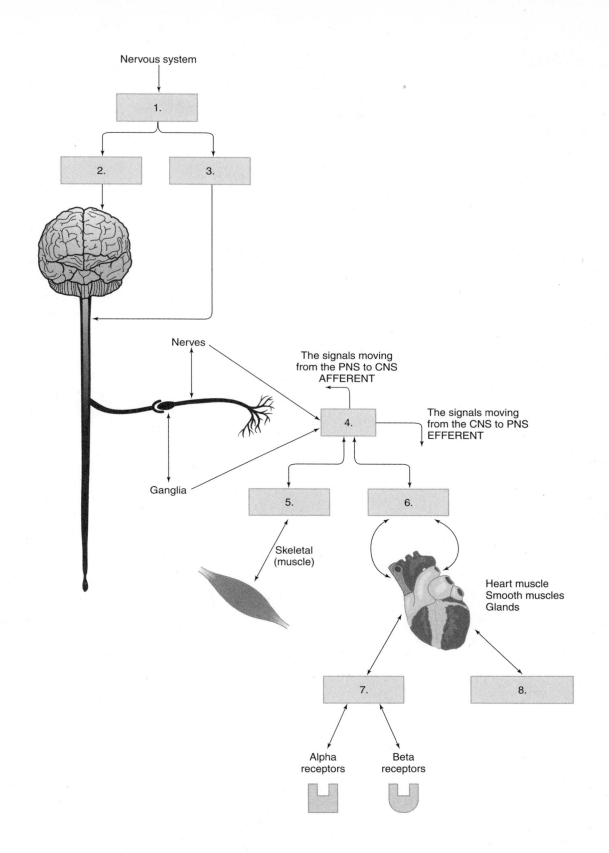

Nervous system

1.

2.

3.

Nerves

The signals moving
from the PNS to CNS
AFFERENT

4.

The signals moving
from the CNS to PNS
EFFERENT

Ganglia

5.

6.

Skeletal
(muscle)

Heart muscle
Smooth muscles
Glands

7.

8.

Alpha
receptors

Beta
receptors

MULTIPLE CHOICE

Complete each question by circling the best answer.

1. The smallest functional part of the CNS is the:
   A. Brain
   B. Synapse
   C. Spinal cord
   D. Neuron

2. The largest area of the brain is the:
   A. Cerebral cortex
   B. Cerebellum
   C. Thalamus
   D. Hypothalamus

3. The midbrain, pons, and medulla oblongata are all part of the:
   A. Cerebrum
   B. Brainstem
   C. Cerebellum
   D. Spinal cord

4. Which of the following is *not* a main neurotransmitter of the sympathetic system?
   A. Dopamine
   B. Epinephrine
   C. Acetylcholine
   D. Norepinephrine

5. Which of the following is an autoimmune disorder that affects nerves within the CNS, and leads to impaired motor function?
   A. Parkinson's disease
   B. Psychosis
   C. Multiple sclerosis
   D. Tardive dyskinesia

6. Dry mouth and inhibition of urine output are side effects of:
   A. Sympathomimetics
   B. Anticholinergics
   C. Adrenergics
   D. Parasympathomimetics

7. Which of the following is not a generalized seizure?
   A. Petit mal
   B. Status epilepticus
   C. Tonic-clonic
   D. None of the above

8. Besides taking medication, individuals with insomnia may be able to help themselves by:
   A. Learning relaxation techniques
   B. Exercising regularly
   C. A and B
   D. None of the above

9. Progressive condition of deteriorating cognitive functions is called:
   A. Epilepsy
   B. Dementia
   C. Seizures
   D. Blood-brain barrier

10. Schedule II medications can be used to treat which of the following conditions?
    A. Alzheimer's disease
    B. Parkinson's disease
    C. Multiple sclerosis
    D. Attention deficit hyperactivity disorder

FILL IN THE BLANKS

Answer each question by completing the statement in the space provided.

1. The three main states of a neuron are _____, _____, and _____.

2. The _____ is responsible for precise movements, such as maintaining balance and posture and coordinating movement.

3. The thin covering that protects the brain and spinal cord from the bony structures of the skull and spinal column is the _____.

4. The two branches of the PNS are called the _____ and _____ nervous systems, which regulate _____ and _____ _____.

5. Drugs that mimic the actions of the sympathetic nervous system are called _____ _____, and drugs that mimic the parasympathetic nervous system are called _____.

6. Alpha$_2$-receptors are mainly located on _____ _____; beta$_1$-receptors are located on the _____, and beta$_2$-receptors are located in the _____ _____ and elsewhere.

7. The function of the sympathetic division is to respond to _____ situations; one of the main functions of the parasympathetic system is to activate the _____ system.

8. The main neurotransmitters of the sympathetic system are _____ and _____, and the main neurotransmitter of the parasympathetic system is _____.

9. The two main types of skeletal muscle relaxants are _____ acting and _____ acting.

10. The main class of drugs used to treat myasthenia gravis is _____.

MATCHING

Matching I
Match the following disease states with their drug treatment classes.

_____ 1. Epilepsy

_____ 2. Alzheimer's disease

_____ 3. Multiple sclerosis

_____ 4. Parkinson's disease

_____ 5. Attention deficit/hyperactivity disorder (ADHD)

A. Interferons
B. Dopamine agonists
C. Acetylcholinesterase inhibitors
D. CNS stimulants
E. Anticonvulsants

279

Matching II

Match the following drugs with the diseases they treat.

_____ 1. Phenytoin

_____ 2. Aricept

_____ 3. Avonex

_____ 4. Sinemet

_____ 5. Mestinon

A. Parkinson's disease
B. Myasthenia gravis
C. Alzheimer's disease
D. Epilepsy
E. Multiple sclerosis

Matching III

Match the drugs with their classifications.

_____ 1. Haldol

_____ 2. Celexa

_____ 3. Cogentin

_____ 4. Xanax

_____ 5. Ambien

A. Anticholinergic
B. Antianxiety agent
C. Antipsychotic
D. Non-benzodiazepine hypnotic
E. SSRI antidepressant

Matching IV

Match the following trade and generic drug names.

_____ 1. Valium

_____ 2. Zoloft

_____ 3. Elavil

_____ 4. Risperdal

_____ 5. Zyprexa

A. Sertraline
B. Olanzapine
C. Diazepam
D. Risperidone
E. Amitriptyline

SHORT ANSWER

Write a short response to each question in the space provided.

1. What are the most common symptoms of Parkinson's disease?

_____

_____

2. What happens to the brain cells in a patient with Alzheimer's disease?

_____

_____

3. Name four drug therapies used in the treatment of insomnia. List an example from each type of drug therapy.

_____

_____

_____

_____

RESEARCH ACTIVITIES

Follow the instructions given in each exercise and provide a response.

1. Access the website *http://en.wikipedia.org/wiki/caffeine* and answer the following questions:

   A. Where is caffeine found in nature?

   B. How does it affect the nervous system?

   C. What health conditions can caffeine possibly help prevent?

   D. Why does the FDA recognize caffeine as generally safe?

   E. Is caffeine safe to consume while pregnant? What limitations are recommended?

2. Access *http://www.alzfdn.org/AboutAlzheimers/treatment.html*. Find and list the latest drugs approved for the treatment of Alzheimer's disease.

CRITICAL THINKING

Reply to each question based on what you have learned in the chapter.

1. It is said that geniuses use approximately 10% of their brain capacity.

   A. About what percentage does the average person use?

   B. What activities can one do to create neuronal connections in the brain?

   C. What role does sleep play in the ability of your brain to function at full capacity?

   D. What is the meaning of the saying, "If you don't use it, you'll lose it?"

2. Many people experience a "rush of adrenaline" or a "natural high" from participating in dangerous sports. What does this mean, and what part of the nervous system is affected?

3. What is contributing to the rise in attention deficit disorder (ADD)/ADHD/OCD in children? Does it have anything to do with preservatives or hormones in food?

LAB SCENARIOS

Therapeutic Agents for the Nervous System

Objective: To review with the pharmacy technician terms associated with the nervous system and review the brand and generic names, indications, contraindications, adverse effects, dosage forms, routes of administration, and recommended daily dosage of medications used to treat disorders of the nervous system.

DID YOU KNOW?

- Epilepsy affects nearly 3 million Americans.
- About 10% of people will experience a seizure at some point during their lifetime.
- Each year 200,000 new cases of epilepsy are diagnosed.
- Epilepsy results in an estimated annual cost of $17.6 billion in medical costs and lost or reduced earnings and production.
- $42 billion a year are spent on anxiety disorders.
- 3.1% of adults are affected by generalized anxiety disorders.
- 1% of adults have OCD, with one third experiencing symptoms in childhood.
- 2.7% of adults suffer from panic disorder, 3.5% from PTSD, 6.8% from social anxiety disorder, and 6.7% from major depressive disorder.
- 5.9 million children 3 to 17 years of age are diagnosed with ADHD.

Lab Activity #15.1: Define the following terms associated with the nervous system.

Equipment needed:

- Medical dictionary
- Pencil/pen

Time needed to complete this activity: 30 minutes

1. Absence seizures _____

2. ADHD _____

3. Akinetic seizures _____

4. Alzheimer's disease _____

5. Anxiety disorder _____

6. Bipolar disorder _____

7. Convulsion _____

8. Dementia _____

9. Depression _____

10. Epilepsy _____

11. Generalized anxiety disorder _____

12. Insomnia _____

13. Mania _____

14. Migraine _____

15. Myoclonic seizures _____

16. OCD _____

17. Panic disorder _____

18. Parkinson's disease _____

19. Partial seizures _____

20. Petit mal seizures _____

21. Phobia _____

22. Polyneuropathy _____

23. Posttraumatic stress disorder (PTSD) _____

24. Psychosis _____

25. Schizophrenia _____

26. Social anxiety disorder _____

27. Status epilepticus _____

28. Tonic-clonic seizures _____

Lab Activity #15.2: Using a drug reference book, identify the generic name, drug classification, indications, contraindications, adverse effects, dosage forms, routes of administration, recommended daily dosage, and drug interactions of medications used to treat conditions affecting the nervous system.

Equipment needed:

■ *Drug Facts and Comparisons* or *Physicians' Desk Reference*
■ Pencil/pen

Time needed to complete this activity: 60 minutes

Brand (Trade) Name	Generic Name	Drug Classification	Indication	List Two Contraindications	List Five Adverse Effects	Dosage Forms Available	Routes of Administration	Recommended Daily Dosage		Drug Interactions	Pregnancy Category	Patient Information
								Adult	Pedi			
Abilify												
Adderall XR												
Ambien CR												
Aricept												
Ativan												
Avonex												
Azilect												
Benadryl												
BuSpar												
Celexa												
Clozaril												
Cogentin												
Concerta												
Copaxone												
Cymbalta												
Depakote												
Depakote ER												
Desyrel												
Dilantin												
Effexor XR												
Eskalith												
Exelon												
Focalin XR												
Gabitril												
Geodon												

Continued

Brand (Trade) Name	Generic Name	Drug Classification	Indication	List Two Contraindications	List Five Adverse Effects	Dosage Forms Available	Routes of Administration	Recommended Daily Dosage		Drug Interactions	Pregnancy Category	Patient Information
								Adult	Pedi			
Halcion												
Haldol												
Imitrex												
Imuran												
Keppra												
Klonopin												
Lamictal												
Lexapro												
Lunesta												
Maxalt												
Maxalt ML												
Mestinon												
Mirapex												
Namenda												
Neurontin												
Pamelor												
Paxil												
Prozac												
Razadyne												
Relpax												
Requip												
Restoril												
Risperdal												
Ritalin												
Seroquel												
Sinemet												
Sinequan												

Brand (Trade) Name	Generic Name	Drug Classification	Indication	List Two Contraindications	List Five Adverse Effects	Dosage Forms Available	Routes of Administration	Recommended Daily Dosage Adult	Pedi	Drug Interactions	Pregnancy Category	Patient Information
Sonata												
Strattera												
Symmetrel												
Tegretol												
Tofranil												
Topamax												
Trileptal												
Valium												
Vyvanse												
Wellbutrin XL												
Xanax												
Zelapar												
Zoloft												
Zomig												
Zonegran												
Zostrix												
Zyprexa												

Lab Activity #15.3: Using a drug reference book, identify MAOIs, food interactions with MAOIs, and auxiliary labels for MAOIs.

Equipment needed:

- *Drug Facts and Comparisons, Physicians' Desk Reference,* or Internet access
- Pencil/pen

Time needed to complete this activity: 30 minutes

1. List the brand and generic names of MAOIs that are used therapeutically.

   _____

   _____

   _____

2. What conditions are MAOIs used to treat?

   _____

   _____

   _____

3. What amino acid should be avoided while taking MAOIs?

   _____

4. Therefore what foods contain the amino acid and should be avoided?

   _____

   _____

   _____

5. What auxiliary labels should be placed on MAOI prescriptions?

   _____

   _____

   _____

6. What can happen if the amino acid is not avoided while taking an MAOI? List signs and symptoms that may indicate a high level of the amino acid.

   _____

   _____

   _____

Record-Keeping and Pharmacy Law for Therapeutic Agents for the Nervous System

Objective: To review with the pharmacy technician recordkeeping and the legal requirements of ordering and receiving Schedule II medications pertaining to drugs used to treat the nervous system.

Lab Activity #15.4: Using DEA Form 222, fill out the form and properly file in the pharmacy.

Equipment needed:

- Sample DEA Form 222
- *Red Book Online* or *the online FDA National Drug Code Directory*
- Blue or black pen

Time needed to complete this activity: 30 minutes

288

Procedure

1. Your pharmacist has asked you to create an order for CII medications. Using a blue or black pen, enter the name of the supplier; the supplier's street address, city, and state; and the date the DEA Form 222 is being filled out.
2. Enter the number of packages, the bottle size, and the name of the medication on the DEA Form 222.
   - 2 bottles of 100 capsules of Adderall XR 10 mg
   - 3 bottles of 100 tablets of Amphetamine salt combo 20 mg
   - 1 bottle of 100 tablets of Dexmethylphenidate HCl 5 mg
   - 3 bottles of 100 tablets of Methylphenidate HCl 20 mg
   - 2 bottles of 100 capsules of Vyvanse 20 mg
   - 2 bottles of 100 capsules of Vyvanse 40 mg
3. Using the *Red Book Online* or the online *FDA National Drug Code Directory,* find the NDC for the drugs being ordered and properly fill in the NDC number on the DEA Form 222.
4. Sign the document.

See Reverse of PURCHASER'S Copy for Instructions		No order form may be issued for Schedule I and II substances unless a completed application form has been received, (21 CFR 1305.04).		OMB APPROVAL No. 1117-0010
TO: *(Name of Supplier)*		STREET ADDRESS		
CITY and STATE		DATE	TO BE FILLED IN BY SUPPLIER	
			SUPPLIERS DEA REGISTRATION No.	

LINE No.	No. of Packages	Size of Package	TO BE FILLED IN BY PURCHASER — Name of Item	National Drug Code	Packages Shipped	Date Shipped
1						
2						
3						
4						
5						
6						
7						
8						
9						
10						

◄ LAST LINE COMPLETED *(MUST BE 10 OR LESS)*   SIGNATURE OF PURCHASER OR ATTORNEY OR AGENT

Date Issued	DEA Registration No.	Name and Address of Registrant
20010101	DEAREGNO	VOID VOID VOID
Schedules		VOID VOID VOID
XXXXXXXXXXXXX		VOID VOID VOID
Registered as a	No. of this Order Form	VOID VOID VOID
XXXXXXXXXXXXX	000000005	VOID VOID VOID

DEA Form -222
(Oct. 2004)

U.S. OFFICIAL ORDER FORMS - SCHEDULES I & II
DRUG ENFORCEMENT ADMINISTRATION
SUPPLIER'S Copy 1

107051797

The pharmacist approved and then sent the CII order. After the order arrived, the pharmacist verified the contents and quantities received and then asked you to properly file the paperwork.

A. What two pieces of paperwork should be filed?

_____

B. How long must these files be retained in your pharmacy?

_____

Lab Activity #15.5: Identify what is missing from the following prescriptions and the measures needed to correct the errors.

Equipment needed:

■ Pen

Time needed to complete this activity: 30 minutes

Rx 1:

Dr. Andre Sheen
1100 Brentwood Blvd, Suite M780
St. Louis, MO 63144
314-527-0000
DEA FS1234563

Michael Smith   January 15, 201X
2624 Main Blvd
St. Louis, MO 63144

DOB: 08/14/62

Rx: Depakote ER

                 ii qd po   Disp #60

Ref x 3   _Andre Sheen, MD_

Identify the missing information and how it can be corrected.

_____

_____

_____

Rx 2:

Dr. Andre Sheen
1100 Brentwood Blvd, Suite M780
St. Louis, MO 63144
314-527-0000

Michael Smith
2624 Main Blvd
St. Louis, MO 63144

DOB:

Rx: Desyrel 50 mg

            i qhs   Disp #30

Ref x 3   _Andre Sheen, MD_

Identify the missing information and how it can be corrected.

_____

_____

_____

Rx 3:

Dr. Andre Sheen
1100 Brentwood Blvd, Suite M780
St. Louis, MO 63144
314-527-0000
DEA FS1234563

2624 Main Blvd
St. Louis, MO 63144

DOB: 08/14/62

Rx: Namenda 10 mg
            i bid   Disp #62

Ref x 3   _Andre Sheen, MD_

Identify the missing information and how it can be corrected.

_____

_____

_____

Rx 4:

Dr. Andre Sheen
1100 Brentwood Blvd, Suite M780
St. Louis, MO 63144
314-527-0000

Michael Smith   January 15, 201X
2624 Main Blvd
St. Louis, MO 63144

DOB:

Rx: Restoril
             i 1° a hs x 10d   Disp #10

Ref x 0   _Andre Sheen, MD_

Identify the missing information and how it can be corrected.

_____

_____

_____

Rx 5:

Dr. Andre Sheen
1100 Brentwood Blvd, Suite M780
St. Louis, MO 63144
314-527-0000
DEA FS1234563

Michael Smith
2624 Main Blvd
St. Louis, MO 63144

DOB: 08/14/62

Rx: Wellbutrin SR

             i bid   Disp #60

Ref x 3   _Andre Sheen, MD_

Identify the missing information and how it can be corrected.

_____

_____

_____

Lab Activity #15.6: Fill out the perpetual inventory log for each of the prescriptions.

Equipment needed:

■ Blue or black pen

Time needed to complete this activity: 30 minutes

Prescription label 1:

Your Friendly Pharmacy
1234 Park Avenue
St. Louis, MO 63144
314-555-1000

Rx: 1001

Michael Smith   Date 01/15/1X
2624 Main Blvd
St. Louis, MO 63144   Dr. A. Sheen

DOB: 08/14/62

Concerta ER 36 mg Tablets
Take one tablet by mouth daily.   30 Tablets

Refills: 0   Manufacturer: McNeil

Fill out the perpetual inventory log for this prescription.

Drug: Concerta ER 36 mg	Manufacturer: McNeil
Dosage Form: Tablets	NDC: 50458-586-01

Date	Rx #	Patient Name	Quantity Dispensed	Balance on Hand	Initials	Verified
				200		

Prescription label 2:

```
                Your Friendly Pharmacy
                   1234 Park Avenue
                  St. Louis, MO 63144
                    314-555-1000

    Rx: 1002

    Michael Smith                          Date 01/15/1X
    2624 Main Blvd
    St. Louis, MO 63144                    Dr. A. Sheen

    DOB: 08/14/62

    Dextroamphetamine, Amphetamine
    (mixed salts) 10 mg Tablets

    Take one tablet by mouth twice daily.      60 Tablets

    Refills: 0                    Manufacturer: CorePharma
```

Fill out the perpetual inventory log for this prescription.

Drug: Dextroamphetamine, Amphetamine (mixed salts) 10 mg	Manufacturer: CorePharma
Dosage Form: Tablets	NDC: 64720-132-10

Date	Rx #	Patient Name	Quantity Dispensed	Balance on Hand	Initials	Verified
				420		

Prescription label 3:

```
                Your Friendly Pharmacy
                   1234 Park Avenue
                  St. Louis, MO 63144
                    314-555-1000

    Rx: 1003

    Michael Smith                          Date 01/15/1X
    2624 Main Blvd
    St. Louis, MO 63144                    Dr. A. Sheen

    DOB: 08/14/62

    Methylphenidate ER 20 mg Tablets

    Take one tablet by mouth twice daily.      60 Tablets


    Refills: 0          Manufacturer: MD Pharmaceuticals
```

Fill out the perpetual inventory log for this prescription.

Drug: Methylphenidate ER 20 mg	Manufacturer: MD Pharmaceuticals
Dosage Form: Tablets	NDC: 43567-562-07

Date	Rx #	Patient Name	Quantity Dispensed	Quantity Remaining	Initials	Verified
				440		

Prescription label 4:

Your Friendly Pharmacy
1234 Park Avenue
St. Louis, MO 63144
314-555-1000

Rx: 1004

Michael Smith   Date 01/15/1X
2624 Main Blvd
St. Louis, MO 63144   Dr. A. Sheen

DOB: 08/14/62

Adderall XR 30 mg Capsules

Take one capsule by mouth daily.   30 Capsules

Refills: 0   Manufacturer: Shire

Fill out the perpetual inventory log for this prescription.

Drug: Adderall XR 30 mg	Manufacturer: Shire
Dosage Form: Capsules	NDC: 54092-391-01

Date	Rx #	Patient Name	Quantity Dispensed	Quantity Remaining	Initials	Verified
				170		

Prescription label 5:

```
                    Your Friendly Pharmacy
                      1234 Park Avenue
                      St. Louis, MO 63144
                        314-555-1000

    Rx: 1005

    Michael Smith                        Date 01/15/1X
    2624 Main Blvd
    St. Louis, MO 63144                  Dr. A. Sheen

    DOB: 08/14/62

    Vyvanse 30 mg Capsules

    Take one capsule by mouth every morning.    30 Capsules


    Refills: 0                     Manufacturer: Shire
```

Fill out the perpetual inventory log for this prescription.

Drug: Vyvanse 30 mg	Manufacturer: Shire
Dosage Form: Capsule	NDC: 59417-0103-10

Date	Rx #	Patient Name	Quantity Dispensed	Quantity Remaining	Initials	Verified
				310		

16 Therapeutic Agents for the Endocrine System

TERMS AND DEFINITIONS

Select the correct term from the following list and write the corresponding letter in the blank next to the statement.

A. Addison's Disease
B. Cretinism
C. Cushing's Disease
D. Diabetes Mellitus
E. Exophthalmos
F. Glucose
G. Goiter
H. Graves' Disease
I. Hormones
J. Hypercalcemia
K. Hypocalcemia
L. Hyperglycemia
M. Hypoglycemia
N. Myxedema
O. Liothyronine
P. Levothyroxine

_____ 1. Condition in which the development of the brain and body is inhibited by a congenital lack of thyroid secretion

_____ 2. Prominence of the eyeball caused by increased thyroid hormone

_____ 3. Low glucose concentration in the bloodstream

_____ 4. An autoimmune disorder caused by hypersecretion of thyroid hormones with diffuse goiter, exophthalmos, and skin changes as symptoms

_____ 5. Increased calcium concentration in the blood

_____ 6. Chronic disease associated with hyperglycemia with two types, Type 1 and Type 2

_____ 7. Simple sugar

_____ 8. Condition resulting in a decrease in levels of adrenocortical hormones such as mineralocorticoids and glucocorticoids, which causes symptoms including muscle weakness and weight loss

_____ 9. Low concentration of calcium in the blood

_____ 10. Known as T_3; contains three ions of iodine

_____ 11. Elevated glucose concentration in the bloodstream

_____ 12. Condition caused by excessive secretion of adrenocorticotropic hormone (ACTH) from the anterior pituitary gland

_____ 13. Chemical substances produced and secreted by an endocrine duct into the bloodstream that results in a physiologic response at a specific target tissue

_____ 14. Condition associated with a decrease in overall thyroid function in adults; also known as hypothyroidism

_____ 15. Condition in which the thyroid is enlarged because of a lack of iodine

_____ 16. Known as T_4; contains four iodine ions

TRUE OR FALSE

Write T or F next to each statement.

_____ 1. The Greek word for hormone means "to excite."

_____ 2. Hormones control women and their moods only.

_____ 3. All hormones are composed of proteins.

_____ 4. Steroids enter and attach to receptor sites inside the cell.

297

_____ 5. Melatonin is a chemical substance that helps control the skin's ability to tan.

_____ 6. The pituitary gland is referred to as the *master gland*.

_____ 7. Calcium is the major mineral found in bones.

_____ 8. The pancreas is not the largest organ of the endocrine system.

_____ 9. Men stop producing sperm at some point during their midlife.

_____ 10. The most well-known condition that can affect the endocrine system is diabetes.

SYSTEM IDENTIFIER

Identify each organ in this system and enter the term next to the corresponding number.

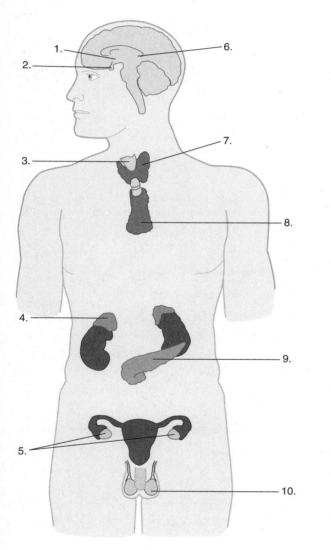

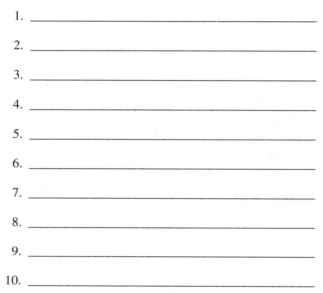

1. _____

2. _____

3. _____

4. _____

5. _____

6. _____

7. _____

8. _____

9. _____

10. _____

MULTIPLE CHOICE

Complete each question by circling the best answer.

1. PTU and methimazole are used for the treatment of:
   A. Diabetes
   B. Osteoporosis
   C. Hyperthyroidism
   D. Estrogen replacement

2. Doxercalciferol and Calcitriol are used for the treatment of:
   A. Diabetes
   B. Hyperparathyroidism
   C. Hyperthyroidism
   D. Estrogen replacement

3. The gland that secretes hormones that help the body keep calcium levels adequate is the:
   A. Thyroid
   B. Parathyroid
   C. Hypothalamus
   D. Pituitary

4. The largest endocrine gland is the _____, which produces insulin and glucagon.
   A. Thyroid
   B. Pituitary
   C. Thymus
   D. Pancreas

5. Which of the following is *not* a system that influences the endocrine system?
   A. Positive feedback
   B. Hormonal chemicals that participate in a chain reaction
   C. Negative feedback
   D. Nervous system

6. Which gland influences water balance, body temperature, appetite, and emotions?
   A. Pancreas
   B. Thymus
   C. Thyroid
   D. Hypothalamus

7. Which glands participate in the activities of the kidneys?
   A. Adrenals
   B. Ovaries
   C. Testes
   D. None of the above

8. Failure of the endocrine system to perform correctly affects what area of the body?
   A. Heart
   B. Kidney
   C. Brain
   D. All of the above

9. A goiter is an enlargement of the:
   A. Prostate gland
   B. Pituitary gland
   C. Thyroid gland
   D. Testes

10. A deficiency of growth hormone in children may result in hypoglycemia and short stature, resulting in:
    A. Diabetes insipidus
    B. Gigantism
    C. Hypopituitary dwarfism
    D. Acromegaly

11. Addison's disease is a rare hormonal disorder that is caused by a deficiency of:
    A. Cortisol
    B. ACTH
    C. Aldosterone
    D. PTH

12. The main categories of insulin used therapeutically include all of the following *except*:
    A. Rapid-acting
    B. Long-acting
    C. Diverse-acting
    D. Intermediate-acting

FILL IN THE BLANKS

Answer each question by completing the statement in the space provided.

1. The _____, _____, and _____ glands, located in the brain, play an important role in hormone production.

2. The _____ links the nervous system to the endocrine system.

3. _____ hormones act on the same cell from which they are secreted, and _____ hormones influence cells that are located farther away.

4. Hormones of the endocrine system are classified as _____, _____, and _____.

5. The _____ _____ is analogous to the control tower of the endocrine system.

6. The two hormones involved in the "fight or flight" response are _____ and _____.

7. The ovaries secrete the hormones _____ and _____, and the testes secrete _____.

8. The hormone _____ stimulates uterine contractions and cervical dilation during birth and lactation.

9. _____, _____, and _____ are three types of hormones produced by the adrenal cortex.

10. The cause of insulin-dependent diabetes mellitus is the inability of the _____ to synthesize and secrete _____.

MATCHING

Matching I

Match the drugs with their indications.

_____ 1. Synthroid

_____ 2. Glucophage

_____ 3. Florinef

_____ 4. Tapazole

_____ 5. Sensipar

A. Addison's disease
B. Hyperthyroidism
C. Thyroid replacement
D. Hypercalcemia
E. Type 2 Diabetes Mellitus

Matching II

Match the trade and generic drug names.

_____ 1. Glucotrol

_____ 2. Rocaltrol

_____ 3. Medrol

_____ 4. Sandostatin

_____ 5. Glucophage

A. Calcitriol
B. Octreotide
C. Metformin
D. Glipizide
E. Methylprednisolone

Matching III

Match the type of insulin with its main category.

_____ 1. Humulin 70/30

_____ 2. Humulin R

_____ 3. Lantus

_____ 4. Novlog

_____ 5. Humulin N

A. Rapid-Acting
B. Short-Acting
C. Intermediate-Acting
D. Long-Acting
E. Pre-Mixed

SHORT ANSWER

Reply to each question based on what you have learned in the chapter.

1. List the three hormones the thyroid gland produces that affect metabolism.

_____

_____

2. List the differences between the endocrine and exocrine glands.

_____

_____

3. List three functions hormones perform throughout the body and how they do it.

_____

_____

_____

_____

Chapter **16** **Therapeutic Agents for the Endocrine System**

4. List the three signaling pathways that influence the endocrine system and the production of hormones.

_____

_____

RESEARCH ACTIVITIES

Follow the instructions given in each exercise and provide a response.

1. Access the website *http://www.drugabuse.gov/publications/drugfacts/anabolic-steroids*. Find information on anabolic steroids that would enable you to answer the following questions:

   A. What are they?

   B. Who uses them and why?

   C. What are the side effects?

   D. In what controlled substance category are they included?

2. Access the website *http://www.ncbi.nlm.nih.gov/pmc/articles/PMC2769828/*. Read the article about Type III diabetes mellitus that would enable you to answer the following questions:

   A. What is Alzheimer's disease (AD)?

   B. What scientific findings lead researchers to link Alzheimer's disease to diabetes mellitus?

   C. How could medications currently used for diabetes mellitus be used to help prevent Alzheimer's disease in the future?

CRITICAL THINKING

Reply to each question based on what you have learned in the chapter.

1. Diabetes mellitus (type 2) has been prevalent in your family for the past few years. What lifestyle choices have you made that could contribute to being diagnosed with this disease? What lifestyle changes can you make to help avoid being diagnosed with this disease?

2. When a young person goes through the adolescence stage of development, the pituitary gland releases hormones that bring about many physical and emotional changes. How many hormones are released, and what parts of the body are affected? What emotional changes take place?

3. The hormone content of meat has been the subject of numerous discussions. Do hormones in meat really affect us physically? If so, how?

RELATE TO PRACTICE

LAB SCENARIOS

Therapeutic Agents for the Endocrine System

Objective: To review with the pharmacy technician the organs of the endocrine system. In addition, to review the brand and generic names, indications, contraindications, adverse effects, dosage forms, routes of administration, and daily dosing of medications used to treat disorders of the endocrine system.

DID YOU KNOW?

- 11.3% of adults 20 years and older suffer from diabetes.
- Approximately 79 million people 20 years of age and older have prediabetes.
- 7 million people suffer from undiagnosed diabetes.
- In 2012, the total cost of diagnosed diabetes was $245 billion.
- More than 70,000 people die each year as the result of diabetes and more than an additional 160,000 people have died from diabetes as a contributing factor.
- Diabetes is the 7th leading cause of death.

Lab Activity #16.1: Define the following terms associated with the endocrine system.

Equipment needed:

- Medical dictionary
- Pencil/pen

Time needed to complete this activity: 30 minutes

1. Diabetes mellitus

   _____

2. Peripheral neuropathy

   _____

3. Gestational diabetes

   _____

4. Graves' disease

   _____

5. Hashimoto's thyroiditis

   _____

6. Hyperglycemia

   _____

7. Hyperthyroidism

   _____

8. Hypoglycemia

   _____

9. Iypothalamus

_____

10. Hypothyroidism

_____

11. Insulin-dependent diabetes mellitus (IDDM)

_____

12. Insulin resistance

_____

13. Non–insulin-dependent diabetes mellitus (NIDDM)

_____

14. Pancreas

_____

15. Thyroid

_____

Lab Activity #16.2: Using a drug reference book, identify the generic name, drug classification, indications, contraindications, adverse effects, dosage forms and routes of administration, recommended daily dosage, and drug interactions of medications used to treat conditions affecting the endocrine system.

Equipment needed:

■ *Drug Facts and Comparisons* or *Physicians' Desk Reference*
■ Pencil/pen

Time needed to complete this activity: 60 minutes

Brand (Trade) Name	Generic Name	Drug Classification	Indication	List Two Contraindications	List Five Adverse Effects	Dosage Forms Available	Routes of Administration	Recommended Daily Dosage Adult	Recommended Daily Dosage Pedi	Drug Interactions	Pregnancy Category	Patient Information
Actoplus Met												
Actos												
Amaryl												
Apidra												
Byetta												
Cytomel												
Declomycin												
Deltasone												
Glucophage												
Glucotrol												
Glucovance												
Humalog												
Humalog Mix 75/25												
Humulin N												
Humulin R												
Humulin 70/30												
Janumet												
Januvia												

Brand (Trade) Name	Generic Name	Drug Classification	Indication	List Two Contraindications	List Five Adverse Effects	Dosage Forms Available	Routes of Administration	Recommended Daily Dosage		Drug Interactions	Pregnancy Category	Patient Information
								Adult	Pedi			
Lantus												
Levemir												
Levothyroid												
Levoxyl												
Micronase												
Novolog												
Novolog 70/30												
Prandin												
Precose												
Rocaltrol												
Starlix												
Sandostatin												
Symlin												
Synthroid												
Tapazole												

Lab Activity #16.3: Using a drug reference, identify the generic name, manufacturer, product size availability, NDC, AWP, and Orange Book code.

Equipment needed:

- Computer with Internet access
- *Red Book Online*
- Pencil/pen

Time needed to complete this activity: 60 minutes

Brand (Trade) Name	Generic Name	Manufacturer	Product Size Availability	NDC	AWP	Orange Book Code
Rapid-Acting Insulin Products						
Humalog						
Humalog KwikPen						
NovoLog						
NovoLog FlexPen						
Apidra						
Apidra SoloStar						
Short-Acting Insulin Products						
Humulin R						
Humulin R Pen						
Novolin R						
Intermediate-Acting Insulin Products						
Humulin N						
Novolin N						
Long-Acting Insulin Products						
Lantus						
Lantus SoloStar						
Levemir						
Levemir FlexPen						

You are to recommend one insulin product from each insulin category for the inpatient pharmacy. Using the information you gathered for the table on the previous page and information learned from previous chapters, answer the following questions to help you determine which product to recommend:

A. For each of the insulin categories, which product (vial or pen) would be most cost effective?

B. List advantages and disadvantages of using a community insulin vial for the inpatient floor.

C. List advantages and disadvantages of using a community insulin pen for the inpatient floor.

D. List advantages and disadvantages of using an insulin vial for each patient.

E. List advantages and disadvantages of using an insulin pen for each patient.

F. Considering the advantages and disadvantages listed, which would be safer to use (vial or pen) for the inpatient setting?

G. For each of the insulin categories, which product would you recommend the inpatient pharmacy to dispense?

Chapter **16 Therapeutic Agents for the Endocrine System**

Using Therapeutic Agents for the Endocrine System

Objective: To review with the pharmacy technician prescription orders, dosage calculations, and sterile product preparation.

Lab Activity #16.4: Answer the questions based on the prescription orders for each question.

Equipment needed:

■ *Drug Facts and Comparisons* or *Physician's Desk Reference*
■ Pencil/pen
■ Calculator

Time needed to complete this activity: 30 minutes

The following are approved DAW codes:

DAW 0: no product selection indicated
DAW 1: substitution not allowed by provider
DAW 2: substitution allowed: patient requested product dispensed
DAW 3: substitution allowed: pharmacist selected product dispensed
DAW 4: substitution allowed: generic drug not in stock
DAW 5: substitution allowed: brand drug dispensed as generic
DAW 6: override
DAW 7: substitution not allowed: brand drug mandated by law
DAW 8: substitution allowed: generic drug not available in marketplace
DAW 9: other

1. Rx 1:
   Humulin-R U-100 insulin, 2 vials
   40 units SC qam and 30 units ac evening meal
   Ref x 3

   A. How much will be dispensed (use metric quantities)? _____

   B. How many days will the medication last? _____

   C. How many refills are permitted on the prescription? _____

   D. What DAW code will be used? _____

   E. Write directions as they would appear on the medication label.

   _____

   _____

   F. What auxiliary label(s) should be affixed to the medication label?

   _____

   _____

   _____

2. Rx 2:
   Lantus insulin, 1 vial
   12 units SC before dinner
   Ref x 1

   A. How much will be dispensed (use metric quantities)? _____

   B. How many days will the medication last? _____

   C. How many refills are permitted on the prescription? _____

   D. What DAW code will be used? _____

E. Write directions as they would appear on the medication label.

_____

_____

F. What auxiliary label(s) should be affixed to the medication label?

_____

_____

_____

3. Rx 3:

Glucophage 500 mg tab, 30 day supply
1 g qam and qpm ac
Ref x 6

A. How much will be dispensed? _____

B. How many days will the medication last? _____

C. How many refills are permitted on the prescription? _____

D. What DAW code will be used? _____

E. Write directions as they would appear on the medication label.

_____

_____

F. What auxiliary label(s) should be affixed to the medication label?

_____

_____

_____

4. Rx 4:

Synthroid 0.1 mg, #30
100 mcg qam, no later than 10am
Ref x3
Brand Name Medically Necessary

A. How much will be dispensed? _____

B. How many days will the medication last? _____

C. How many refills are permitted on the prescription? _____

D. What DAW code will be used? _____

E. Write directions as they would appear on the medication label.

_____

_____

F. What auxiliary label(s) should be affixed to the medication label?

_____

_____

_____

5. Rx 5:

Prednisone 10 mg tablets
i qid × 2d; i tid × 2d; i bid × 2d; i qd × 2d; ss qd × 2d
Ref

A. How much will be dispensed? _____

B. How many days will the medication last? _____

C. How many refills are permitted on the prescription? _____

D. What DAW code will be used? _____

E. Write directions as they would appear on the medication label.

_____

_____

F. What auxiliary label(s) should be affixed to the medication label?

_____

_____

_____

Lab Activity #16.5: Calculate the quantity of the ingredients needed to prepare the following dilutions.

Equipment needed:

- Calculator
- Pencil/pen
- Paper

Time needed to complete this activity: 30 minutes

1. Dilution #1

   A. The pharmacy has in stock a 10 mL vial of Humulin R insulin with a concentration of 100 units/mL. How much of the 100 units/mL Humulin R insulin and how much diluent are needed to prepare 10 mL of a dilution with a concentration of 10 units/mL?

   Humulin R Insulin 100 units/mL: _____

   Diluent: _____

   B. Using the dilution made in part A, how much Humulin R insulin 10 units/mL and how much diluent are needed to prepare 30 mL of a second dilution with a concentration of 1unit/mL?

   Humulin R Insulin 10 units/mL: _____

   Diluent: _____

2. The pharmacy has in stock hydrocortisone 100 mg/2mL. How much of the hydrocortisone 100 mg/2mL and how much diluent are needed to prepare 8 mL of a 5 mg/mL hydrocortisone solution?

   Hydrocortisone 100 mg/2mL: _____

   Diluent: _____

Lab Activity #16.6: Using the calculations from Lab Activity 16.5, question 1, prepare a dilution of insulin using sterile compounding procedures.

Equipment needed:

- Alcohol swabs
- Diluent
- Laminar airflow hood
- Empty Sterile 10 mL vial
- Empty Sterile 30 mL vial
- PPEs
- Sharps container
- Humulin R Insulin 10 mL vial
- Sink with running hot and cold water
- Syringes with needles
- Vented needles
- Labels

Procedure

1. Gather all materials needed for activity.
2. Wash hands properly.
3. Don PPEs in the proper sequence.
4. Clean laminar flow workbench in the proper manner, using the correct supplies and techniques.
5. Collect the medication to be compounded.
6. Check expiration dates on both the vial and sterile vials.
7. Place ingredients in the laminar flow hood.
8. Swab the rubber top of the diluent and empty sterile vial with alcohol. Allow the alcohol to dry.
9. Make sure the needle is firmly attached to the syringe.
10. Prepare the syringe by adding the amount of air that will be equal to the amount of diluent to be withdrawn into the syringe.
11. Hold the syringe with the thumb and the index and middle fingers.
12. Remove cap from needle.
13. Insert the needle at a 45-degree angle into the rubber stopper of the vial with beveled part of the needle facing upward.
14. Hold the vial with the hand opposite the hand that is holding the syringe.
15. Invert the vial.
16. Push the plunger, forcing the air in the syringe into the vial, and release gently, allowing the fluid to be drawn into the syringe.
17. Tap the syringe to force air bubbles out of it.
18. Draw up the correct amount of diluent needed to dilute the insulin to correct concentration.
19. Pull back on the plunger to clear the neck of the syringe. Remove the needle, and replace with a vented needle.
20. Remove all excess air from syringe.
21. Insert vented needle of the syringe at a 45-degree angle into the rubber top of the empty sterile vial and transfer the diluent.
22. Swab the rubber top of the insulin vial and sterile vial (with diluent in it) with alcohol. Allow the alcohol to dry.
23. Make sure the needle is firmly attached to the syringe.
24. Prepare the syringe by adding the amount of air that will be equal to the amount of insulin to be withdrawn into the syringe.
25. Hold the syringe with the thumb and the index and middle fingers.
26. Remove cap from needle.
27. Insert the needle at a 45-degree angle into the rubber stopper of the vial with beveled part of the needle facing upward.
28. Hold the vial with the hand opposite the hand that is holding the syringe.
29. Invert the vial.
30. Push the plunger, forcing the air in the syringe into the vial, and release gently, allowing the fluid to be drawn into the syringe.
31. Tap the syringe to force air bubbles out of it.
32. Draw up the correct amount of insulin needed to dilute the insulin to correct concentration.
33. Pull back on the plunger to clear the neck of the syringe. Remove the needle, and replace with a vented needle.

34. Remove all excess air from syringe.
35. Insert vented needle of the syringe at a 45-degree angle into the rubber top of the sterile vial and transfer the insulin.
36. Gently swirl to mix.
37. Discard syringes into sharps container.
38. Properly label vial with correct concentration and expiration date.
39. Repeat steps 5 through 38 to perform the second dilution to 1 unit/mL.
40. Remove PPEs in the proper sequence, and discard.
41. Record initials, date, and time on the cleaning log.

Time needed to complete this activity: 45 minutes

Glucose Testing

Objective: To introduce glucose monitors and related supplies to the pharmacy technician and the procedure for testing blood glucose levels. To review and apply information learned about diabetes mellitus.

Lab Activity #16.7: Answer the following questions to predict a normal, high, or low blood glucose level.

Equipment needed:

- Pencil/pen
- Paper

Time needed to complete this activity: 15 minutes

1. At what time did you eat your last meal/snack? _____

2. Do you smoke? _____

3. Have you had coffee or other caffeine today? If so, at what time? _____

4. Do you have any medical conditions? _____

   A. If you have diabetes, what medications are you currently on and have you taken them today?

   B. If you have high blood pressure, what medications are you currently on and have you taken them today?

5. Are you currently taking any OTC or herbal products or prescription medications? If so, which ones?

   _____

   _____

   _____

6. Based on your answers from the previous questions and your knowledge of foods, medications, and health conditions that affect blood glucose, do you think your blood glucose level will be normal, high, or low if you checked it right now? Why?

   _____

   _____

   _____

Lab Activity #16.8: Using a glucose monitor, test your blood glucose level. Answer the questions based on the information given in Lab Activity #16.7 and your glucose reading.

Equipment needed:

- Glucose monitor
- Glucose strips
- Lancet device
- Lancets
- Alcohol swabs
- Gauze/cotton balls
- Bandage
- Sharps container
- Pencil/pen

Procedure

1. Clean workspace in proper manner, using correct supplies and techniques.
2. Gather all materials needed for activity.
3. Wash hands properly.
4. Assemble equipment.
5. Select puncture site.
6. Gently rub finger to promote circulation.
7. Clean site with alcohol swab and allow to dry.
8. Firmly grasp finger.
9. Hold lancet device at a 90-degree angle (perpendicular) to patient's finger and make a rapid, deep puncture on the fingertip.
10. Wipe away 1st drop of blood with a clean gauze/cotton ball.
11. Apply gentle pressure to cause blood to flow freely.
12. Collect sample.
13. Clean site with clean gauze/cotton ball.
14. Apply pressure with clean gauze/cotton ball.
15. Record reading.
16. Check for bleeding, then apply bandage.
17. Dispose of material in proper containers.
18. Clean work area.
19. Properly wash hands using correct procedures and techniques

Time needed to complete this activity: 30 minutes

Optimal Blood Glucose Level	Category
70-130 mg/dL	Fasting
Less than 180 mg/dL	1-2 hours after a meal

1. Glucose reading: _____ mg/dL

2. Is your blood glucose level within the optimal blood glucose guidelines?

   _____

3. What factors may have contributed to your blood glucose level?

   _____

   _____

   _____

4. Was your prediction from Lab Activity #16.7, question 6 correct? Why or why not?

_____

_____

_____

5. As a pharmacy technician, how could you help those with diabetes mellitus while working in a pharmacy?

_____

_____

_____

17 Therapeutic Agents for the Musculoskeletal System

TERMS AND DEFINITIONS

Select the correct term from the following list and write the corresponding letter in the blank next to the statement.

A. Analgesic
B. Antipyretic
C. Arthroplasty
D. Bone Fracture
E. Bone Marrow
F. Cancellous Bone
G. Compact Bone
H. Cyclooxygenase (COX)
I. Euphoria
J. Fascicles
K. Gout
L. Ligament
M. Motor Nerve
N. Muscle Fiber
O. Neuromuscular Junction
P. Opioid Analgesics
Q. Prostaglandin
R. Reye's Syndrome
S. Spongy Bone
T. Subchondral Bone
U. Synovium
V. Tendon
W. Uric Acid

_____ 1. Bone located below the cartilage, particularly within a joint

_____ 2. Fatty network of connective tissue that fills the cavities of bones

_____ 3. Junction between a nerve fiber and the muscle it supplies

_____ 4. Feeling or state of intense excitement and happiness

_____ 5. Disease characterized by defective metabolism of uric acid that leads to arthritis and acute pain

_____ 6. Thin membrane in synovial (freely moving) joints that lines the joint capsule and secretes synovial fluid

_____ 7. Water-insoluble end product of purine metabolism; deposition of it as crystals in the joints and kidneys causes gout

_____ 8. Drug that acts to relieve pain

_____ 9. Flexible but inelastic cord of strong fibrous collagen tissue attaching a muscle to a bone

_____ 10. Mediator responsible for inflammation features such as swelling, pain, stiffness, redness, and warmth

_____ 11. Either of two related enzymes that control the production of prostaglandins

_____ 12. Nerve carrying impulses from the brain or spinal cord to a muscle or gland

_____ 13. Surgical reconstruction or replacement of a joint

_____ 14. Meshwork of spongy bone typically found at the core of vertebral bones in the spine and the ends of long bones, also known as cancellous bone

_____ 15. Meshwork of spongy bone, also known as spongy bone, typically found at the core of vertebral bones in the spine and the ends of long bones

_____ 16. Break or rupture of a bone

_____ 17. Bundle of structures, such as muscle fibers

_____ 18. Drug used to prevent or reduce fever

_____ 19. Analgesic medication that activates opioid receptors

_____ 20. Fibrous connective tissue that connects to bones

_____ 21. Rigid bone, also known as cortical bone, constituting most of the skeleton

_____ 22. Muscle cell

_____ 23. Life-threatening metabolic disorder in young children of uncertain cause, but sometimes precipitated by aspirin use

TRUE OR FALSE

Write T or F next to each statement.

_____ 1. The bark from the willow tree is effective as a pain, fever, and inflammation reducer.

_____ 2. Opioid analgesics play an important role in helping the skeletal muscles relax.

_____ 3. Acetaminophen is not an antiinflammatory agent.

_____ 4. The first company to market aspirin was St. Joseph's.

_____ 5. Nonsteroidal antiinflammatory drugs (NSAIDs) all work the same; if one brand does not work, neither will another brand.

_____ 6. Steroids have an important role in the maintenance of the body system.

_____ 7. Osteoarthritis is the most common form of joint disease.

_____ 8. The prognosis of osteoporosis can be good when treated with dietary changes, exercise, and medication.

_____ 9. Weight loss, abstaining from alcohol, and adopting a low purine diet can be particularly beneficial for those with gout.

_____ 10. Individuals with liver disease may take 4000 mg of acetaminophen daily.

SYSTEM IDENTIFIER

Label the following parts of the structure of a typical bone and the internal structure of a long bone.

1. _____

2. _____

3. _____

4. _____

5. _____

6. _____

7. _____

8. _____

9. _____

10. _____

11. _____

12. _____

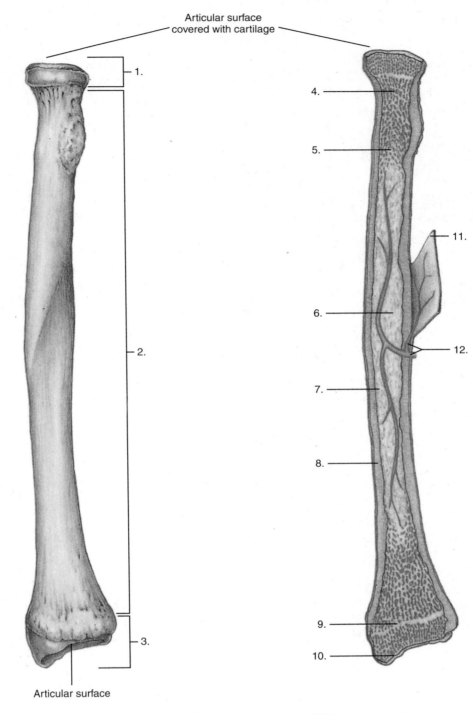

Articular surface
covered with cartilage

1.

2.

3.

Articular surface

4.

5.

11.

6.

12.

7.

8.

9.

10.

(A) The structure of a typical long bone.

(B) Internal structure of a long bone.

Label the following parts of the muscle.

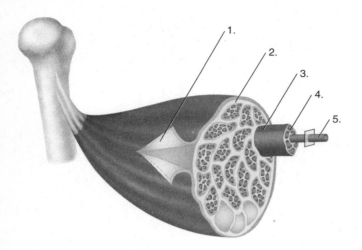

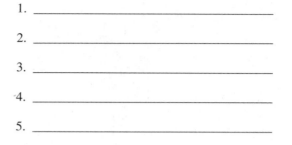

1. _____

2. _____

3. _____

4. _____

5. _____

MULTIPLE CHOICE

Complete each question by circling the best answer.

1. Aspirin is used to treat:
   A. Thromboembolism
   B. Inflammation
   C. Fever
   D. All of the above

2. Aspirin should not be given to children because its use in that age group has been linked to:
   A. Toxic shock syndrome
   B. Reye's syndrome
   C. Chickenpox
   D. Sudden infant death syndrome (SIDS)

3. Which of the following is true about NSAIDs?
   A. All NSAIDs are available in lesser strengths over the counter (OTC)
   B. They are highly addictive
   C. They reduce fever
   D. They increase inflammation

4. Relafen and Toradol are both:
   A. NSAIDs
   B. Corticosteroids
   C. Antihistamines
   D. Bronchodilators

5. Which of the following is *not* a potential side effect of corticosteroids?
   A. Inflammation
   B. Increased blood sugar
   C. High blood pressure
   D. Fluid retention

6. NSAIDs are used to treat many different types of conditions and chronic illnesses, including:
   A. Muscle pain
   B. Rheumatoid arthritis (RA)
   C. Joint pain such as in osteoarthritis
   D. All of the above

7. Which of the following can be used topically to help treat muscle strains and osteoarthritis?
   A. Benadryl
   B. Duragesic
   C. Tiger balm
   D. Motrin

8. The maximum daily dosage of acetaminophen is
   A. 4 mg
   B. 4 g
   C. 4000 g
   D. 40 g

9. The drug _____ is used only for treatment of osteoporosis.
   A. Miacalcin
   B. Evista
   C. Forteo
   D. Caltrate

10. Oral bisphosphonate medications should be taken:
    A. With milk
    B. With a meal
    C. On an empty stomach
    D. With orange juice

FILL IN THE BLANKS

Answer each question by completing the statement in the space provided.

1. Aspirin should be used cautiously in combination with _____ such as warfarin.

2. NSAIDs suppress inflammation by inhibiting the enzyme _____, which is responsible for prostaglandin synthesis.

3. _____ _____ can also be helpful in the management of osteoarthritis and muscle strains.

4. Analgesia with opioids is mediated through changes in the perception of _____ at the level of the spinal cord and CNS.

5. Opioid medications are _____ _____, with the schedule depending on the agent and formulation.

6. Fractures of the _____ and _____ _____ are associated with the most morbidity and mortality.

7. _____ helps to increase bone density.

8. _____ _____ _____ are often used for injuries of the musculoskeletal system and work by decreasing muscle tone.

9. _____ capsules and tablets vary enough to cause differences in efficacy and side effects if changing between dosage forms.

10. Neuromuscular blocking agents are used with _____ when a patient is undergoing surgery.

Chapter **17** **Therapeutic Agents for the Musculoskeletal System**

Write a short response to each question in the space provided.

1. Explain how the enzyme cyclooxygenase affects the body.

   _____

   _____

2. What is Reye's syndrome?

   _____

   _____

3. What three properties do aspirin and NSAIDs have?

   A. _____

   B. _____

   C. _____

4. What three problems can be caused by the overuse of NSAIDs?

   A. _____

   B. _____

   C. _____

5. What is the difference between a cyclooxygenase (COX)-1 inhibitor and a COX-2 inhibitor?

   _____

   _____

   _____

   _____

   _____.

MATCHING

Matching I

Match the following trade and generic drug names.

_____ 1. Motrin	A. Allopurinol	
_____ 2. Duragesic	B. Baclofen	
_____ 3. Ultram	C. Ibuprofen	
_____ 4. Naprosyn	D. Naproxen	
_____ 5. Fosamax	E. Fentanyl	
_____ 6. Zyloprim	F. Alendronate	
_____ 7. Flexeril	G. Methocarbamol	
_____ 8. Soma	H. Cyclobenzaprine	
_____ 9. Lioresal	I. Tramadol	
_____10. Robaxin	J. Carisoprodol	

Matching II

Match the drugs with their classifications.

_____ 1. Aspirin

_____ 2. Indocin

_____ 3. Celebrex

_____ 4. Percocet

_____ 5. Narcan

_____ 6. Actonel

_____ 7. Miacalcin

_____ 8. Zyloprim

_____ 9. Prolia

_____10. Forteo

A. Opioid antagonist
B. Calcitonin hormone analogue
C. Monoclonal antibody
D. NSAID
E. Opioid analgesic
F. Bisphosphonate
G. Salicylate
H. Xanthine oxidase
I. Cox-2 inhibitor
J. Parathyroid hormone analogue

RESEARCH ACTIVITIES

Follow the instructions given in each exercise and provide a response.

1. Access the website *http://www.fda.gov/Drugs/DrugSafety/ucm310469.htm.*

   A. What is the maximum daily dosage for acetaminophen?

   B. What are the potential effects if more than the maximum daily dosage is taken over an extended period of time?

   C. What is the recommended labeling verbiage on acetaminophen-containing products to warn consumers of this dangerous effect?

2. Access the website *http://pubs.niaaa.nih.gov/publications/Medicine/medicine.htm.*

   A. List the medications used for the musculoskeletal system that interact with alcohol.

   B. For each of the medications listed, what is the possible reaction when taken with alcohol?

CRITICAL THINKING

Reply to each question based on what you have learned in the chapter.

1. TV advertisements sometimes can be deceiving. Picture this: A man is rowing a boat across a lake, and his arms become sore. He comes over to the dock, where his friend awaits him. The rower complains about his arms, and the friend recommends Tylenol for his sore muscles. What is wrong with this picture?

2. Osteoporosis occurs most commonly in postmenopausal women. What change occurred to help cause this? What can women do to help prevent this?

RELATE TO PRACTICE

LAB SCENARIOS

Therapeutic Agents for the Skeletal System

Objective: To review with the pharmacy technician terms associated with the musculoskeletal system and review the brand and generic names, indications, contraindications, adverse effects, dosage forms, routes of administration, and recommended daily dosage of medications used to treat disorders of the musculoskeletal system.

DID YOU KNOW?

- 2% of men (0.8 million) greater than 50 years of age have osteoporosis of the hip.
- 10% of women (4.5 million) greater than 50 years of age have osteoporosis of the hip.
- Arthritis affects approximately 50 million adults.
- Osteoarthritis is the most common form of arthritis.
- 13.9% of adults aged 25 and older and 33.6% of those greater than 65 years of age have osteoarthritis.
- 55% of all arthritis-related hospitalizations were due to osteoarthritis.

Lab Activity #17.1: Define the following terms associated with the musculoskeletal system.

Equipment needed:

- Medical dictionary
- Pencil/pen

Time needed to complete this activity: 30 minutes

1. Amyotrophic lateral sclerosis (ALS) _____

2. Cerebral palsy _____

3. Gout _____

4. Hyperuricemia _____

5. Multiple sclerosis _____

6. Muscle strain _____

7. Myasthenia gravis _____

8. Myoglobin _____

9. Myositis _____

10. Osteoarthritis _____

11. Osteoblasts _____

12. Osteoclasts _____

13. Osteopenia _____

14. Osteoporosis _____

15. Paget's disease _____

16. Paralysis _____

17. Rhabdomyolysis _____

18. Rheumatoid arthritis _____

19. Spasticity _____

20. Systemic lupus erythematosus _____

21. Trigeminal neuralgia _____

Lab Activity #17.2: Using a drug reference book, identify the generic name, drug classification, indications, contraindications, adverse effects, dosage forms, routes of administration, and recommended daily dosage of medications used to treat conditions affecting the musculoskeletal system.

Equipment needed:

- *Drug Facts & Comparisons* or *Physicians' Desk Reference*
- Pencil/pen

Time needed to complete this activity: 60 minutes

Brand (Trade) Name	Generic Name	Drug Classification	Indication	List Two Contraindications	List Five Adverse Effects	Dosage Forms Available	Routes of Administration	Recommended Daily Dosage — Adult	Recommended Daily Dosage — Pedi	Drug Interactions	Pregnancy Category	Patient Information
Actonel												
Aleve												
Anectine												
Benuryl												
Boniva												
Celebrex												
Colcrys												
Demerol												
Didronel												
Dilaudid												
Duragesic												
Ecotrin												
Evista												
Flexeril												
Fosamax												
Indocin												
Lodine												
Lioresal												
Lortab												

Brand (Trade) Name	Generic Name	Drug Classification	Indication	List Two Contraindications	List Five Adverse Effects	Dosage Forms Available	Routes of Administration	Recommended Daily Dosage		Drug Interactions	Pregnancy Category	Patient Information
								Adult	Pedi			
Miacalcin												
Mobic												
Motrin												
MS Contin												
Naprosyn												
Narcan												
Norco												
Norcuron												
OxyContin												
Pavulon												
Percocet												
Robaxin												
Roxicodone												
Skelaxin												
Soma												
Tylenol												
Ultram												
Vicodin												
Voltaren												
Zanaflex												
Zemuron												
Zyloprim												

327

Lab Activity #17.3: Using a drug reference book, identify the generic name, storage requirements, and expiration date (at room temperature) for neuromuscular blocking agents.

Equipment needed:

- *Handbook on Injectable Drugs*
- Pencil/pen

Time needed to complete this activity: 30 minutes

Brand Name	Generic Name	Storage Requirements	Expiration Date
Anectine			
Nimbex			
Norcuron			
Zemuron			
Tracrium			
Pavulon			

Using Therapeutic Agents for the Musculoskeletal System

Objective: To review with the pharmacy technician prescription orders and dosage calculations.

Lab Activity #17.4: Answer the questions based on the prescription orders for each question.

Equipment needed:

- *Drug Facts and Comparisons* or *Physicians' Desk Reference*
- Pencil/pen
- Calculator

Time needed to complete this activity: 30 minutes

The following are approved DAW codes:

DAW 0: no product selection indicated
DAW 1: substitution not allowed by provider
DAW 2: substitution allowed: patient requested product dispensed
DAW 3: substitution allowed: pharmacist selected product dispensed
DAW 4: substitution allowed: generic drug not in stock
DAW 5: substitution allowed: brand drug dispensed as generic
DAW 6: override
DAW 7: substitution not allowed: brand drug mandated by law
DAW 8: substitution allowed: generic drug not available in marketplace
DAW 9: other

1. Rx 1:
   Mobic 7.5 mg #30
   i tab po qd
   Ref

   A. How much will be dispensed? _____

   B. How many days will the medication last? _____

   C. How many refills are permitted on the prescription? _____

   D. What DAW code will be used? _____

   E. Write directions as they would appear on the medication label.

   _____

   _____

F. What auxiliary label(s) should be affixed to the medication label?

_____

_____

_____

2. Rx 2:
   Zanaflex 4 mg #21
   i tab po q8h
   Ref

   A. How much will be dispensed? _____

   B. How many days will the medication last? _____

   C. How many refills are permitted on the prescription? _____

   D. What DAW code will be used? _____

   E. Write directions as they would appear on the medication label.

   _____

   _____

   F. What auxiliary label(s) should be affixed to the medication label?

   _____

   _____

   _____

3. Rx 3:
   Actonel 35 mg #4
   i tab po weekly
   Ref

   A. How much will be dispensed? _____

   B. How many days will the medication last? _____

   C. How many refills are permitted on the prescription? _____

   D. What DAW code will be used? _____

   E. Write directions as they would appear on the medication label.

   _____

   _____

   F. What auxiliary label(s) should be affixed to the medication label?

   _____

   _____

   _____

4. Rx 4:

Skelaxin 800 mg #42

i tab po q8h

Ref

Brand Name Medically Necessary

A. How much will be dispensed? _____

B. How many days will the medication last? _____

C. How many refills are permitted on the prescription? _____

D. What DAW code will be used? _____

E. Write directions as they would appear on the medication label.

_____

_____

F. What auxiliary label(s) should be affixed to the medication label?

_____

_____

_____

5. Rx 5:

Flexeril 10 mg

i tab po tid x2 weeks

Ref

A. How much will be dispensed? _____

B. How many days will the medication last? _____

C. How many refills are permitted on the prescription? _____

D. What DAW code will be used? _____

E. Write directions as they would appear on the medication label.

_____

_____

F. What auxiliary label(s) should be affixed to the medication label?

_____

_____

_____

6. Rx 6:

Soma 350 mg

i tab po tid and hs x1 week

Ref

A. How much will be dispensed? _____

B. How many days will the medication last? _____

C. How many refills are permitted on the prescription? _____

D. What DAW code will be used? _____

E. Write directions as they would appear on the medication label.

_____

_____

F. What auxiliary label(s) should be affixed to the medication label?

_____

_____

_____

7. Rx 7:

Robaxin 500 mg #56
ii tab po qid
Ref

A. How much will be dispensed? _____

B. How many days will the medication last? _____

C. How many refills are permitted on the prescription? _____

D. What DAW code will be used? _____

E. Write directions as they would appear on the medication label.

_____

_____

F. What auxiliary label(s) should be affixed to the medication label?

_____

_____

_____

8. Rx 8:

Motrin 600 mg #15
i tab po tid
Ref

A. How much will be dispensed? _____

B. How many days will the medication last? _____

C. How many refills are permitted on the prescription? _____

D. What DAW code will be used? _____

E. Write directions as they would appear on the medication label.

_____

_____

F. What auxiliary label(s) should be affixed to the medication label?

_____

_____

_____

Chapter **17 Therapeutic Agents for the Musculoskeletal System**

9. Rx 9:

Naprosyn 500 mg #90

i tab po tid

Ref x 5

   A. How much will be dispensed? _____

   B. How many days will the medication last? _____

   C. How many refills are permitted on the prescription? _____

   D. What DAW code will be used? _____

   E. Write directions as they would appear on the medication label.

   _____

   _____

   F. What auxiliary label(s) should be affixed to the medication label?

   _____

   _____

   _____

10. Rx 10:

Fosamax #4

i tab po weekly

Ref x6

   A. How much will be dispensed? _____

   B. How many days will the medication last? _____

   C. How many refills are permitted on the prescription? _____

   D. What DAW code will be used? _____

   E. Write directions as they would appear on the medication label.

   _____

   _____

   F. What auxiliary label(s) should be affixed to the medication label?

   _____

   _____

   _____

18 Therapeutic Agents for the Cardiovascular System

TERMS AND DEFINITIONS

Select the correct term from the following list and write the corresponding letter in the blank next to the statement.

A. Vena Cava
B. Artery
C. Capillary
D. Coagulation
E. Diuretic
F. Endocardium
G. Enzyme
H. Thrombin
I. Thrombolytic
J. Vein
K. Syndrome
L. Pericardium
M. Embolus
N. Epicardium
O. Myocardium

_____ 1. Medication used to break up a thrombus or blood clot

_____ 2. A vessel that carries oxygenated blood from the heart to the tissues of the body

_____ 3. Thin membrane that lines the interior of the heart

_____ 4. An agent that increases urine output and excretion of water from the body

_____ 5. A vessel that carries deoxygenated blood to the heart

_____ 6. To solidify or change from a fluid state to a solid state as in forming a blood clot

_____ 7. Protein that speeds up a reaction by reducing the amount of energy required to initiate a reaction

_____ 8. Large veins that bring deoxygenated blood from the upper and lower part of the body to the right atrium of the heart

_____ 9. An enzyme formed in coagulating blood that forms blood clots

_____ 10. Extremely small vessel that connects the ends of the smallest arteries to the smallest veins; where the exchange of nutrients and waste, oxygen, and carbon dioxide occurs

_____ 11. Set of conditions that occur together

_____ 12. Muscle tissue layer of the heart

_____ 13. A clump of material, often a blood clot, that travels from one part of the body to another ending up obstructing a blood vessel

_____ 14. Fluid-filled membrane that surrounds the heart

_____ 15. Inner layer of the pericardium

TRUE OR FALSE

Write T or F next to each statement.

_____ 1. A normal heart beats 160 to 200 times per minute.

_____ 2. The right atrium receives oxygenated blood from the lungs and pumps it out to the body.

_____ 3. The cardiac conduction system provides the electrical charge that makes the heart pump.

_____ 4. Most of the body's blood supply is cycled through the heart in 1 minute.

_____ 5. Heart failure (HF) is a condition in which the heart cannot pump as vigorously as necessary to deliver blood throughout the body.

_____ 6. The good cholesterol is known as *LDL*.

_____ 7. High blood pressure is also known as the "silent killer" because it has no obvious signs.

_____ 8. Sublingual nitroglycerin must be kept in a dry area and in the original light-protected glass container.

_____ 9. A person suffering from hypotension has high blood pressure.

_____ 10. Diet and exercise can lower lipid content.

SYSTEM IDENTIFIER

Identify each component in the heart system and enter the term next to the corresponding number.

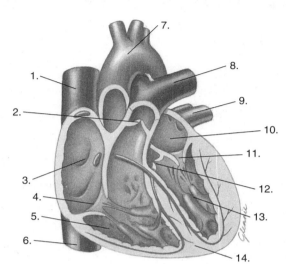

1. _____

2. _____

3. _____

4. _____

5. _____

6. _____

7. _____

8. _____

9. _____

10. _____

11. _____

12. _____

13. _____

14. _____

MULTIPLE CHOICE

Complete each question by circling the best answer.

1. Tenormin, Inderal, and Lopressor are all classified as:
   A. Angiotensin-converting enzyme (ACE) inhibitors
   B. Beta blockers
   C. Calcium channel blockers
   D. Diuretics

2. Which of the following is *not* a main layer of the heart?
   A. Endocardium
   B. Myocardium
   C. Subcardium
   D. Epicardium

3. Pain and pressure in the chest caused by a lack of blood flow and oxygenation of the heart muscle are primary features of:
   A. Angina pectoris
   B. Arrhythmia
   C. Hyperlipidemia
   D. High blood pressure

4. Which of the following is *not* a greater risk factor for hypertension?
   A. Age
   B. Gender
   C. Race
   D. None of the above

5. Rapid heart rate, usually greater than 100 beats per minute is:
   A. Tachycardia
   B. Bradycardia
   C. Hypertension
   D. Hypotension

6. Gemfibrozil, simvastatin, and ezetimibe are classified as:
   A. Antihypertensives
   B. Antiarrhythmics
   C. Anticoagulants
   D. Antihyperlipidemics

7. A dry, hacking cough that does not resolve over time is a side effect of:
   A. Calcium channel blockers
   B. ARBs
   C. ACE inhibitors
   D. Beta-blockers

8. An antidote for an overdose of Lanoxin is:
   A. Digoxin
   B. Digibind
   C. Digitalis
   D. Digitonin

9. In addition to treating hypertension, _____ can be is used for migraine prophylaxis and treatment of some tremors.
   A. Amlodipine
   B. Midodrine
   C. Propranolol
   D. Cholestyramine

10. Nitrostat tablets should be administered by which route?
    A. PO
    B. SL
    C. SubQ
    D. PR

FILL IN THE BLANKS

Answer each question by completing the statement in the space provided.

1. The main arteries that supply blood to the heart muscle are called _____ _____.

2. _____ is a syndrome that affects arterial blood vessels.

3. A thrombus in the heart can cause a _____ _____.

4. Cholesterol is important for the making of _____ _____ and _____

_____.

5. When niacin is used at therapeutic doses it can cause the characteristic _____ _____, which can result in headaches, pain, and pruritus in some people.

6. A category of drugs available over the counter (OTC) that can increase blood pressure are the _____.

7. Nitrates are used in the treatment of _____.

8. If plaque increases to form a blood clot, a _____ is created. This eventually may close off the vessel, causing a _____.

9. _____ and/or _____ are two side effects of hypotension.

10. _____ is a B vitamin that can help lower cholesterol.

MATCHING

Match the classes of drugs.

_____ 1. Antihyperlipidemics

_____ 2. Arrhythmic agents

_____ 3. Antiplatelet agents

_____ 4. Antihypertensives

_____ 5. Anticoagulants

A. Quinidine, procainamide, amiodarone
B. Heparin, warfarin
C. ACE inhibitors, beta blockers, calcium channel blockers
D. Bile acid sequestrants, HMG-CoA reductase inhibitors
E. Clopidogrel, aspirin

DRUG NAMES

Give the generic names for the following drugs.

1. Mevacor _____

2. Norpace _____

3. Lanoxin _____

4. Dyrenium _____

5. Lotensin _____

6. Hytrin _____

7. Quinidex _____

8. Zestril _____

9. Cozaar _____

10. Cardizem _____

SHORT ANSWER

Reply to each question in the space provided.

1. What are four common classifications of agents used to treat heart conditions?

   _____

   _____

2. Which antihyperlipidemic drug is also used to treat type 2 diabetes?

   _____

3. How do angiotensin receptor blockers (ARBs) work?

   _____

   _____

   _____

4. How do ACE inhibitors help reduce blood pressure?

   _____

   _____

   _____

5. How do calcium channel blockers (CCBs) work?

   _____

   _____

   _____

RESEARCH ACTIVITIES

Follow the instructions given in each exercise and provide a response.

1. Access the website *www.americanheart.org*. What is tPA? How does this drug help stroke victims recover?

2. Access the website *http://jama.jamanetwork.com/article.aspx?articleid=*1791497. From the article, what are the recommendations for the management of hypertension? What evidence led researchers to these recommendations?

CRITICAL THINKING

Reply to each question based on what you have learned in the chapter.

1. "An aspirin a day keeps a heart attack away." What are some everyday activities people can do to "keep a heart attack away?"

2. You have just finished your lunch, which consisted of a double cheeseburger, extra large fries, and a cola. Name all the body systems that will be affected by that "yummy" meal.

3. "I feel like I'm having a heart attack," someone says to you. How do you know for sure? What symptoms do you look for?

RELATE TO PRACTICE

LAB SCENARIOS

Therapeutic Agents for the Cardiovascular System

Objective: To review with the pharmacy technician terms associated with the cardiovascular system and review the brand and generic names, indications, contraindications, adverse effects, dosage forms, routes of administration, and recommended daily dosage of medications used to treat disorders of the cardiovascular system.

DID YOU KNOW?

- In 2010, 787,650 people died of cardiovascular disease, which was 31.9% of all deaths.
- Heart disease is the leading cause of death for both men and women.
- Coronary heart disease is the most common type of heart disease and caused 379,559 deaths in 2010.
- In 2010, the United States spent $315.4 billion on heart disease. This total includes the cost of health care services, medications, and lost productivity.
- 44% of African Americans have hypertension, the highest prevalence in the world.
- 33% of all adults age 20 and older are diagnosed with hypertension.
- 31.9 million adults age 20 years and older suffer from high serum cholesterol ($\geq$240 mg/dL).
- In 2010, on average, someone had a stroke every 40 seconds and every 4 minutes someone died from a stroke.

Lab Activity #18.1: Define the following terms associated with the cardiovascular system.

Equipment needed:

- Medical dictionary
- Pencil/pen

Time needed to complete this activity: 45 minutes

1. Aneurysm _____

2. Angina _____

338

3. Anoxia _____

4. Aorta _____

5. Arrhythmia _____

6. Arteriosclerosis _____

7. Atherosclerosis _____

8. Atrial fibrillation _____

9. Atrial flutter _____

10. Bradycardia _____

11. Cardiomyopathy _____

12. Deep vein thrombosis (DVT) _____

13. Diastolic blood pressure _____

14. Embolic stroke _____

15. Endocarditis _____

16. Heart failure (HF) _____

17. Hemorrhagic stroke _____

18. Hyperkalemia _____

19. Hyperlipidemia _____

20. Hypernatremia _____

21. Hypertension _____

22. Hypokalemia _____

23. Hyponatremia _____

24. Hypotension _____

25. Hypoxia _____

26. Infarction _____

27. Ischemia _____

28. Mitral valve prolapse _____

29. Mitral valve stenosis _____

30. Myocardial infarction (MI) _____

Chapter **18** **Therapeutic Agents for the Cardiovascular System**

31. Orthostatic hypotension _____

32. Peripheral vascular disease _____

33. Phlebitis _____

34. Plaque _____

35. Prehypertension _____

36. Raynaud's disease _____

37. Rheumatic heart disease _____

38. Stable angina _____

39. Stroke _____

40. Supraventricular tachycardia _____

41. Systolic blood pressure _____

42. Tachycardia _____

43. Thrombophlebitis _____

44. Thrombosis _____

45. Thrombotic stroke _____

46. Thrombus _____

47. Transient ischemic attack (TIA) _____

48. Unstable angina _____

49. Variant _____

50. Ventricular fibrillation _____

51. Ventricular tachycardia _____

Lab Activity #18.2: Using a drug reference book, identify the generic name, drug classification, indications, contraindications, adverse effects, dosage forms, routes of administration, and recommended daily dosage of medications used to treat conditions affecting the cardiovascular system.

Equipment needed:

- *Drug Facts & Comparisons* or *Physicians' Desk Reference*
- Pencil/pen

Time needed to complete the exercise: 60 minutes

Brand (Trade) Name	Generic Name	Drug Classification	Indication	List Two Contraindications	List Five Adverse Effects	Dosage Forms Available	Routes of Administration	Recommended Daily Dosage Adult	Recommended Daily Dosage Pedi	Drug Interactions	Pregnancy Category	Patient Information
Aggrenox												
Aldactone												
Altace												
Atacand												
Avapro												
Benicar												
Benicar HCT												
Bumex												
Bystolic												
Caduet												
Calan												
Cardizem												
Cardura												
Catapres-TTS												
Cordarone												
Coreg CR												
Coumadin												
Covera												
Cozaar												
Crestor												
Diovan												
Diovan HCT												
Dyazide												
Hytrin												
Hyzaar												

Continued

Chapter **18 Therapeutic Agents for the Cardiovascular System**

Brand (Trade) Name	Generic Name	Drug Classification	Indication	List Two Contraindications	List Five Adverse Effects	Dosage Forms Available	Routes of Administration	Recommended Daily Dosage Adult	Recommended Daily Dosage Pedi	Drug Interactions	Pregnancy Category	Patient Information
Imdur												
Inderal												
Isoptin SR												
Isordil												
Jantoven												
Klor-Con												
Lanoxin												
Lasix												
Lipitor												
Lovenox												
Lozol												
Maxzide												
Mevacor												
Micardis												
Micardis HCT												
Niaspan												

Brand (Trade) Name	Generic Name	Drug Classification	Indication	List Two Contraindications	List Five Adverse Effects	Dosage Forms Available	Routes of Administration	Recommended Daily Dosage		Drug Interactions	Pregnancy Category	Patient Information
								Adult	Pedi			
Nitrostat												
Norpace												
Norvasc												
Plavix												
Prinivil												
Procardia												
Sectral												
Tambocor												
Tenormin												
Toprol XL												
TriCor												
Trilipix												
Vasotec												
Vytorin												
WelChol												
Zestril												
Zetia												
Zocor												

Lab Activity #18.3: Using information learned and resources available, identify OTC products that can affect blood pressure and products available for those with hypertension.

Equipment needed:

- *Drug Facts & Comparisons* or *Pocket Guide for Nonprescription Product Therapeutics*
- Pencil/pen

Time needed to complete the exercise: 45 minutes

1. Which OTC products can affect blood pressure?

2. As a pharmacy technician, how can you help those with hypertension ensure they do not take OTC products that can affect blood pressure?

3. List available decongestant OTC products available specifically for those with hypertension.

Using Therapeutic Agents for the Cardiovascular System
Objective: To review with the pharmacy technician prescription orders and dosage calculations.
Lab Activity #18.4: Answer the questions based on the prescription orders for each questions.

Equipment needed:

- Calculator
- *Drug Facts and Comparisons* or *Physicians' Desk Reference*
- Pencil/pen

Time needed to complete this activity: 30 minutes

The following are approved DAW codes:

DAW 0: no product selection indicated
DAW 1: substitution not allowed by provider
DAW 2: substitution allowed: patient requested product dispensed
DAW 3: substitution allowed: pharmacist selected product dispensed
DAW 4: substitution allowed: generic drug not in stock
DAW 5: substitution allowed: brand drug dispensed as generic
DAW 6: override
DAW 7: substitution not allowed: brand drug mandated by law
DAW 8: substitution allowed: generic drug not available in marketplace
DAW 9: other

1. Rx 1:
   Crestor 20 mg #30
   i tab po qd
   Ref x5

   A. How much will be dispensed? _____

   B. How many days will the medication last? _____

   C. How many refills are permitted on the prescription? _____

D. What DAW code will be used? _____

E. Write directions, as they would appear on the medication label.

_____

_____

F. What auxiliary label(s) should be affixed to the medication label?

_____

_____

_____

2. Rx 2:

   Mevacor 40 mg #30
   i tab po qpm
   Ref x3

   A. How much will be dispensed? _____

   B. How many days will the medication last? _____

   C. How many refills are permitted on the prescription? _____

   D. What DAW code will be used? _____

   E. Write directions as they would appear on the medication label.

   _____

   _____

   F. What auxiliary label(s) should be affixed to the medication label?

   _____

   _____

   _____

3. Rx 3:

   Coreg 25 mg #60
   i tab po bid
   Ref x2

   A. How much will be dispensed? _____

   B. How many days will the medication last? _____

   C. How many refills are permitted on the prescription? _____

   D. What DAW code will be used? _____

   E. Write directions as they would appear on the medication label.

   _____

   _____

   F. What auxiliary label(s) should be affixed to the medication label?

   _____

   _____

   _____

Chapter **18** **Therapeutic Agents for the Cardiovascular System**

4. Rx 4:

   Zocor 40 mg #31

   i tab po qpm

   Ref x5

   Brand Name Medically Necessary

   A. How much will be dispensed? _____

   B. How many days will the medication last? _____

   C. How many refills are permitted on the prescription? _____

   D. What DAW code will be used? _____

   E. Write directions as they would appear on the medication label.

   _____

   _____

   F. What auxiliary label(s) should be affixed to the medication label?

   _____

   _____

   _____

5. Rx 5:

   Trilipix 45 mg #30

   i tab po qd

   Ref x5

   A. How much will be dispensed? _____

   B. How many days will the medication last? _____

   C. How many refills are permitted on the prescription? _____

   D. What DAW code will be used? _____

   E. Write directions as they would appear on the medication label.

   _____

   _____

   F. What auxiliary label(s) should be affixed to the medication label?

   _____

   _____

   _____

6. Rx 6:

   Lopressor 100 mg #30

   i tab po qd

   Ref x5

   A. How much will be dispensed?_____

   B. How many days will the medication last? _____

   C. How many refills are permitted on the prescription? _____

   D. What DAW code will be used? _____

E. Write directions as they would appear on the medication label.

_____

_____

F. What auxiliary label(s) should be affixed to the medication label?

_____

_____

_____

7. Rx 7:

Diovan 80 mg #31
i tab po daily
Ref x3

A. How much will be dispensed? _____

B. How many days will the medication last? _____

C. How many refills are permitted on the prescription? _____

D. What DAW code will be used? _____

E. Write directions as they would appear on the medication label.

_____

_____

F. What auxiliary label(s) should be affixed to the medication label?

_____

_____

_____

8. Rx 8:

Zestril 2.5 mg #32
i tab po qd
Ref x5

A. How much will be dispensed? _____

B. How many days will the medication last? _____

C. How many refills are permitted on the prescription? _____

D. What DAW code will be used? _____

E. Write directions as they would appear on the medication label.

_____

_____

F. What auxiliary label(s) should be affixed to the medication label?

_____

_____

_____

9. Rx 9:

Bystolic 20 mg #31

i tab po daily

Ref x2

A. How much will be dispensed?_____

B. How many days will the medication last? _____

C. How many refills are permitted on the prescription? _____

D. What DAW code will be used? _____

E. Write directions as they would appear on the medication label.

_____

_____

F. What auxiliary label(s) should be affixed to the medication label?

_____

_____

_____

10. Rx 10:

Prinivil 20 mg #31

i tab po qd

Ref x2

A. How much will be dispensed? _____

B. How many days will the medication last? _____

C. How many refills are permitted on the prescription? _____

D. What DAW code will be used? _____

E. Write directions as they would appear on the medication label.

_____

_____

F. What auxiliary label(s) should be affixed to the medication label?

_____

_____

_____

Cholesterol Testing

Objective: To introduce cholesterol monitors and related supplies to the pharmacy technician and the procedure for testing total blood cholesterol levels. To review and apply information learned about hyperlipidemia.

Lab Activity #18.5: Using a cholesterol monitor, test your total blood cholesterol level. Answer the questions based on your cholesterol reading.

Equipment needed:

- Alcohol swabs
- Bandage
- Cholesterol monitor
- Cholesterol testing strips

348

- Gauze/cotton balls
- Lancet device
- Lancets
- Sharps container
- Pencil/pen

Procedure

1. Clean workspace in proper manner, using correct supplies and techniques.
2. Gather all materials needed for activity.
3. Wash hands properly
4. Assemble equipment.
5. Select puncture site.
6. Gently rub finger to promote circulation.
7. Clean site with alcohol swab and allow to dry.
8. Firmly grasp finger.
9. Hold lancet device at a 90-degree angle (perpendicular) to patient's finger and make a rapid, deep puncture on the fingertip.
10. Wipe away the first drop of blood with a clean gauze/cotton ball.
11. Apply gentle pressure to cause blood to flow freely.
12. Collect sample.
13. Clean site with clean gauze/cotton ball.
14. Apply pressure with clean gauze/cotton ball.
15. Record reading.
16. Check for bleeding, then apply bandage.
17. Dispose of material in proper containers.
18. Clean work area.
19. Properly wash hands using correct procedures and techniques.

Time needed to complete this activity: 30 minutes

Total Cholesterol Level (mg/dL)	Category
<200	Recommended
200-239	Borderline high
≥240	High

1. Total cholesterol reading: _____ mg/dL

2. Is your total blood cholesterol level recommended, borderline high, or high? _____

3. What factors may have contributed to your total blood cholesterol level?

   _____

   _____

   _____

4. As a pharmacy technician, how could you help those with hyperlipidemia while working in a pharmacy?

   _____

   _____

   _____

TERMS AND DEFINITIONS

Select the correct term from the following list and write the corresponding letter in the blank next to the statement.

A. Antitussive
B. Aspiration
C. Asthma
D. Chronic Obstructive Pulmonary Disease (COPD)
E. Cough Reflex
F. Decongestant
G. Dyspnea
H. Expectorant
I. Expiration
J. Inspiration
K. Metered Dose Inhaler (MDI)
L. Prophylaxis
M. Sputum
N. Viscosity

_____ 1. Fluid coughed up from the lungs and bronchial tissues

_____ 2. The thickness of a solution or fluid

_____ 3. Response of the body intended to clear air passages of foreign substances and mucus by forceful expiration

_____ 4. Difficult or labored breathing

_____ 5. Medication that prevents or relieves coughing

_____ 6. A method of supplying medication to the lungs through a pressurized inhalation

_____ 7. The act of breathing in; inhalation

_____ 8. Drugs that reduce swelling of the mucous membranes by constricting dilated blood vessels, diminishing blood flow to nasal tissues, and thereby reducing nasal congestion

_____ 9. The drawing of a foreign substance into the respiratory tract during inhalation

_____ 10. A disease process in which the lungs have a decreased capacity for gas exchange; three types are *emphysema*, *chronic bronchitis* and *asthma*

_____ 11. Preventive treatment

_____ 12. Agent able to break up thick mucus secretions of the lungs or bronchi so that they can be easily expelled from the respiratory tract by coughing

_____ 13. A condition in which inflammation and narrowing of the airways impedes breathing

_____ 14. The act of breathing out; exhalation

TRUE OR FALSE

Write T or F next to each statement.

_____ 1. The respiratory rate of a child and an adult are the same.

_____ 2. Cartilage around the larynx is usually only visible in men.

_____ 3. The left bronchus is bigger than the right bronchus.

_____ 4. The diaphragm separates the chest cavity from the abdominal area.

_____ 5. Breathing is an involuntary mechanism.

_____ 6. The most common bacterial organism causing community-acquired pneumonia is *Mycobacterium tuberculosis*.

_____ 7. Older adults are at a high risk for pneumonia, especially after an injury.

_____ 8. Asthma is a chronic inflammatory condition that affects the airways.

_____ 9. Tuberculosis is a leading cause of morbidity and mortality worldwide.

_____ 10. Individuals who have high blood pressure should take Sudafed regularly.

SYSTEM IDENTIFIER

Identify each anatomical part in this system and enter the term next to the corresponding number.

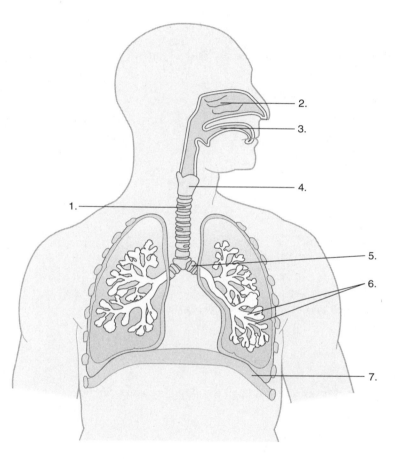

1. _____   5. _____

2. _____   6. _____

3. _____   7. _____

4. _____

Complete each question by circling the best answer.

1. The body's pH level must remain close to:
   A. 1.7
   B. 5.6
   C. 6.5
   D. 7.4

2. Where does the exchange of gases take place?
   A. Trachea
   B. Bronchi
   C. Bronchioles
   D. Alveolar sacs

3. Which of the following is *not* a part of the upper respiratory system?
   A. Trachea
   B. Larynx
   C. Pharynx
   D. Nose

4. The windpipe is called the:
   A. Trachea
   B. Larynx
   C. Pharynx
   D. Nose

5. The voice box is called the:
   A. Trachea
   B. Larynx
   C. Pharynx
   D. Nose

6. Which of the following is *not* a part of the lower respiratory tract?
   A. Larynx
   B. Trachea
   C. Bronchioles
   D. Lungs

7. To loosen mucus so that it can be expelled through coughing, a patient can take a (an):
   A. Antitussive
   B. Expectorant
   C. Antihistamine
   D. Decongestant

8. Some medications, like _____, can suppress the respiratory rate.
   A. Bronchodilators
   B. Corticosteroids
   C. Opioids
   D. Xanthines

9. *Rhinorrhea* is the medical name for a (an):
   A. Allergy
   B. Cold
   C. Sore throat
   D. Runny nose

10. Emphysema can be caused by:
    A. Exposure to environmental hazards
    B. Smoking
    C. Genetic disposition
    D. All of the above

FILL IN THE BLANKS

Answer each question by completing the statement in the space provided.

1. The respiratory control center, located in the _____ within the brainstem, automatically controls the rate and depth of breathing depending on the oxygen needs of the body.

2. The _____ of the lungs allows the capacity to vary widely depending on the need for oxygen.

3. The functions of nasal mucous membranes are to _____ and _____ inhaled air.

4. The function of the _____ is to distribute air throughout the lungs and into the alveoli.

5. The main function of the lungs is breathing and facilitation of _____ _____.

6. The exchange of oxygen and carbon dioxide also helps keep the _____ of our blood balanced.

7. Symptoms of a respiratory illness are noticeable because of the _____ _____ and _____ symptoms that typically accompany such conditions.

8. Gargling with _____ _____ can help provide relief from a sore throat.

9. Common symptomatic treatments for a cold include _____, _____, _____, and _____.

10. For severe influenza, _____ may be prescribed at the early onset of symptoms to help shorten the course or lessen the severity of the illness.

MATCHING

Matching I

Match the following classes of drugs with their mechanisms of action.

_____ 1. Antitussives

_____ 2. Mucolytics

_____ 3. Decongestants

_____ 4. Corticosteroids

_____ 5. Anticholinergics

A. Help clear respiratory passages
B. Act as antiinflammatory agents
C. Break up mucus in patients with COPD
D. Inhibit the action of acetylcholine
E. Suppress coughing

Matching II

Match the disease states with their drug treatments.

_____ 1. Tuberculosis (TB)

_____ 2. Chronic asthma

_____ 3. Cold

_____ 4. COPD

_____ 5. Cough

A. Pseudoephedrine
B. Guaifenesin
C. Isoniazid
D. Triamcinolone acetonide
E. Ipratropium bromide

Matching III

Match the brand name with the generic name.

_____ 1. Nasonex

_____ 2. Singulair

_____ 3. Flovent

_____ 4. TheoDur

_____ 5. Ventolin HFA

A. Theophylline
B. Mometasone
C. Albuterol
D. Montelukast
E. Fluticasone

SHORT ANSWER

Reply to each question based on what you have learned in the chapter.

1. List the common symptoms of a cold and two preventative efforts to help ward off a cold.

   _____

   _____

2. List common types of drugs used to treat the common symptoms of a cold.

   _____

   _____

3. List two drugs used for the treatment of non-small cell lung cancer.

   _____

   _____

RESEARCH ACTIVITIES

Follow the instructions given in each exercise and provide a response.

1. Visit the website *http://www.lung.org/stop-smoking/about-smoking/health-effects/secondhand-smoke.html*. What are the effects of secondhand smoke in children?

2. Access the website *http://www.cdc.gov/flu/about/viruses/change.htm*. What is "antigenic drift"? Why does this allow for reoccurrence of the flu? How can an "antigenic shift" cause a flu pandemic?

CRITICAL THINKING

Reply to each question based on what you have learned in the chapter.

1. Smoking has increased dramatically among teenagers over the years. What do you think has been a contributing factor to the increase?

2. Electronic cigarettes (e-cigarettes) have become very popular among smokers. What are potential benefits and hazards of e-cigarettes? Do you think this is a better option than cigarettes?

3. What are the health benefits of having plants in your home and office?

4. While having dinner in a restaurant, you see a person who may be choking. You quickly go over to help. What is the first question you should ask the person? Why?

5. Pseudoephedrine now must be sold by a pharmacist, and customers must fill out a log book for their purchase. Why is the sale of pseudoephedrine now controlled?

6. Why do some people become ill with the flu even if they have received the flu vaccine?

LAB SCENARIOS

Therapeutic Agents for the Respiratory System

Objective: To review with the pharmacy technician terms associated with the respiratory system and review the brand and generic names, indications, contraindications, adverse effects, dosage forms, routes of administration, and recommended daily dosage of medications used to treat disorders of the respiratory system.

DID YOU KNOW?

- In 2011, an estimated 12.7 million adults had COPD.
- 10.1 million adults were diagnosed with chronic bronchitis in 2011.
- 4.7 million adults have been diagnosed with emphysema.
- 6.5 million children have asthma in the United States.
- 15.5 million adults suffer from asthma.

Lab Activity #19.1: Define the following terms associated with the respiratory system.

Equipment needed:

- Medical dictionary
- Pencil/pen

Time needed to complete this activity: 30 minutes

1. Acute bronchitis _____

2. Allergic asthma _____

3. Allergic rhinitis _____

4. Anaphylaxis _____

5. Asthma _____

6. Bronchiolitis _____

7. COPD _____

8. Emphysema _____

9. Hypersensitivity pneumonitis _____

10. Influenza _____

11. Severe acute respiratory syndrome (SARS) _____

Lab Activity #19.2: Using a drug reference book, identify the generic name, drug classification, indications, contraindications, adverse effects, dosage forms, routes of administration, and recommended daily dosage of medications used to treat conditions affecting the respiratory system.

Equipment needed:

- *Drug Facts & Comparisons* or *Physicians' Desk Reference*
- Pencil/pen

Time needed to complete this activity: 60 minutes

Brand (Trade) Name	Generic Name	Drug Classification	Indication	List Two Contraindications	List Five Adverse Effects	Dosage Forms Available	Routes of Administration	Recommended Daily Dosage Adult	Recommended Daily Dosage Pedi	Drug Interactions	Pregnancy Category	Patient Information
Accolate												
Advair Diskus												
Allegra												
Allegra-D												
Astelin												
Atrovent												
Azmacort												
Clarinex												
Combivent												
Flonase												
Flovent HFA												
Intal												
Mucomyst												
Nasacort AQ												
Nasarel												
Nasonex												
Patanase												
ProAir HFA												
Proventil HFA												
Pulmicort Respules												
Rhinocort Aqua												
Rifadin												
Serevent												

Continued

357

Chapter **19** **Therapeutic Agents for the Respiratory System**

Brand (Trade) Name	Generic Name	Drug Classification	Indication	List Two Contraindications	List Five Adverse Effects	Dosage Forms Available	Routes of Administration	Recommended Daily Dosage		Drug Interactions	Pregnancy Category	Patient Information
								Adult	Pedi			
Singulair												
Spiriva												
Symbicort												
TheoDur												
Ventolin												
Veramyst												
Xopenex												
Xopenex HFA												
Zyflo												

Using Therapeutic Agents for the Respiratory System

Objective: To review with the pharmacy technician prescription orders and dosage calculations.

Lab Activity #19.3: Answer the questions based on the prescription orders for each question.

Equipment needed:

- *Drug Facts and Comparisons* or *Physician's Desk Reference*
- Pencil/pen
- Calculator

Time needed to complete this activity: 30 minutes

The following are approved DAW codes:

DAW 0: no product selection indicated
DAW 1: substitution not allowed by provider
DAW 2: substitution allowed: patient requested product dispensed
DAW 3: substitution allowed: pharmacist selected product dispensed
DAW 4: substitution allowed: generic drug not in stock
DAW 5: substitution allowed: brand drug dispensed as generic
DAW 6: override
DAW 7: substitution not allowed: brand drug mandated by law
DAW 8: substitution allowed: generic drug not available in marketplace
DAW 9: other

1. Rx 1:

    Flonase Nasal Spray (120 sprays)
    i spr to each nost bid
    Ref x 5

    A. How much will be dispensed (use metric quantities)? _____

    B. How many days will the medication last? _____

    C. How many refills are permitted on the prescription? _____

    D. What DAW code will be used? _____

    E. Write directions as they would appear on the medication label.

    _____

    _____

    F. What auxiliary label(s) should be affixed to the medication label?

    _____

    _____

    _____

2. Rx 2:

    Nasacort AQ Nasal Spray (120 sprays)
    i spr to each nost qd
    Ref x 6

    A. How much will be dispensed (use metric quantities)? _____

    B. How many days will the medication last? _____

    C. How many refills are permitted on the prescription? _____

    D. What DAW code will be used? _____

E. Write directions as they would appear on the medication label.

_____

_____

F. What auxiliary label(s) should be affixed to the medication label?

_____

_____

_____

3. Rx 3:

Nasonex (120 sprays)

ii spr to each nost daily

Ref x 2

A. How much will be dispensed (use metric quantities)? _____

B. How many days will the medication last? _____

C. How many refills are permitted on the prescription? _____

D. What DAW code will be used? _____

E. Write directions as they would appear on the medication label.

_____

_____

F. What auxiliary label(s) should be affixed to the medication label?

_____

_____

_____

4. Rx 4:

Albuterol (200 actuations)

i to ii inhalations q 4 to 6 h prn SOB and 15 min before exercise

Ref x 3

A. How much will be dispensed (use metric quantities)? _____

B. How many days will the medication last? _____

C. How many refills are permitted on the prescription? _____

D. What DAW code will be used? _____

E. Write directions as they would appear on the medication label.

_____

_____

F. What auxiliary label(s) should be affixed to the medication label?

_____

_____

_____

5. Rx 5:

Combivent (200 actuations)

ii inhalations qid

Ref x 6

   A. How much will be dispensed (use metric quantities)? _____

   B. How many days will the medication last? _____

   C. How many refills are permitted on the prescription? _____

   D. What DAW code will be used? _____

   E. Write directions as they would appear on the medication label.

     _____

     _____

   F. What auxiliary label(s) should be affixed to the medication label?

     _____

     _____

     _____

6. Rx 6:

Flovent HFA (120 metered doses)

ii inhalations bid

Ref x 3

   A. How much will be dispensed (use metric quantities)? _____

   B. How many days will the medication last? _____

   C. How many refills are permitted on the prescription? _____

   D. What DAW code will be used? _____

   E. Write directions as they would appear on the medication label.

     _____

     _____

   F. What auxiliary label(s) should be affixed to the medication label?

     _____

     _____

     _____

7. Rx 7:

Azmacort (240 actuations)

ii inhalations qid

Ref x 2

   A. How much will be dispensed (use metric quantities)? _____

   B. How many days will the medication last? _____

   C. How many refills are permitted on the prescription? _____

   D. What DAW code will be used? _____

E. Write directions as they would appear on the medication label.

_____

_____

F. What auxiliary label(s) should be affixed to the medication label?

_____

_____

_____

8. Rx 8:

Beconase AQ (180 metered sprays)
ii spr in each nost bid
Ref x 3

A. How much will be dispensed (use metric quantities)? _____

B. How many days will the medication last? _____

C. How many refills are permitted on the prescription? _____

D. What DAW code will be used? _____

E. Write directions as they would appear on the medication label.

_____

_____

F. What auxiliary label(s) should be affixed to the medication label?

_____

_____

_____

9. Rx 9:

Advair Diskus 250/50 (60 blisters)
i inhalation qam and qpm
Ref x 5

A. How much will be dispensed (use metric quantities)? _____

B. How many days will the medication last? _____

C. How many refills are permitted on the prescription? _____

D. What DAW code will be used? _____

E. Write directions as they would appear on the medication label.

_____

_____

F. What auxiliary label(s) should be affixed to the medication label?

_____

_____

_____

10. Rx 10:

Pulmicort Respules 0.25 mg, 2 cartons (30 respules/carton)

i respule in neb bid

Ref x 3

A. How much will be dispensed? _____

B. How many days will the medication last? _____

C. How many refills are permitted on the prescription? _____

D. What DAW code will be used? _____

E. Write directions as they would appear on the medication label.

_____

_____

F. What auxiliary label(s) should be affixed to the medication label?

_____

_____

_____

20 Therapeutic Agents for the Gastrointestinal System

TERMS AND DEFINITIONS

Select the correct term from the following list and write the corresponding letter in the blank next to the statement.

A. Absorption
B. Amino Acids
C. Antiemetic
D. Carbohydrates
E. Chyme
F. Digestion
G. Emesis
H. Excretion
I. Fistula
J. Ingestion
K. Peristalsis
L. Surface Area

_____ 1. Amount of an object's surface that is in contact with its surroundings

_____ 2. Molecules that make up proteins

_____ 3. A drug effective in the treatment of nausea and vomiting

_____ 4. Vomiting

_____ 5. The movement of nutrients, fluids, and medications from the GI tract into the bloodstream

_____ 6. The soupy consistency of food after it has mixed with stomach acids and as it passes into the small intestine

_____ 7. Chemical substances made up of only carbon, hydrogen, and oxygen (e.g., sugars, starches, and cellulose)

_____ 8. To take in food, liquid, or other substances (medications)

_____ 9. A permanent abnormal passageway between two organs in the body or between an organ and the exterior of the body

_____ 10. Elimination of waste products through stools and urine

_____ 11. The mechanical, chemical, and enzymatic action of breaking down food into molecules that can be used in metabolism

_____ 12. The contraction and relaxation of the tubular muscles of the esophagus, stomach, and intestines that move substances from the mouth to the anus

TRUE OR FALSE

Write T or F next to each statement.

_____ 1. All medications used to treat symptoms of the digestive tract and intestines are prescription only.

_____ 2. The GI system is controlled by the sympathetic system.

_____ 3. The pharynx connects the mouth to the esophagus.

_____ 4. The small intestine is about 6 feet in length.

_____ 5. Intestinal secretions have a more alkaline pH when compared with the stomach, allowing for good absorption of nutrients.

_____ 6. The gallbladder aids digestion by releasing bile.

_____ 7. The colon is the shortest section of the intestinal tract.

_____ 8. Carbohydrates arrive in the stomach as small sugar molecules and are converted into polysaccharides for easy digestion.

_____ 9. Some medications need to be administered parenterally to bypass the stomach and its acidic environment.

_____ 10. Most antiemetics require a prescription.

SYSTEM IDENTIFIER

Identify each organ/anatomical part in this system and enter the term next to the corresponding number.

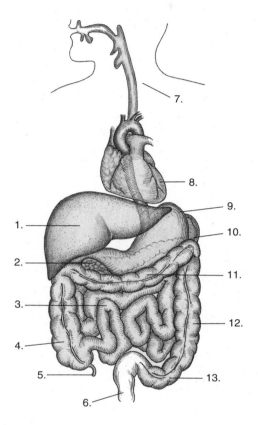

7.
8.
9.
10.
11.
12.
13.
1.
2.
3.
4.
5.
6.

1. _____

2. _____

3. _____

4. _____

5. _____

6. _____

7. _____

8. _____

9. _____

10. _____

11. _____

12. _____

13. _____

Complete each question by circling the best answer.

1. Which of the following is *not* a main function of the GI system?
   A. Digestion
   B. Absorption
   C. Metabolism
   D. Bioavailability

2. Which of the following is *not* a salivary gland?
   A. Subcutaneous
   B. Sublingual
   C. Submandibular
   D. Parotid

3. Absorption primarily takes place in the:
   A. Stomach
   B. Large intestine
   C. Pancreas
   D. Small intestine

4. Which of the following is *not* part of the large intestine?
   A. Cecum
   B. Rectum
   C. Ileum
   D. Colon

5. Which of the following is *not* a common condition that affects the GI system?
   A. Heartburn
   B. Appendicitis
   C. Constipation
   D. Diarrhea

6. Simethicone is indicated for:
   A. Flatulence
   B. Diarrhea
   C. Heartburn
   D. Constipation

7. Aluminum can cause:
   A. Flatulence
   B. Diarrhea
   C. Heartburn
   D. Constipation

8. Which of the following is a prescription drug for diarrhea?
   A. Pepto-Bismol
   B. Lomotil
   C. Kaopectate
   D. Imodium AD

9. First-line recommendations for *H. pylori* in patients who are allergic to penicillin include:
   A. A PPI, clarithromycin, and metronidazole
   B. A PPI, clarithromycin, and amoxicillin
   C. A PPI, bismuth salicylate, tetracycline and metronidazole
   D. Bismuth salicylate, clarithromycin, and metronidazole

10. If a patient is vomiting, the physician may prescribe:
    A. Axid
    B. Colace
    C. Compazine
    D. Lomotil

FILL IN THE BLANKS

Answer each question by completing the statement in the space provided.

1. The level of acidity is important in the _____ of many drugs and minerals.

2. The environment of the stomach is a more _____ pH, and the environment of the intestines is a more _____ pH.

3. The _____ begins the process of digestion by physically breaking down food into smaller pieces through the act of chewing.

4. High acid content of stomach fluids commonly contributes to _____ _____ , _____ or _____.

5. _____ are normally used for occasional dyspepsia or heartburn because they decrease the acidity of the stomach.

6. _____ _____ _____ are used primarily in the treatment of GERD and peptic ulcer.

7. *H. pylori* is treated with a combination of _____ and _____-_____ medications.

8. _____ are one of the most common causes of diarrhea or constipation, along with other GI side effects.

9. OTC drugs used to manage _____ include medications such as Kaopectate, FiberCon, and Pepto-Bismol.

10. A common side effect of chemotherapy is _____.

MATCHING

Matching I
Match the following trade and generic drug names.

_____ 1. Pepcid

_____ 2. Prevacid

_____ 3. Dulcolax

_____ 4. Imodium

_____ 5. Compazine

_____ 6. Tagamet

_____ 7. Protonix

_____ 8. Lomotil

_____ 9. MiraLAX

_____ 10. Colace

A. Bisacodyl
B. Loperamide
C. Famotidine
D. Prochlorperazine
E. Lansoprazole
F. Polyethylene glycol
G. Cimetidine
H. Docusate sodium
I. Atropine/diphenoxylate
J. Pantoprazole

Matching II

Match the following drug classes with the correct example.

_____ 1. Tagamet

_____ 2. Prilosec

_____ 3. Fibercon

_____ 4. Reglan

_____ 5. Ipecac

A. Antidiarrheal
B. Antiemetic
C. H$_2$-antagonist
D. Emetic
E. Proton pump inhibitor

SHORT ANSWER

Write a short response to each question in the space provided.

1. What is the sequence of organs in the GI tract?

_____

_____

_____

2. List the vitamins and minerals that can interact with the absorption of medications in the GI tract.

_____

_____

_____

RESEARCH ACTIVITIES

Follow the instructions given in each exercise and provide a response.

1. Many prescription medications for GI upset and heartburn have been changed to OTC status. Visit the website *www .fda.gov*. Locate *Drugs@FDA* under the *Approvals and Clearances* link; type in OTC and make a list of the GI medications that were prescription only and are now available over the counter.

2. Access the website *http://www.accessdata.fda.gov/scripts/cdrh/cfdocs/cfCFR/CFRSearch.cfm?fr=201.308*. What new label requirement must be in red letters on bottles of Ipecac syrup? Why must this label be a part of the labeling requirements for this product?

CRITICAL THINKING

Reply to each question based on what you have learned in the chapter.

1. It has been stated that you must chew your food "32 times." How does not chewing your food affect digestion in the stomach?

2. A hectic and stressful lifestyle can contribute to many "stomach problems" such as indigestion and acid reflux. What lifestyle changes can be made to reduce these problems?

3. What constitutes good oral hygiene? Is flossing that important? How can flossing impact the GI system?

4. Chemotherapy and radiation can have many adverse effects on patients, including GI system effects (eating, swallowing, saliva production). What prescription and OTC products are available to help with these unwanted effects? As a pharmacy technician, how could you help support these patients?

5. Is bulimia a psychological or a physical condition? Why?

LAB SCENARIOS

Therapeutic Agents for the Gastrointestinal System

Objective: To review with the pharmacy technician terms associated with the GI system and review the brand and generic names, indications, contraindications, adverse effects, dosage forms, routes of administration, and recommended daily dosage of medications used to treat disorders of the GI system.

DID YOU KNOW?

- 60 to 70 million people are affected by a digestive disease.
- In 2010, 48.3 million ambulatory care visits were made for digestive system–related care.
- In 2010, 21.7 million people were hospitalized for digestive system–related problems.
- In 2009, 245,921 digestive disease–related deaths occurred.
- In 2007, 12% of all inpatient procedures were for digestive system care.
- 20% of the population suffers from GERD.
- Chronic constipation represents the highest prevalence of GI related problems, with 63 million people reporting having suffered from it.

Lab Activity #20.1: Define the following terms associated with the GI system.

Equipment needed:

- Medical dictionary
- Pencil/pen

Time needed to complete this activity: 30 minutes

1. Appendicitis _____

2. Constipation _____

3. Diarrhea _____

4. Duodenal ulcer _____

5. Crohn's disease _____

6. Fistula _____

7. Gastric ulcer _____

8. Gastritis _____

9. Gastroesophageal reflux disease (GERD) _____

10. Hiatal hernia _____

11. Inflammatory bowel syndrome (IBS) _____

12. Intrinsic factor (IF) _____

13. Irritable bowel disease (IBD) _____

14. Laryngopharyngeal reflux _____

15. Lipids _____

16. Peptic ulcer _____

17. Peptic ulcer disease (PUD) _____

18. Reflux _____

19. Stomatitis _____

20. Ulcer _____

21. Ulcerative colitis _____

22. Villus _____

23. Xerostomia _____

Lab Activity #20.2: Using a drug reference book, identify the generic name, drug classification, indications, contraindications, adverse effects, dosage forms, routes of administration, and recommended daily dosage of medications used to treat conditions affecting the GI system.

Equipment Needed:

- *Drug Facts & Comparisons* or *Physicians' Desk Reference*
- Pencil/pen

Time needed to complete this activity: 60 minutes

Brand (Trade) Name	Generic Name	Drug Classification	Indication	List Two Contraindications	List Five Adverse Effects	Dosage Forms Available	Routes of Administration	Recommended Daily Dosage		Drug Interactions	Pregnancy Category	Patient Information
								Adult	Pedi			
AcipHex												
Asacol												
Axid												
Azulfidine												
Bentyl												
Cytotec												
Dipentum												
Imuran												
Lomotil												
Pentasa												
Pepcid												
Prevacid												
Prevpac												
Protonix												
Reglan												
Tagamet												
Zantac												

Lab Activity #20.3: Using resources available, complete the following table of OTC drug products for the GI system.

Equipment needed:

- Computer with Internet access
- Paper
- Pencil/pen
- *Pocket Guide for Nonprescription Product Therapeutics*

Time needed to complete this activity: 60 minutes

Brand Name	Active Ingredient(s)	Dosage Forms Available	Mechanism of Action	Interactions	Cautions	Patient Information	Adult Dose	Child Dose	Rx Strength Availability
Oral and GI Problems									
Alka-Seltzer									
Axid AR									
Gaviscon									
Milk of Magnesia									
Mylanta									
Pepcid									
Pepto-Bismol									
Prevacid									
Prilosec									
Tagamet HB									
Zantac 75									
Motion Sickness									
Bonine									
Dramamine									
Intestinal Discomfort									
Beano									
Gas-X									
Lactaid									
Mylicon									

Brand Name	Active Ingredient(s)	Dosage Forms Available	Mechanism of Action	Interactions	Cautions	Patient Information	Adult Dose	Child Dose	Rx Strength Availability
Constipation									
Benefiber									
Castor Oil									
Colace									
Dulcolax									
FiberCon									
Fleet									
Metamucil									
Senokot									
Surfak									
Diarrhea									
Imodium AD									
Pedialyte									

Using Therapeutic Agents for the Gastrointestinal System

Objective: To review with the pharmacy technician medication orders, dosage calculations, and sterile product preparation.

Lab Activity #21.4: Prepare a small-volume parenteral.

Equipment needed:

- 100 mL NS IV bag
- Alcohol swabs
- Diluent (NS)
- Labels
- Laminar airflow hood
- Protonix 40 mg IV for injection vial
- PPEs
- Sharps container
- Sink with running hot and cold water
- Syringes with needles
- Vented needles

Med Order:

The doctor has ordered a Protonix 40 mg IV infusion, 7 mg/min, in 100 mL of NS. Your pharmacy has in stock Protonix 40 mg IV for injection vial, which should be reconstituted with 10 mL of NS for a concentration of 4 mg/mL.

A. How many mL of Protonix will be needed to make this IV infusion?

B. How many vials will you need to make this IV infusion?

C. How long will this IV infusion last?

Procedure

1. Gather all materials needed for manipulation.
2. Wash hands properly.
3. Don PPEs.
4. Clean laminar flow workbench in the proper manner, using the correct supplies and techniques.
5. Check the expiration date on the Protonix vial, diluent, and IV bag.
6. Place ingredients in the laminar flow hood.
7. Select syringe of proper size.
8. Swab the rubber tops of Protonix and diluent with alcohol. Allow the alcohol to dry.
9. Make sure the needle is firmly attached to the syringe.
10. Prepare the syringe by adding the amount of air that will be equal to the amount of diluent to be withdrawn into the syringe.

11. Hold the syringe with the thumb and the index and middle fingers.
12. Remove cap from needle.
13. Insert the needle at a 45-degree angle into the rubber stopper of the vial with beveled part of the needle facing upward.
14. Hold the vial with the hand that is opposite the hand holding the syringe.
15. Push the plunger, forcing the air in the syringe into the vial, and release, gently allowing the fluid to be drawn into the syringe.
16. Tap the syringe to force air bubbles out of it.
17. Draw up the correct amount of diluent needed for reconstitution.
18. Pull the back on the plunger to clear the neck of the syringe. Remove the needle and replace with a vented needle.
19. Remove all excess air from syringe.
20. Insert vented needle of the syringe at a 45-degree angle into the rubber top of the powdered vial.
21. Gently shake or swirl to dissolve. The powder must dissolve completely.
22. Place needle and syringe into the sharps container.
23. Swab the rubber top of the reconstituted Protonix vial with alcohol. Allow the alcohol to dry.
24. Make sure the needle is firmly attached to the syringe.
25. Prepare the syringe by adding the amount of air that will be equal to the amount of pantoprazole to be withdrawn into the syringe.
26. Hold the syringe with the thumb and the index and middle fingers.
27. Remove cap from needle.
28. Insert the needle at a 45-degree angle into the rubber stopper of the vial with beveled part of the needle facing upward.
29. Hold the vial with the hand opposite the hand that is holding the syringe.
30. Invert the vial.
31. Push the plunger, forcing the air in the syringe into the vial, and release gently, allowing the fluid to be drawn into the syringe.
32. Tap the syringe to force air bubbles out of it.
33. Draw up the correct amount of Protonix by slowly pulling the syringe's plunger back.
34. Remove the needle from the vial once the correct amount of drug has been measured.
35. Remove air bubbles from syringe.
36. Recap the syringe.
37. Clean IV bag port with alcohol swab.
38. Inject medication into IV bag.
39. Mix thoroughly after the medication has been injected into the IV bag.
40. Check for any particulate matter.
41. Clean the outside of the IV bag with moist gauze, as well as all IV ports.
42. Place a small piece of foil around the medication port.
43. Label final product.
44. Place used syringe and needle into sharps container.
45. Remove PPEs in proper sequence, and place in a hazardous waste container.
46. Record initials, date, and time on the cleaning log.

Time needed to complete this activity: 30 minutes

REINFORCE KEY CONCEPTS

TERMS AND DEFINITIONS

Select the correct term from the following list and write the corresponding letter in the blank next to the statement.

A. Acidification
B. Acidosis
C. Alkalosis
D. Dialysis
E. Dialysate
F. Diuretic
G. Edema
H. Lithotripsy
I. Micturition
J. Nephrons
K. Osmosis
L. Peritonitis
M. Tubular Reabsorption
N. Tubular Secretion
O. Urethritis
P. Urolithiasis

_____ 1. Diffusion of water from low solute concentrations to higher solute concentrations, across a semipermeable membrane

_____ 2. Treatment with ultrasound shock waves to break a kidney stone into small particles

_____ 3. Solid mineral deposits that form stones in the urinary tract

_____ 4. Filtering unit of the kidneys

_____ 5. Agent that increases urine output and excretion of water from the body

_____ 6. Fluid into which material passes by way of the membrane in dialysis

_____ 7. Inflammation of the urethra

_____ 8. Urination

_____ 9. Passage of a solute through a semipermeable membrane to remove toxic materials/wastes and to maintain fluid, electrolyte, and pH levels of the body system

_____ 10. Conversion of urine to a more acidic state

_____ 11. Conservation of protein, glucose, bicarbonate, and water from the glomerular filtrated by the tubules

_____ 12. Condition characterized by an excess of watery fluid collection in the cavities or tissues of the body

_____ 13. Increase of alkalinity of the blood resulting from the accumulation of alkali or reduction of acid content

_____ 14. Increase of acid content of the blood resulting from the accumulation of acid or loss of bicarbonate

_____ 15. Inflammation of the peritoneum, typically caused by bacterial infection

_____ 16. Function of the nephron in which ions, toxins, and water are secreted into the collecting duct to be excreted

TRUE OR FALSE

Write T or F next to each statement.

_____ 1. The shape of the kidneys is similar to the shape of a kidney bean.

_____ 2. When the kidney is full, the person feels the need to urinate.

_____ 3. The body excretes approximately 1000 mL of urine per day.

_____ 4. Each kidney contains millions of microscopic nephrons.

_____ 5. The ureters lead to the bladder.

_____ 6. It is impossible for people to survive without two functioning kidneys.

_____ 7. Drinking plenty of water is one of the most effective ways to take care of the urinary system.

_____ 8. Younger adults suffer from acute renal failure more often than older people.

_____ 9. Chloride is an important electrolyte that helps conduct nerve impulses and balance fluid in the body

_____ 10. Incontinence tends to affect women more than men.

SYSTEM IDENTIFIER

Identify each main organ/anatomical part in the urinary system and enter the term next to the corresponding number.

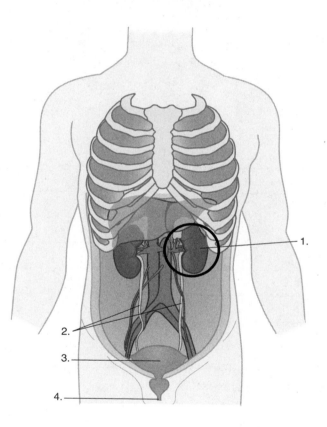

1. _____   3. _____

2. _____   4. _____

Label the parts of the kidney.

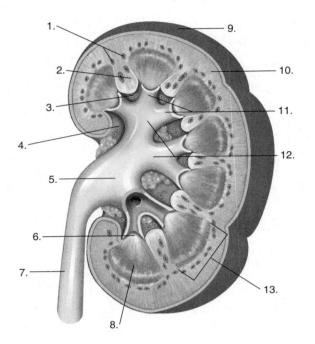

1. _____   8. _____

2. _____   9. _____

3. _____   10. _____

4. _____   11. _____

5. _____   12. _____

6. _____   13. _____

7. _____

MULTIPLE CHOICE

Complete each question by circling the best answer.

1. The bladder can store almost _____ of fluid.
   A. 2000 mL
   B. 1000 mL
   C. 500 mL
   D. 100 mL

2. What volume of blood products do the kidneys filter each day?
   A. 1 gallon
   B. 5 gallons
   C. 45 gallons
   D. 100 gallons

3. Albumins and antibodies are components of:
   A. Plasma
   B. Blood
   C. Hemoglobin
   D. All of the above

4. The one-way reabsorption of sodium and chloride from the loop of Henle is called:
   A. Ion exchange
   B. Osmosis
   C. Active transport
   D. Tubular secretion

5. The kidneys are also responsible for the production of _____, which helps maintain water balance in the body.
   A. Erythropoietin
   B. Aldosterone
   C. Renin
   D. Hilus

6. Those that have end-stage renal disease (ESRD) may be prescribed _____ to help overcome anemia.
   A. Calcitriol
   B. Sevelamer
   C. Vitamin D
   D. Epogen

7. A nosocomial infection is an infection:
   A. Of the nose
   B. Acquired in the hospital or health care setting
   C. Acquired while in a coma
   D. None of the above

8. Which of the following is *not* a means of cleansing the blood of patients with ESRD?
   A. Hemodialysis
   B. Peritoneal dialysis
   C. Nocturnal dialysis
   D. Oxydialysis

9. The most common side effect of all thiazide-like agents is:
   A. Frequent urination
   B. Infrequent urination
   C. Increased thiamine levels
   D. Decreased thiamine levels

10. Kegel exercises are done to help overcome:
    A. Stress
    B. Incontinence
    C. CHF
    D. UTIs

FILL IN THE BLANKS

Answer each question by completing the statement in the space provided.

1. The four major metabolic functions of the body are _____, _____, _____, and _____.

2. _____ occurs when too many free hydrogen ions are present, and _____ occurs when there is either retention of bicarbonate or excessive loss of hydrogen ions.

381

Chapter **21 Therapeutic Agents for the Renal System**

3. _____ are primarily responsible for the regulation of fluids, solutes, and wastes within the body.

4. Two important functions of the nephron are _____ _____ and _____ _____.

5. The acid content in urine is between a pH of _____ and _____.

6. An example of a buffer is _____.

7. Two general types of peripheral edema are _____ and _____.

8. The most common cause of a UTI is the bacterium _____ _____ from the colon.

9. People receiving dialysis must watch their _____ and _____ intake.

10. The mechanism of action for thiazides and thiazide-like agents is that they equally _____ the urinary excretion of the ions _____ and _____.

MATCHING

Matching I

Match the following medical terms with their definitions.

_____ 1. Anuria

_____ 2. Cystitis

_____ 3. Urethritis

_____ 4. Hypokalemia

_____ 5. Pyelonephritis

A. Inflammation of the urethra
B. Inflammation of the kidney
C. Excessive decrease in potassium in the blood
D. Lack of urine formation
E. Inflammation of the bladder

Matching II

Match the following trade names with their generic drug names.

_____ 1. Thalitone

_____ 2. Lasix

_____ 3. Aldactone

_____ 4. Diamox

_____ 5. Macrobid

_____ 6. Demadex

_____ 7. Osmitrol

_____ 8. Pyridium

_____ 9. Midamor

_____ 10. Vesicare

A. Spironolactone
B. Acetazolamide
C. Chlorthalidone
D. Nitrofurantoin
E. Furosemide
F. Amiloride
G. Mannitol
H. Solifenacin
I. Torsemide
J. Phenazopyridine

Matching III

Match the following drugs with their classification.

_____ 1. Bumex

_____ 2. Dyrenium

_____ 3. Zaroxolyn

_____ 4. Ditropan

_____ 5. Diamox

A. Potassium-sparing diuretic
B. Carbonic anhydrase inhibitor
C. Loop diuretic
D. Thiazide-like diuretic
E. Antimuscarinic

SHORT ANSWER

Write a short response to each question in the space provided.

1. Name the six main classes of diuretics used to treat edema.

_____

_____

_____

_____

_____

2. What are the symptoms of a kidney stone?

_____

_____

_____

3. Who is at high risk for renal failure?

_____

_____

_____

RESEARCH ACTIVITIES

Follow the instructions given in each exercise and provide a response.

1. Visit the website *http://www.mayoclinic.com/health/water/NU00283*. Investigate how much water you should drink in a day.

   A. How much water is recommended for men and women on a daily basis? How does this differ from the "eight glasses per day" recommendation?

B. What are the health benefits of water?

C. What factors affect daily water intake?

D. What foods can you eat to help meet the recommended daily water intake?

E. Is it possible to drink too much water? Why or why not?

2. Visit the website *http://www.nlm.nih.gov/medlineplus/dialysis.html*. Investigate what dialysis is and how it works.

A. What are the two types of kidney dialysis discussed?

B. What does dialysis help the kidneys do?

C. How does each type of dialysis work?

CRITICAL THINKING

Reply to each question based on what you have learned in the chapter.

1. Nosocomial urinary tract infections are a very common hospital-acquired infection. Who would be more at risk for acquiring this type of infection? What are some ways to prevent the spread of this type of infection?

2. If a UTI is left untreated, how will the infection progress?

    A. What are some common symptoms of a UTI?

    B. What drug therapy (prescription, OTC, and alternative medications) could be used to help treat a UTI?

3. Diabetes can be complicated by hypertension and kidney failure. A change in the patient's diet is always recommended. Apply your knowledge of the disease and devise a list of lifestyle changes that would benefit a diabetic patient.

LAB SCENARIOS

Therapeutic Agents for the Renal and Urologic Systems

Objective: To review with the pharmacy technician the organs of the renal and urologic system. In addition, to review the brand and generic names, indications, contraindications, adverse effects, dosage forms, routes of administration, and daily dosing of medications used to treat disorders of the renal and urologic system.

DID YOU KNOW?

- 4.4 million (1.9%) adults are diagnosed with kidney disease.
- Kidney disease is the eighth leading cause of death.
- More than 10% of adults greater than 20 years of age have chronic kidney disease.
- More than 35% of adults greater than 20 years of age with diabetes have chronic kidney disease.
- More than 20% of adults greater than 20 years of age with hypertension have chronic kidney disease.
- In 2007, approximately 110,000 patients began treatment (dialysis or kidney transplant) for end-stage renal disease.

Lab Activity #21.1: Define the following terms associated with the urinary system.

Equipment needed:

- Medical dictionary
- Pencil/pen

Time needed to complete this activity: 45 minutes

1. Anion _____

2. Anuria _____

3. Benign prostatic hyperplasia (BPH) _____

4. Blood urea nitrogen (BUN) _____

5. Cation _____

6. Chronic kidney disease _____

7. Collecting duct _____

8. Dehydration _____

9. Electrolyte _____

10. End-stage renal disease _____

11. Erythropoietin _____

12. Excretion _____

13. Hyperchloremia _____

14. Hyperkalemia _____

15. Hypernatremia _____

16. Hyperphosphatemia _____

17. Hypocalcemia _____

18. Hypochloremia _____

19. Hypokalemia _____

20. Hyponatremia _____

21. Hypophosphatemia _____

22. Incontinence _____

23. Interstitial space _____

24. Ions _____

25. Kidney stones _____

26. Nosocomial infection _____

27. Oliguria _____

28. Plasma _____

29. Polyuria _____

30. Prostate disease _____

31. Renal osteodystrophy _____

32. Renin _____

33. Stress incontinence _____

34. Uremia _____

35. Ureteroscopy _____

36. Urge incontinence _____

Lab Activity #21.2: Using a drug reference book, identify the generic name, drug classification, indications, contraindications, adverse effects, dosage forms, routes of administration, and recommended daily dosage of medications used to treat conditions affecting the renal and urologic system.

Equipment needed:

- *Drug Facts & Comparisons* or *Physicians' Desk Reference*
- Pencil/pen

Time needed to complete this activity: 60 minutes

Brand (Trade) Name	Generic Name	Drug Classification	Indication	List Two Contraindications	List Five Adverse Effects	Dosage Forms Available	Routes of Administration	Recommended Daily Dosage		Drug Interactions	Pregnancy Category	Patient Information
								Adult	Pedi			
Avodart												
Bumex												
Cardura												
Caverject												
Cialis												
Flomax												
Hytrin												
Klor-Con												
Lasix												
Levitra												
Proscar												
Uroxatral												
Viagra												

Lab Activity #21.3: Using a drug reference, identify the generic name, manufacturer, product size availability, NDC, AWP, and Orange Book code.

Equipment needed:

- Computer with Internet access
- Pencil/pen
- *Red Book Online*

Time needed to complete this activity: 60 minutes

Brand (Trade) Name	Generic Name	Manufacturer	Product Size Availability (oral)	NDC	AWP	Orange Book Code
Loop Diuretics						
Bumex						
Demadex						
Lasix						
Potassium-Sparing Diuretics						
Aldactone						
Dyrenium						
Midamor						
Thiazide and Thiazide-Like Diuretics						
Microzide						
Thalitone						
Zaroxolyn						

You are to recommend one diuretic product from each diuretic category for the inpatient pharmacy. Using the information you gathered for the above table and information learned from previous chapters, answer the following questions to help you determine which product to recommend.

A. For each of the diuretic categories, which product would be most cost-effective?

B. For each of the diuretic categories, which product would you recommend the inpatient pharmacy to dispense? (Also consider the dosing schedule.)

Using Therapeutic Agents for the Renal and Urologic System

Objective: To review with the pharmacy technician medication orders, dosage calculations, and sterile product preparation.

Lab Activity #21.4: Prepare a small-volume parenteral.

Equipment needed:

- Alcohol swabs
- Diluent
- Furosemide 10 mg/mL, 10 mL vial
- Labels
- Laminar airflow hood
- 50 mL NS IV bag
- PPEs
- Sharps container
- Sink with running hot and cold water
- Syringes with needles

Med Order:

1. The doctor has ordered a Lasix 480 mg IV drip, 20 mg/h, in 50 mL of NS. Your pharmacy has in stock furosemide 10 mg/mL, 10 mL vials.

   A. How many mL of furosemide 10 mg/mL will be needed to make this IV drip?

   B. How many vials will you need to make this drip?

   C. How long will this IV drip last?

Procedure

1. Gather all materials needed for activity.
2. Wash hands properly.
3. Don PPEs in the proper sequence.
4. Clean laminar flow workbench in the proper manner, using the correct supplies and techniques.
5. Collect the medication to be compounded.
6. Check expiration dates on both the vial and sterile vials.
7. Place ingredients in the laminar flow hood.
8. Swab the rubber top of the furosemide vial with alcohol. Allow the alcohol to dry.
9. Make sure the needle is firmly attached to the syringe.
10. Prepare the syringe by adding the amount of air that will be equal to the amount of furosemide to be withdrawn into the syringe.

11. Hold the syringe with the thumb and the index and middle fingers.
12. Remove cap from needle.
13. Insert the needle at a 45-degree angle into the rubber stopper of the vial with beveled part of the needle facing upward.
14. Hold the vial with the hand opposite the hand that is holding the syringe.
15. Invert the vial and pull back on the plunger.
16. Push the plunger, forcing the air in the syringe into the vial, and release gently, allowing the fluid to be drawn into the syringe.
17. Tap the syringe to force air bubbles out of it.
18. Draw up the correct amount of furosemide by slowly pulling the syringe's plunger back.
19. Remove the needle from the vial once the correct amount of drug has been measured.
20. Remove air bubbles from syringe.
21. Recap the syringe.
22. Clean IV bag port with alcohol swab.
23. Inject medication into IV bag.
24. Mix thoroughly after the medication that has been injected into the IV bag.
25. Check for any particulate matter.
26. Clean the outside of the IV bag with moist gauze, as well as all IV ports.
27. Place a small piece of foil around the medication port.
28. Label final product.
29. Place used syringe and needle into sharps container.
30. Remove PPEs in proper sequence, and place in a hazardous waste container.
31. Record initials, date, and time on the cleaning log.

Time needed to complete this activity: 30 minutes

22 Therapeutic Agents for the Reproductive System

REINFORCE KEY CONCEPTS

TERMS AND DEFINITIONS

Select the correct term from the following list and write the corresponding letter in the blank next to the statement.

A. Abortifacient
B. Androgen
C. Benign Prostatic Hyperplasia (BPH)
D. Chloasma
E. Depot
F. Erectile Dysfunction
G. Estrogen
H. Inert Ingredient
I. Negative Feedback
J. Nocturia
K. Palliative
L. Spermatogenesis
M. Spermicide
N. Teratogen

_____ 1. Brings relief but does not cure

_____ 2. Enlargement of the prostate

_____ 3. An agent that kills sperm

_____ 4. An ingredient that has little or no effect on body functions

_____ 5. The development of sperm within the testes

_____ 6. Any agent causing abnormal embryonic or fetal development

_____ 7. Any of a group of anabolic sex hormones that promote the development and maintenance of female sexual characteristics

_____ 8. Urination at night

_____ 9. A self-regulating mechanism in which the output of a system has input or control over the process

_____ 10. Inability of a man to maintain an erection sufficient for satisfying sexual activity

_____ 11. Any treatment that causes abortion of a fetus

_____ 12. Male hormone

_____ 13. Area of the body in which a substance can accumulate or be stored for later distribution

_____ 14. Hyperpigmentation of skin, limited or confined to a certain area

TRUE OR FALSE

Write T or F next to each statement.

_____ 1. The reproductive system is not interdependent with other body systems.

_____ 2. The gonads provide characteristics of both males and females.

_____ 3. Enzymes largely control the functions of the reproductive system.

_____ 4. All women produce several ova every month.

_____ 5. The female uterus houses the fertilized ovum.

_____ 6. Mammary gland tissue is regulated by hormonal secretions.

_____ 7. The hypothalamus can distinguish between natural and synthetic hormones.

_____ 8. Natural testosterone used for medicinal purposes is obtained from the testes of horses.

_____ 9. Oral contraceptives provide protection from sexually transmitted diseases.

_____ 10. The morning-after pill is a high-dose oral contraceptive.

Male Reproductive System

Identify each component in this system and enter the term next to the corresponding number.

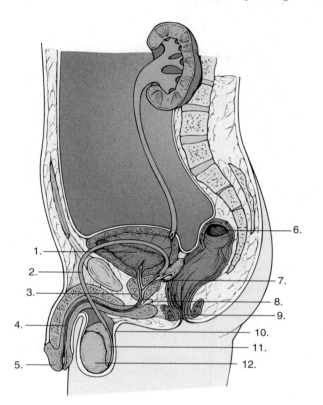

1. _____

2. _____

3. _____

4. _____

5. _____

6. _____

7. _____

8. _____

9. _____

10. _____

11. _____

12. _____

Female Reproductive System

Identify each component in this system and enter the term next to the corresponding number.

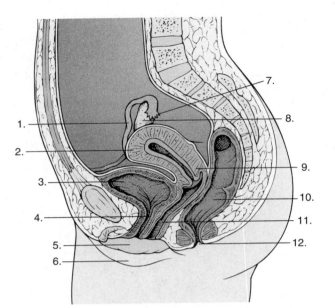

1. _____   7. _____

2. _____   8. _____

3. _____   9. _____

4. _____   10. _____

5. _____   11. _____

6. _____   12. _____

MULTIPLE CHOICE

Complete each question by circling the best answer.

1. The gonads or reproductive organs are responsible for:
   A. Secretion of hormones
   B. Production of sex cells
   C. Gender characteristics of males only
   D. A and B

2. Sperm production in males begins before the age of puberty and continues:
   A. To midlife
   B. Until age 70
   C. Throughout the lifetime
   D. None of the above

3. The most abundant androgen is:
   A. Estrogen
   B. Testosterone
   C. Progesterone
   D. Inhibin

4. The ovum is most commonly fertilized in the:
   A. Uterus
   B. Fallopian tube
   C. Ovary
   D. Cervix

5. Oral contraceptives are formulated in which of the following combinations?
   A. Monophasic
   B. Biphasic
   C. Triphasic
   D. All of the above

6. The goal of treatment for benign prostatic hypertrophy is to:
   A. Relieve hesitancy of urination
   B. Decrease nocturia
   C. Prevent the development of urinary tract infections
   D. All of the above

7. Which of the following hormones is used to treat abnormal uterine bleeding, abnormal ovulation, and infertility?
   A. Progesterone
   B. Estrogen
   C. Testosterone
   D. Follicle-stimulating hormone

8. For the treatment of oligospermia, which of the following can be used?
   A. Proscar
   B. Avodart
   C. Clomid
   D. Mirena

9. Palliative treatment of metastatic breast cancer may include:
   A. Methitest
   B. Menest
   C. Implanon
   D. Lupron depot

10. For osteoporosis prophylaxis, which of the following can be used?
    A. Menest
    B. Ogen
    C. Premarin
    D. All of the above

FILL IN THE BLANKS

Answer each question by completing the statement in the space provided.

1. Patients taking _____ should not take sildenafil or related drugs for erectile dysfunction (ED) concurrently because of the potential for dangerous decreases in blood pressure.

2. When using testosterone gel products it is important to cover the _____ _____ and not hold small children where transfer of the testosterone may occur.

Chapter **22 Therapeutic Agents for the Reproductive System**

3. _____ is also available in a 1-mg dose for the treatment of male pattern baldness.

4. Because 5-alpha reductase inhibitors may cause _____ _____, a woman who is pregnant or trying to become pregnant should avoid contact with these drugs because they can penetrate through the skin.

5. _____ acts as an antagonist to progesterone and prevents the maintenance of the pregnancy.

6. The barrier types of contraceptives for females include _____, _____ _____, and _____.

7. Some of the risks of combination _____ _____ include thromboembolism, myocardial infarction, and stroke.

8. The side effects of _____ include weight gain, stomach pain, and stomach cramping.

9. Oil-based injectable estrogen medications are called _____ medications and are prepared to prolong the medication's action.

10. Left untreated, some sexually transmitted diseases (STDs) can cause irreversible _____, _____, and even _____.

MATCHING

Matching I
Match the following trade and generic drug names.

_____ 1. Proscar

_____ 2. Flomax

_____ 3. Premarin

_____ 4. Ogen

_____ 5. Provera

A. Conjugated estrogens
B. Estropipate
C. Finasteride
D. Medroxyprogesterone
E. Tamsulosin

Matching II
Match the following trade and generic drug names.

_____ 1. Parlodel

_____ 2. Ortho Tri-Cyclen

_____ 3. Lo Ovral

_____ 4. Hytrin

_____ 5. Viagra

A. Ethinyl estradiol/norgestrel
B. Sildenafil
C. Terazosin
D. Bromocriptine
E. Ethinyl estradiol/norgestimate

Matching III

Match the following drugs with their indication.

_____ 1. Lupron

_____ 2. Clomid

_____ 3. Prempro

_____ 4. Ortho-Cept

_____ 5. Doxycycline

_____ 6. AndroGel

_____ 7. Cardura

_____ 8. Muse

_____ 9. Zoladex

_____ 10. Android

A. Androgen supplement
B. Oral contraceptive
C. Endometriosis
D. Breast cancer
E. Pelvic inflammatory disease
F. Infertility
G. Prostate cancer
H. Benign prostatic hypertrophy
I. Erectile dysfunction
J. Hormone replacement therapy

SHORT ANSWER

Reply to each question based on what you have learned in the chapter.

1. List the available dosage forms of estrogen.

_____

_____

2. List six types of non-oral contraceptives and their available dosage forms.

_____

_____

3. List six types of androgens and their available dosage forms.

_____

_____

RESEARCH ACTIVITIES

Follow the instructions given in each exercise and provide a response.

1. Access the website *http://www.niaid.nih.gov/topics/pelvicInflammatoryDisease/Pages/default.aspx* and read about pelvic inflammatory disease (PID).

   A. Who is at risk for PID?

   B. What causes PID?

C. What are the symptoms of PID?

D. What drug therapy is used to treat PID?

2. Access the website *http://www.nlm.nih.gov/medlineplus/ency/article/000369.htm* and read about polycystic ovarian syndrome (PCOS).

A. What are the effects of PCOS?

B. What drug therapy is used to help treat the symptoms of PCOS?

REFLECT CRITICALLY

CRITICAL THINKING

Reply to each question based on what you have learned in the chapter.

1. Women have been told for many years that when menopause occurs, they will need hormonal replacement therapy (HRT). However, recently released information indicates that long-term HRT is more harmful than beneficial. If you were the pharmacist, what advice would you give women on this subject?

2. Birth control has been taught in middle schools and high schools for many years in an attempt to curb teen pregnancy. Why is the rate of teen pregnancy still high?

3. Propecia was approved by the Food and Drug Administration (FDA) for the treatment of hair loss. The active ingredient in Propecia is finasteride, which is the same drug used to treat benign prostatic hypertrophy, under the brand name Proscar. What is the difference in strength between Propecia and Proscar, and what are the side effects of finasteride?

LAB SCENARIOS

Therapeutic Agents for the Reproductive System

Objective: To review with the pharmacy technician terms associated with the organs of the reproductive system and review the brand and generic names, indications, contraindications, adverse effects, dosage forms, routes of administration, and recommended daily dosage of medications used to treat disorders of the reproductive system.

DID YOU KNOW?

- 17.1% of women ages 15 to 44 currently use oral contraceptives.
- 10.4% of women ages 15 to 44 currently use a patch for contraception.
- 6.2% of women ages 15 to 44 currently rely on their partners having a vasectomy as their main form of contraception.
- 6.7 million (10.9%) women ages 15 to 44 have impaired ability to have children.
- In 2008, more than 110 million men and women were reported to have a sexually transmitted infection.
- In 2010, a total of $16 billion dollars were spent on medical costs because of sexually transmitted infections.
- The most common sexually transmitted infection is HPV, with more than 79 million men and women affected nationwide.

Lab Activity #22.1: Define the following terms associated with the reproductive system.

Equipment needed:

- Medical dictionary
- Pencil/pen

Time needed to complete this activity: 30 minutes

1. Amenorrhea _____

2. Anabolic steroid _____

3. Dysfunctional uterine bleeding (DUB) _____

4. Dysmenorrhea _____

5. Endometriosis _____

6. Erectile dysfunction _____

7. Hypogonadism _____

8. Hysterectomy _____

9. Infertility _____

10. Kallmann's syndrome _____

11. Klinefelter's syndrome _____

12. Pelvic inflammatory disease (PID) _____

13. Polycystic ovarian syndrome (PCOS) _____

14. Pregnancy _____

15. Premenstrual syndrome (PMS) _____

16. Salpingitis _____

17. Stein-Leventhal syndrome _____

18. Tubal ligation _____

19. Vasectomy _____

20. Vaginitis _____

Lab Activity #22.2: Using a drug reference book, identify the generic name, drug classification, indication, contraindications, adverse effects, dosage forms, routes of administration, and recommended daily dosage of medications used to treat conditions affecting the reproductive system.

Equipment needed:

■ *Drug Facts & Comparisons* or *Physicians' Desk Reference*
■ Pencil/pen

Time needed to complete this activity: 60 minutes

Brand (Trade) Name	Generic Name	Drug Classification	Indication	List Two Contraindications	List Five Adverse Effects	Dosage Forms Available	Routes of Administration	Recommended Daily Dosage	Drug Interactions	Pregnancy Category	Patient Information
Alesse											
Androderm											
Apri											
Avodart											
Cialis											
Climara											
Clomid											
Danocrine											
Demulen											
Depo-Provera											
Desogen											
Diflucan											
Estrace											
Estraderm											
Femhrt											
Fertinex											
Flagyl											
Flomax											
Junel Fe											
Levitra											
Loestrin 24 Fe											
Lunelle											
Lupron											
Micronor											

Continued

401

Brand (Trade) Name	Generic Name	Drug Classification	Indication	List Two Contraindications	List Five Adverse Effects	Dosage Forms Available	Routes of Administration	Recommended Daily Dosage	Drug Interactions	Pregnancy Category	Patient Information
NuvaRing											
Ortho-Est											
Ortho Evra											
Ortho Novum											
Ortho-Cyclen											
Ortho Tri-Cyclen Lo											
Ovral											
Ovrette											
Parlodel											
Plan B											
Premarin											
Prempro											
Prometrium											
Proscar											
Provera											
Tri-Levlen											
Triphasil											
Tri-Sprintec											
Vagistat											
Valtrex											
Viagra											
Vivelle-Dot											
Yasmin 28											
Zoladex											
Zovirax											

Using Therapeutic Agents for the Reproductive System

Objective: To review with the pharmacy technician dosage calculations and extemporaneous compounding.

Lab Activity #22.3: Compounding a cream.

Prepare 1 ounce of the following formula:

Testosterone	60 mg
Glycerin	
Dermabase cream	qs 30 g

Equipment needed:

- 1 Ounce jar or tube for dispensing
- Auxiliary labels
- Calculator
- Dermabase cream
- Disinfecting agent/cleanser
- Electronic balance or torsion balance with metric weights
- Glycerin
- Label
- Latex gloves
- Mortar card
- Ointment slab, parchment paper, or glass mortar and pestle
- Pen
- Sink with running hot and cold water
- Spatula
- Testosterone powder
- Weighing boats or weighing papers
- Ziploc bag (if desired)

Procedure

1. Wash hands and dry thoroughly.
2. Gather all necessary supplies.
3. Double check recipe and calculations.
4. Put gloves on.
5. Weigh testosterone powder on electronic balance or torsion balance.
6. Levigate testosterone powder with a few drops of glycerin to form a smooth paste.
7. Using geometric dilution, incorporate Dermabase cream; qs to 30 g.
8. Check product for uniformity and appearance.
9. Using a Ziploc bag, package the cream ensuring pharmaceutical elegance.
10. Label product with all necessary information, including the levigating agent and auxiliary labels.
11. Document procedure and all necessary information on compounding log.
12. Clean equipment and put away.
13. Clean work area.

Packaging: light-resistant container
Labeling: For external use only. Use only as directed.
BUD: The shorter of 6 months or the expiration date of any ingredients used
Storage: Room temperature

Time needed to complete this activity: 45 minutes

Pharmacy Compounding Log						
Drug Name	Lot Number	Mfg. Expiration Date	Quantity Prepared	Measured By	Verified By	Beyond-Use Date

23 Therapeutic Agents for the Immune System

TERMS AND DEFINITIONS

Select the correct term from the following list and write the corresponding letter in the blank next to the statement.

A. Anaphylaxis
B. Antigen
C. Attenuated
D. Cytokine
E. Immunity
F. Immunization
G. Immunoglobulin
H. Lymph Node
I. Lymphocyte
J. Monocyte
K. Phagocyte
L. Plasma Cell
M. Systemic
N. Toxoid
O. Virion
P. Virus

_____ 1. Mononuclear leukocyte found in the blood, lymph, and lymphoid tissues

_____ 2. Type of resistance to infection caused by an immune response from the body following exposure to antigens or administration of vaccines

_____ 3. Cell of the immune system that secretes antibodies

_____ 4. Type of vaccine where a toxin has been rendered harmless but still invokes an antigenic response, improving immunity against the active toxin at some future date

_____ 5. Antibody

_____ 6. Cell of the immune system that engulfs cells, debris and antigens

_____ 7. Substance that prompts the production of antibodies producing an immune response

_____ 8. Microscopic nonliving particle that replicates exclusively inside the host's cell, using parts of the host cell including DNA, ribosomes, and proteins

_____ 9. Structure that consists of many small, oval nodules that filter lymphatic fluid and fight infection; site of lymphocyte, monocyte, and plasma cell production

_____ 10. Virus particle

_____ 11. Proteins that signal cells of the immune system

_____ 12. Phagocytic leukocyte

_____ 13. Extreme, potentially life-threatening allergic reaction

_____ 14. Altered or weakened live vaccine made from the disease organism against which the vaccine protects

_____ 15. Pertaining to the entire organism: "widespread" in contrast to "local."

_____ 16. Act of conferring immunity, such as with vaccination

TRUE OR FALSE

Write T or F next to each statement.

_____ 1. The thymus is much larger in children than in adults.

_____ 2. Eosinophils are the most abundant leukocyte in adults

_____ 3. There are two types of immunity, inactive and passive.

_____ 4. With live vaccines, the risk of contracting the full-blown infection from the vaccine is high.

_____ 5. Tetanus vaccine should be given every 6 years for the first 20 years of life.

_____ 6. Vaccines are unavailable for malaria and fungal infections.

_____ 7. Use of sunscreen to minimize exposure to ultraviolet light may be helpful as well as increased physical activity when treating SLE.

_____ 8. With strict drug and physical therapy, RA will resolve itself.

_____ 9. Methotrexate should be administered once weekly.

_____ 10. Thyroid hormone replacement agents need to be taken for life (one dose a day) owing to the chronic nature of the condition.

SYSTEM IDENTIFIER

Identify each component of the lymphatic system and enter the term next to the corresponding number.

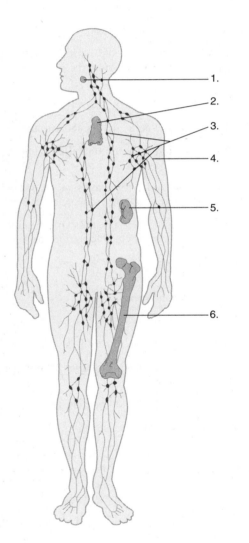

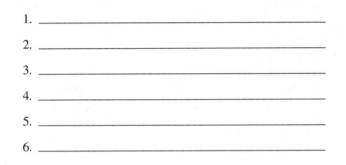

1. _____

2. _____

3. _____

4. _____

5. _____

6. _____

MULTIPLE CHOICE

Complete each question by circling the best answer.

1. Which of the following may be given to help treat rheumatoid arthritis and juvenile rheumatoid arthritis?
   A. Propylthiouracil
   B. Orencia
   C. Tapazole
   D. Rapamune

2. To help prevent kidney transplant rejection, _____ can be given intravenously.
   A. Novantrone
   B. Betaseron
   C. Rapamune
   D. Nulojix

3. To help treat multiple sclerosis, _____ can be given weekly by intramuscular injection.
   A. Campath
   B. Rebif
   C. Avonex
   D. Benlysta

4. Therapy for Graves' disease includes:
   A. Propylthiouracil
   B. Radioactive iodine
   C. Methimazole
   D. All of the above

5. _____ can be used in the management of SLE.
   A. Orthoclone
   B. Imuran
   C. Avonex
   D. Copaxone

6. Varicella, MMR, and hepatitis B are all examples of which type of vaccine?
   A. Immune globulin
   B. Antivenins
   C. Viral
   D. Toxoids

7. One vaccine that protects against meningitis is called:
   A. Prevnar 13
   B. Pentacel
   C. Varivax
   D. Havrix

8. _____ is a subunit vaccine that is grown in yeast cells and then is given as a vaccine.
   A. Hepatitis B
   B. Influenza
   C. Yellow fever
   D. Rotavirus

9. Which of the following is an acellular vaccine?
   A. Pertussis
   B. Tetanus
   C. Diphtheria
   D. All of the above

10. _____ is a newer type of vaccine that is based on using an antibody that is shaped like the antigen which can make it possible to kill deadly viruses such as human immunodeficiency virus.
   A. Transplant vaccine
   B. Subunit vaccine
   C. Antiidiotypic vaccine
   D. Acellular vaccine

FILL IN THE BLANKS

Answer each question by completing the statement in the space provided.

1. The body has a built-in _____ _____ that helps protect it from invading organisms.

2. Medications that inhibit the effects of _____ can be used to treat conditions associated with chronic inflammation like rheumatoid arthritis.

3. Inflammation is a necessary response to _____ _____.

4. _____ is the most severe case of an allergic reaction, which can be deadly if not treated immediately.

5. For the most severe reactions that cause swelling of the airways, _____ is administered.

6. In the treatment of many autoimmune disorders, therapies aimed at _____ the immune system are often used.

7. Medications used to treat _____ _____ include NSAIDs, analgesics, corticosteroids, and DMARDs.

8. Most vaccines should be stored in the _____.

9. Antivenins are also given to counteract _____ from creatures such as snakes and spiders.

10. Common _____ include those for diphtheria, rabies, and botulism.

MATCHING

Matching I

Match the following trade and generic drug names.

_____ 1. CellCept

_____ 2. Imuran

_____ 3. Prograf

_____ 4. Sandimmune

_____ 5. Rapamune

_____ 6. Copaxone

_____ 7. Humira

_____ 8. Orencia

_____ 9. Avonex

_____ 10. Novantrone

A. Glatiramer
B. Interferon beta-1a
C. Tacrolimus
D. Mycophenolate
E. Mitoxantrone
F. Adalimumab
G. Azathioprine
H. Abatacept
I. Sirolimus
J. Cyclosporine

Matching II

Match the following vaccine with their availability as a live or inactivated vaccine.

_____ 1. Anthrax

_____ 2. DTaP

_____ 3. Hepatitis B

_____ 4. Herpes zoster

_____ 5. Measles, mumps, rubella (MMR)

_____ 6. Polio

_____ 7. Rabies

_____ 8. Rotavirus

_____ 9. Varicella

_____ 10. Yellow fever

A. Live
B. Inactivated

SHORT ANSWER

Reply to each question based on what you have learned in the chapter.

1. List two types of vaccines available for human papillomavirus (HPV) and who may receive each type.

_____

_____

2. List three types of vaccines for meningitis and who may receive each type.

_____

_____

_____

3. List two types of vaccines for pneumonia and who may receive each type.

_____

_____

4. List the vaccine(s) that are recommended for those in the military.

_____

_____

RESEARCH ACTIVITIES

Follow the instructions given in each exercise and provide a response.

1. Access the website *http://wwwnc.cdc.gov/travel/*.

   A. Choose a country to travel to and list the vaccines you will need to receive before going on your trip.

   B. Choose one of the Travel Health Notices posted. List the necessary precautions you would need to take if you were planning to travel there.

2. Access the website *http://www.cdc.gov/vaccines/vac-gen/shortages/default.htm*. List any vaccine delay or shortage. For each one listed, what is the anticipated date of availability?

3. Access the website *http://www2a.cdc.gov/nip/StateVaccApp/statevaccsApp/default.asp*.

   A. What vaccinations does your state require hospital employees to have?

   B. What vaccinations does your state require hospital inpatients to be offered?

C. What vaccinations does your state require ambulatory care employees to have?

D. Does your state allow for opting out of receiving vaccinations? If so, in what circumstances may one opt out?

REFLECT CRITICALLY

CRITICAL THINKING

Reply to each question based on what you have learned in the chapter.

1. Human immunodeficiency virus (HIV) infection can be a devastating disease. What type of lymphocyte is most important for patients with HIV infection? Why?

2. In the United States, sanitization and hygiene are stressed, yet people still frequently become ill. Does constant sanitization bring about a healthier immune system or does it weaken it?

3. Botulinum toxin (example: Botox) is the latest product being used to "reduce or eliminate wrinkles." Can repeated Botox injections harm the recipients or cause them to build up a resistance to the toxin?

4. The World Health Organization (WHO) has been working tirelessly to eradicate infectious diseases throughout the world, with much success. What would happen to the planet's population if all infectious diseases were eradicated and vaccinations were not needed?

5. Many people decide every year to not receive the flu vaccine because "they always get the flu when they get the vaccine." What could you say to help convince them that they are unable to get the flu from the vaccine? List reasons why they may still come down with the flu even though they received the vaccine.

LAB SCENARIOS

Therapeutic Agents for the Immune System

Objective: To review with the pharmacy technician terms associated with the components of the immune system and review the brand and generic names, indications, contraindications, adverse effects, dosage forms, routes of administration, and recommended daily dosage of medications used to treat disorders of the immune system.

DID YOU KNOW?

- A person with the flu can spread it to others up to 6 feet away when they cough and sneeze.
- An estimated 79,000 hospitalizations were prevented in the 2012–2013 flu season from the flu vaccine.
- In 2012, not all children between the ages of 19 and 35 months old received the necessary vaccinations; 85% received diphtheria, tetanus, and pertussis vaccine, 94% received the polio vaccine, 92% received the MMR vaccine, 91% received the varicella vaccine.
- 1.3 million adults suffer from rheumatoid arthritis.
- 294,000 people have juvenile arthritis.
- Approximately 161,000 to 322,000 adults have systemic lupus erythematosus.

Lab Activity #23.1: Define the following terms associated with the immune system.

Equipment needed:

- Medical dictionary
- Pencil/pen

Time needed to complete this activity: 30 minutes

1. Antibodies complex _____

2. Antigen presenting cell _____

3. Biological response modifier _____

4. Hashimoto's thyroiditis _____

5. Hematopoiesis _____

6. Humoral immunity _____

7. Inflammation _____

8. Innate immunity _____

9. Juvenile rheumatoid arthritis (JRA) _____

10. Leukocyte _____

11. Multiple sclerosis (MS) _____

12. Rheumatoid arthritis (RA) _____

13. Systemic lupus erythematosus _____

14. Transplant rejection _____

15. Vaccine _____

Lab Activity #23.2: Using a drug reference book, identify the generic name, drug classification, indications, contraindications, adverse effects, dosage forms, routes of administration, and recommended daily dosage of medications used to treat conditions affecting the immune system.

Equipment needed:

■ *Drug Facts & Comparisons* or *Physicians' Desk Reference*
■ Pencil/pen

Time needed to complete this activity: 60 minutes

Brand (Trade) Name	Generic Name	Drug Classification	Indication	List Two Contraindications	List Five Adverse Effects	Dosage Forms Available	Routes of Administration	Recommended Daily Dosage		Drug Interactions	Pregnancy Category	Patient Information
								Adult	Pedi			
Actemra												
Avonex												
Azulfidine												
Benlysta												
Betaseron												
Campath												
CellCept												
Cimzia												
Copaxone												
Decadron												
Deltasone												
Enbrel												
Gengraf												
Humira												
Imuran												
Kineret												
Novantrone												

Brand (Trade) Name	Generic Name	Drug Classification	Indication	List Two Contraindications	List Five Adverse Effects	Dosage Forms Available	Routes of Administration	Recommended Daily Dosage		Drug Interactions	Pregnancy Category	Patient Information
								Adult	Pedi			
Nulojix												
Orapred												
Orencia												
Orthoclone												
Prograf												
Rapamune												
Rebif												
Remicade												
Rheumatrex												
Rituxan												
Sandimmune												
Simponi												
Simulect												
Tysabri												
Zortress												

415

Using Therapeutic Agents for the Immune System

Objective: To introduce the pharmacy technician to the use of vaccines in the practice of pharmacy.

Lab Activity #23.3: Using the Centers for Disease Control and Prevention website, *www.cdc.gov/flu*, answer the following questions regarding seasonal influenza.

Equipment needed:

■ Computer with Internet connection
■ Paper
■ Pencil/pen

Time needed to complete this activity: 45 minutes

1. Who should be vaccinated for seasonal influenza?

_____

_____

_____

2. What are some of the symptoms of seasonal influenza?

_____

_____

_____

_____

3. Who is at risk for contacting the flu?

_____

_____

_____

4. How does the flu spread from individual to individual?

_____

_____

_____

_____

5. What are three ways to protect one from getting seasonal influenza?

_____

_____

_____

_____

6. What is the composition of the current flu vaccine?

_____

_____

_____

7. At what temperature should the flu vaccine be stored?

_____

_____

_____

8. Which month do we experience the greatest number of cases of the flu?

_____

9. What antiviral medications may be used in the treatment of seasonal influenza?

_____

10. Complete the following table.

Trade Name	Manufacturer	Presentation	Mercury Content	Age Group	Number of Doses	Route of Administration	Storage Requirement
Fluzone		0.25 mL prefilled syringe					
		0.5 mL prefilled syringe					
		0.5 mL vial					
		5.0 mL multi-dose vial					
Fluvirin		5.0 mL multi-dose vial					
		0.5 mL prefilled syringe					
Agriflu		0.5 mL prefilled syringe					
Fluarix		0.5 mL prefilled syringe					
FluLaval		5.0 mL multi-dose vial					
Afluria		0.5 mL prefilled syringe					
Fluzone High-Dose		0.5 mL prefilled syringe					
FluMist		0.2 mL sprayer					

Chapter 23 Therapeutic Agents for the Immune System

Objective: Obtain information on immunization training requirements within your state.

Lab Activity #23.4: Use the Internet to research information on the criteria to immunize customers (patients) in your state, and complete the following table.

Equipment needed:

- Computer with Internet connection
- Pencil/pen

Time needed to complete this activity: 30 minutes

What is the name of your state?	
Who may immunize pharmacy customers?	
What immunizations may they perform?	
What age group may be immunized at the pharmacy? List any restrictions or special circumstances.	
Describe the training required to be able to immunize a customer.	
Does an individual require clinical training before being permitted to immunize patients?	
Does an individual need to register with a regulatory agency in the state? If yes, which agency?	
Does an individual need to be licensed to immunize customers?	
What does it cost to be able to immunize customers?	
Does an individual need continuing education for the renewal of his or her registration or license? If so, how many CEUs are needed annually?	

Objective: Retail pharmacy visit.

Lab Activity #23.5: Visit a retail pharmacy that offers flu shots or other immunizations to their customers. Ask for a copy of the paperwork that the patient must fill out before receiving an immunization.

Equipment needed:

- None

Time needed to complete this activity: 30 minutes

1. Compare and contrast the information found on the sheet with other members of your class. What is the same? What is different?

_____

_____

_____

_____

2. Does medical or prescription drug coverage pay for the immunization?

_____

_____

_____

3. What documentation must the pharmacy keep and for how long?

_____

_____

_____

Lab Activity #23.6: Use the Centers for Disease Control and Prevention (CDC) website *www.cdc.gov/vaccines/* to identify the generic name, indications, contraindications, adverse effects, and the routes of administration of the vaccines listed in the following table.

Equipment needed:

- Computer with Internet connection
- Pencil/pen

Time needed to complete this activity: 60 minutes

Brand (Trade) Name	Generic Name	Indication	List Two Contraindications	List Five Adverse Effects	Routes of Administration	Storage Requirements	Can It Be Administered at the Pharmacy?
Adacel							
BioThrax							
Boostrix							
Cervarix							
Daptacel							
Dryvax							
Engerix-B							
Gardasil							
Havrix							
Imovax Rabies							
Infanrix							
IPOL							
Ixiaro							
JE-VAX							
Kinrix							
Menactra							
Menomune							
Menveo							
M-M-R II							
Pediarix							
Pentacel							
Pneumovax 23							
Prevnar							

Continued

Brand (Trade) Name	Generic Name	Indication	List Two Contraindications	List Five Adverse Effects	Routes of Administration	Storage Requirements	Can It Be Administered at the Pharmacy?
ProQuad							
Recombivax HB							
Rotarix							
Twinrix							
Varivax							
Vivotif							
YF-Vax							
Zostavax							

24 Therapeutic Agents for the Eyes, Ears, Nose, and Throat

TERMS AND DEFINITIONS

Select the correct term from the following list and write the corresponding letter in the blank next to the statement.

A. Aqueous Humor
B. Auditory Canal
C. Auditory Ossicles
D. Auricles
E. Cones
F. Conjunctiva
G. Cornea
H. Eustachian Tube
I. Lens
J. Miosis
K. Mydriasis
L. Ophthalmic
M. Orbit
N. Otic
O. Rods
P. Sclera
Q. Tinnitus
R. Tympanic membrane

_____ 1. The transparent tissue covering the anterior portion of the eye

_____ 2. Pertaining to the ear

_____ 3. Flexible, clear tissue that focuses images

_____ 4. Dilation of the pupil

_____ 5. Pertaining to the eye

_____ 6. Photoreceptors responsible for color

_____ 7. Transparent protective mucus membrane that lines the underside of the eyelid

_____ 8. A 1-inch segment of tube that runs from the external ear to the middle ear

_____ 9. A membranous skin that separates the external ear from the middle ear

_____ 10. Eye socket

_____ 11. Contraction of the pupil

_____ 12. Photoreceptors responsible for black and white colors that respond to dim light

_____ 13. Small bones of the middle ear that transmit sound from the eardrum to the inner ear

_____ 14. The fluid found in the anterior chamber of the eye, in front of the lens

_____ 15. White of the eyes

_____ 16. Ringing or buzzing in the ears

_____ 17. A tubular structure in the middle ear that runs to the nasopharynx (throat)

_____ 18. The outer protecting portion of the ear

TRUE OR FALSE

Write T or F next to each statement.

_____ 1. The cornea contains blood vessels that provide nourishment to the eye.

_____ 2. The iris is responsible for the color of the eye.

_____ 3. Glaucoma can cause blindness.

_____ 4. Corrective lenses can be used for glaucoma treatment.

_____ 5. Lacrimal glands are activated by the sympathetic nervous system.

_____ 6. Ophthalmic erythromycin comes in many dosage forms.

_____ 7. The Eustachian tube is located in the middle ear.

_____ 8. The human ear is only responsible for hearing.

_____ 9. An ophthalmic medication commonly is prescribed to treat an otic condition.

_____ 10. Most infections of the ear are caused by bacterial infections.

SYSTEM IDENTIFIER

Identify the components of the eye and eyelid and enter the term next to the corresponding number.

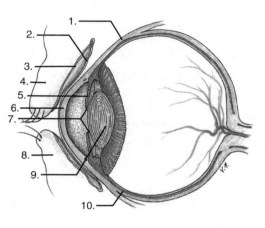

1. _____

2. _____

3. _____

4. _____

5. _____

6. _____

7. _____

8. _____

9. _____

10. _____

Identify the components of the ear and enter the term next to the corresponding number.

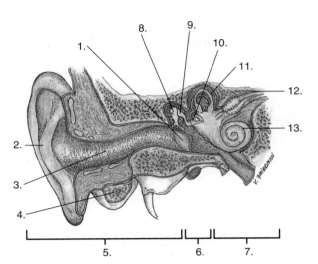

1. _____   8. _____

2. _____   9. _____

3. _____   10. _____

4. _____   11. _____

5. _____   12. _____

6. _____   13. _____

7. _____

MULTIPLE CHOICE

Complete each question by circling the best answer.

1. Alteration of which two senses can most dramatically change a life?
   A. Sight and touch
   B. Smell and taste
   C. Hearing and sight
   D. Smell and hearing

2. A person who is trained to perform an eye examination is called an:
   A. Optician
   B. Optometrist
   C. Optimist
   D. Ophthalmologist

3. Agents indicated for the treatment of glaucoma include all of the following *except*:
   A. Pilocar
   B. Xalatan
   C. Azopt
   D. Bleph-10

Chapter **24** Therapeutic Agents for the Eyes, Ears, Nose, and Throat

4. Glaucoma is caused by:
   A. Viral infections
   B. Bacterial infections
   C. Increased pressure within the eye
   D. Allergies

5. Which of the following is *not* a cause of conjunctivitis?
   A. Virus
   B. Bacterial infections
   C. Postoperative ocular inflammation
   D. Allergies

6. Which drug would be indicated for conjunctivitis?
   A. Patanol
   B. Tobrex
   C. Lumigan
   D. Restasis

7. A possible side effect of Xalatan is:
   A. Drowsiness
   B. Nausea and vomiting
   C. Diarrhea
   D. Changes in iris color

8. What are the two major functions of the eardrum?
   A. To produce cerumen
   B. To protect the middle ear from foreign objects
   C. To transmit sound toward the middle ear
   D. B and C

9. The part of the eye that contains antimicrobial enzymes that help protect the eye from infection is the:
   A. Retina
   B. Sclera
   C. Lacrimal gland
   D. Conjunctiva

10. The _____ contain(s) the photoreceptive cells for vision.
    A. Choroids
    B. Cornea
    C. Vitreous body
    D. Retina

FILL IN THE BLANKS

Answer each question by completing the statement in the space provided.

1. An alternative to wearing glasses is _____ surgery.

2. Three common ophthalmic dosage forms are _____, _____, and _____.

3. Carbonic anhydrase inhibitors are used as a long-term treatment for _____ _____ _____ and short-term preoperatively for individuals with _____ _____ _____.

4. Most of the agents used to reduce inflammation of the eyes or the ears are _____ and _____ (dosage forms).

424

5. Decongestants, antihistamines, and mast cell stabilizers are used to combat _____.

6. Three common viral infections of the eye are _____ _____, _____ and _____.

7. The three main functions of the ear are _____, _____ and _____.

8. The fluid-filled inner ear is called the _____, which transmits sound via _____ _____ to the brain.

9. Pediatricians or ear, nose, and throat doctors (ENTs) insert _____ _____ in the ears of children who suffer from chronic _____ _____.

10. In addition to antiinfectives, _____, _____ and _____ are often used to treat the symptoms of otitis media.

MATCHING

Matching I
Match the following trade and generic drug names.

_____ 1. Trusopt	A. Latanoprost
_____ 2. Xalatan	B. Dexamethasone
_____ 3. Voltaren	C. Tobramycin
_____ 4. Maxidex	D. Dorzolamide
_____ 5. Tobrex	E. Diclofenac
_____ 6. Diamox	F. Phenylephrine
_____ 7. Timoptic	G. Moxifloxacin
_____ 8. Vigimox	H. Antipyrine/benzocaine
_____ 9. Neo-Synephrine	I. Acetazolamide
_____10. Auralgan	J. Timolol

Matching II
Match the following medications or products with the conditions they treat.

_____ 1. Swim-Ear	A. Allergy of the eyes
_____ 2. Zaditor	B. Otitis media
_____ 3. Cerumenex	C. Eye infection
_____ 4. Erythromycin	D. Ear wax softening
_____ 5. Omnicef	E. Swimmer's ear

Matching III

Match the following medications with their drug classification.

_____ 1. Lumigan
_____ 2. Ocupress
_____ 3. Azopt
_____ 4. Ciloxin
_____ 5. PredForte
_____ 6. Pilocar
_____ 7. Opticrom
_____ 8. Acular
_____ 9. Genoptic
_____10. OcuClear

A. Antiviral
B. Cholinergic
C. Beta-adrenergic blocker
D. Mast cell stabilizer
E. NSAID
F. Prostaglandin agonist
G. Antibiotic
H. Corticosteroid
I. Adrenergic agonist
J. Carbonic anhydrase inhibitor

SHORT ANSWER

Reply to each question based on what you have learned in the chapter.

1. List two ways those with allergies can minimize symptoms without drug therapy.

   _____

   _____

2. List the side effects of ophthalmic antiviral medications.

   _____

   _____

3. List several ways to help avoid conjunctivitis.

   _____

   _____

4. List available ophthalmic dosage forms for treating glaucoma.

   _____

   _____

5. Besides antiinfectives, list other types of medications that may be used to treat the symptoms of otitis media.

   _____

   _____

6. In addition to antibiotic therapy, list other medications that can be used for symptom management of bacterial sinusitis.

   _____

   _____

RESEARCH ACTIVITIES

Follow the instructions given in each exercise and provide a response.

1. Visit a local pharmacy and locate the eye- and ear-care sections.

   A. What is the active ingredient in most OTC eye drops?

   B. What is the active ingredient in most OTC ear drops?

   C. What is the active ingredient in nasal saline spray?

2. Access the website *http://www.glaucoma.org/research/*. What are the latest developments in the treatment of glaucoma?

REFLECT CRITICALLY

CRITICAL THINKING

Reply to each question based on what you have learned in the chapter.

1. You been working in the intravenous (IV) room all day and your eyes are feeling very dry. What is the reason for your "dry eyes" and what can you do to resolve the situation?

2. Night blindness is often caused by a lack of vitamin A. What food(s) can you eat to help prevent night blindness?

3. Your child came home from school with "pinkeye." How can you prevent yourself from getting this contagious eye infection?

4. Why is sodium chloride (NaCl) an ingredient in every artificial tear product?

5. How is having an inner ear infection different from having a middle ear infection?

RELATE TO PRACTICE

LAB SCENARIOS

Therapeutic Agents for the Eyes, Ears, Nose, and Throat

Objective: To review with the pharmacy technician terms associated with the eyes, ears, nose, and throat and review the brand and generic name, indications, contraindications, adverse effects, dosage forms, routes of administration, and recommended daily dosage of medications used to treat disorders affecting the eyes, ears, nose and throat.

DID YOU KNOW?

- Glaucoma is the leading cause of blindness in the United States and second-leading cause in the world.
- Over 2.2 million Americans have glaucoma and are not aware of it.
- More than 10 million physician visits are made yearly for glaucoma.

Lab Activity #24.1: Define the following terms associated with the eyes, ears, nose, and throat.

Equipment needed:

- Medical dictionary
- Pencil/pen

Time needed to complete this activity: 30 minutes

1. Auralgia _____

2. Blepharitis _____

3. Closed-angle glaucoma _____

4. Conjunctivitis _____

5. Cytomegalovirus _____

6. Herpes simplex keratitis _____

7. Herpes zoster ophthalmicus _____

8. Iritis _____

9. Keratitis _____

10. Ocular toxoplasmosis _____

11. Open-angle glaucoma _____

12. Otalgia _____

13. Otitis externa _____

14. Otitis media _____

15. Otorrhea _____

16. Otosclerosis _____

17. Photopsia _____

18. Stye _____

19. Uveitis _____

20. Vertigo _____

Lab Activity #24.2: Using a drug reference book, identify the generic name, drug classification, indications, contraindications, adverse effects, dosage forms, routes of administration, and recommended daily dosage of medications used to treat conditions affecting the eyes, ears, nose, and throat.

Equipment needed:

- *Drug Facts & Comparisons* or *Physicians' Desk Reference*
- Pencil/pen

Time needed to complete this activity: 60 minutes

Brand (Trade) Name	Generic Name	Drug Classification	Indication	List Two Contraindications	List Five Adverse Effects	Dosage Forms Available	Routes of Administration	Recommended Daily Dosage Adult	Recommended Daily Dosage Pedi	Drug Interactions	Pregnancy Category	Patient Information
Alphagan P												
Antivert												
Cerumenex												
Ciloxan												
Ciprodex Otic												
Cortisporin Otic												
Cosopt												
Cytovene												
Foscavir												
Iopidine												
Lumigan												
Maxitrol												
Neosporin Ophthalmic												
Patanol												
Restasis												
Sulamyd												
Timoptic												
TobraDex												
Transderm Scop												
Travatan												
Trusopt												
Xalatan												

Using Therapeutic Agents for the Eyes, Ears, Nose, and Throat

Objective: To review with the pharmacy technician prescription orders, dosage calculations, and reconstituting a solid.

Lab Activity #24.3: Answer the questions based on the prescription orders for each question.

Equipment needed:

■ *Drug Facts and Comparisons* or *Physician's Desk Reference*
■ Pencil/pen
■ Calculator

Time needed to complete this activity: 30 minutes

The following are approved DAW codes:
    DAW 0: no product selection indicated
    DAW 1: substitution not allowed by provider
    DAW 2: substitution allowed: patient requested product dispensed
    DAW 3: substitution allowed: pharmacist selected product dispensed
    DAW 4: substitution allowed: generic drug not in stock
    DAW 5: substitution allowed: brand drug dispensed as generic
    DAW 6: override
    DAW 7: substitution not allowed: brand drug mandated by law
    DAW 8: substitution allowed: generic drug not available in marketplace
    DAW 9: other

1. Rx 1:
Ciloxin Ophthalmic Solution 10 ml
gtts i to ii ou q2h while awake x2d, gtts i to ii q4h while awake x5d

    A. How much will be dispensed (use metric quantities)? _____

    B. How many days will the medication last? _____

    C. How many refills are permitted on the prescription? _____

    D. What DAW code will be used? _____

    E. Write directions as they would appear on the medication label.

    _____

    _____

    F. What auxiliary label(s) should be affixed to the medication label?

    _____

    _____

    _____

2. Rx 2:
Acetasol HC Otic Solution 10 ml
gtts iii to v q4-6h utd
Ref

    A. How much will be dispensed (use metric quantities)? _____

    B. How many days will the medication last? _____

    C. How many refills are permitted on the prescription? _____

D. What DAW code will be used?

_____

E. Write directions as they would appear on the medication label.

_____

_____

F. What auxiliary label(s) should be affixed to the medication label?

_____

_____

_____

3. Rx 3:
Cortisporin Otic Suspension 10 ml
gtts ii to iii au q4h for ear infection
Ref

A. How much will be dispensed (use metric quantities)? _____

B. How many days will the medication last? _____

C. How many refills are permitted on the prescription? _____

D. What DAW code will be used?

_____

E. Write directions as they would appear on the medication label.

_____

_____

F. What auxiliary label(s) should be affixed to the medication label?

_____

_____

_____

4. Rx 4:
A/B Otic Solution 10 ml
gtts iii to v q2h prn p
Ref

A. How much will be dispensed (use metric quantities)? _____

B. How many days will the medication last? _____

C. How many refills are permitted on the prescription? _____

D. What DAW code will be used?

_____

E. Write directions as they would appear on the medication label.

_____

_____

F. What auxiliary label(s) should be affixed to the medication label?

_____

_____

_____

5. Rx 5:
   Vigamox 3 ml
   gtts i os tid x7d
   Ref

   A. How much will be dispensed (use metric quantities)? _____

   B. How many days will the medication last? _____

   C. How many refills are permitted on the prescription? _____

   D. What DAW code will be used?

   _____

   E. Write directions as they would appear on the medication label.

   _____

   _____

   F. What auxiliary label(s) should be affixed to the medication label?

   _____

   _____

   _____

6. Rx 6:
   Vexol 1% Ophthalmic Suspension
   gtts ii ou qid x2 weeks
   Ref

   A. How much will be dispensed (use metric quantities)? _____

   B. How many days will the medication last? _____

   C. How many refills are permitted on the prescription? _____

   D. What DAW code will be used?

   _____

Chapter **24** Therapeutic Agents for the Eyes, Ears, Nose, and Throat

E. Write directions as they would appear on the medication label.

_____

_____

F. What auxiliary label(s) should be affixed to the medication label?

_____

_____

_____

7. Rx 7:
   Azopt 1% Ophthalmic Suspension 2.5 ml
   gtt i od tid
   Ref x 2

   A. How much will be dispensed (use metric quantities)? _____

   B. How many days will the medication last? _____

   C. How many refills are permitted on the prescription? _____

   D. What DAW code will be used?

   _____

   E. Write directions as they would appear on the medication label.

   _____

   _____

   F. What auxiliary label(s) should be affixed to the medication label?

   _____

   _____

   _____

8. Rx 8:
   Lumigan 0.03% Ophthalmic Solution 2.5 ml
   gtt i ou qpm
   Ref x 1

   A. How much will be dispensed (use metric quantities)? _____

   B. How many days will the medication last? _____

   C. How many refills are permitted on the prescription? _____

   D. What DAW code will be used?

   _____

   E. Write directions as they would appear on the medication label.

   _____

   _____

F. What auxiliary label(s) should be affixed to the medication label?

_____

_____

_____

9. Rx 9:
   Patanol 5 ml
   gtt i ou bid
   Ref x 5

   A. How much will be dispensed (use metric quantities)? _____

   B. How many days will the medication last? _____

   C. How many refills are permitted on the prescription? _____

   D. What DAW code will be used?

   _____

   E. Write directions as they would appear on the medication label.

   _____

   _____

   F. What auxiliary label(s) should be affixed to the medication label?

   _____

   _____

   _____

10. Rx 10:
    Timoptic 0.5% Ophthalmic Solution 10 ml
    gtt i ou bid
    Ref x 3

    A. How much will be dispensed (use metric quantities)? _____

    B. How many days will the medication last? _____

    C. How many refills are permitted on the prescription? _____

    D. What DAW code will be used?

    _____

    E. Write directions as they would appear on the medication label.

    _____

    _____

Chapter **24** **Therapeutic Agents for the Eyes, Ears, Nose, and Throat**

F. What auxiliary label(s) should be affixed to the medication label?

_____

_____

_____

11. Rx 11:
    Genoptic 5 ml
    gtt ii ou q4h
    Ref

    A. How much will be dispensed (use metric quantities)? _____

    B. How many days will the medication last? _____

    C. How many refills are permitted on the prescription? _____

    D. What DAW code will be used?

    _____

    E. Write directions as they would appear on the medication label.

    _____

    _____

    F. What auxiliary label(s) should be affixed to the medication label?

    _____

    _____

    _____

12. Rx 12:
    Xalatan 2.5 ml
    gtt i ou qpm
    Ref x 6

    A. How much will be dispensed (use metric quantities)? _____

    B. How many days will the medication last? _____

    C. How many refills are permitted on the prescription? _____

    D. What DAW code will be used?

    _____

    E. Write directions as they would appear on the medication label.

    _____

    _____

    F. Where should this medication be stored? _____

G. What auxiliary label(s) should be affixed to the medication label?

_____

_____

_____

Lab Activity #24.4: Reconstituting an antibiotic.

Equipment needed:

- Reconstitution tube
- Distilled water (diluent)
- Amoxicillin 250 mg/5 ml, 100 ml
- Disinfecting agent/cleanser
- "Shake well" label
- Storage label
- Expiration date label
- Lint-free paper towels
- Pen
- Calculator

Time needed to complete this activity: 20 minutes

13. Rx 13:
    Amoxicillin 250 mg/5 ml, 100 ml
    200 mg bid x10 d for ear infection
    No Refills

    A. How many mLs of Amoxicillin 250 mg/5 ml suspension will the patient take at each dose?

    B. Using the dose on the prescription, how much leftover medication will remain after the 10-day regimen?

    C. What should the patient be advised to do with the remaining medication in the bottle after the 10-day regimen?

Procedure

1. Gather supplies necessary to reconstitute the antibiotic for this prescription.
2. Wash hands.
3. Make sure the lower clamp on the reconstitution tube is clamped closed by pinching the clamp until it clicks shut.
4. Open the upper clamp on the reconstitution tube by clicking the clamp open.
5. Allow the amount of distilled water needed (on antibiotic bottle) to flow into the reconstitution tube. When the tube is filled to that amount, close the upper clamp by pinching it shut.
6. Shake the antibiotic power to loosen it, then remove bottle top.
7. Place the tip of the lower tube of the reconstitution tube into the mouth of the antibiotic bottle.
8. Open the lower clamp to allow approximately ⅔ of the water to enter the antibiotic bottle. Close lower clamp.
9. Place bottle top back on the bottle and shake well.
10. Remove bottle top and place the tip of the reconstitution tube into the mouth of the amber bottle and add remaining water into the antibiotic bottle.
11. Tightly recap the bottle and shake well.
12. Label with necessary auxiliary labels—beyond-use date, storage requirements, shake well.
13. Clean work area
14. Complete compounding log.

Pharmacy Compounding Log						
Drug Name	Lot Number	Mfg. Expiration Date	Quantity Prepared	Measured By	Verified By	Beyond-Use Date

25 Therapeutic Agents for the Dermatologic System

TERMS AND DEFINITIONS

Select the correct term from the following list and write the corresponding letter in the blank next to the statement.

A. Acne Vulgaris
B. Alopecia
C. Antiseptic
D. Comedone
E. Eczema
F. Emollient
G. Eschar
H. Exfoliation
I. Hirtusim
J. Keratolytic
K. Melanin
L. Metastasize
M. Nodule
N. Onychomycosis
O. Papule
P. Pustule
Q. Pruritus
R. Seborrhea
S. Sebum
T. Uticaria
U. Xerosis

_____ 1. A substance that slows or stops the growth of microorganisms on surfaces such as skin

_____ 2. Oily/waxy substance that lubricates the skin and keeps water in to provide moisture

_____ 3. A medical condition in which patches of skin become rough and inflamed

_____ 4. A small swelling or aggregation of cells in the body

_____ 5. Abnormal dryness of the skin, eyes, or mucous membranes

_____ 6. Itching

_____ 7. Excessive discharge of sebum from the sebaceous glands

_____ 8. Also known as hives; red welts that arise on the surface of the skin, often attributable to an allergic reaction but may have nonallergic causes

_____ 9. A small blister or pimple on the skin containing pus

_____ 10. The process by which cancer spreads from the place of origin as a primary tumor to distant locations in the body

_____ 11. A small, raised, solid pimple on the skin

_____ 12. Commonly known as pimples, this condition occurs when the pores of the skin are clogged with oil or bacteria

_____ 13. A drug that causes shedding of the outer layer of the skin

_____ 14. The peeling off of dead skin

_____ 15. A preparation that softens the skin

_____ 16. A dark brown to black pigment occurring in the hair, skin, and iris of the eye

_____ 17. Blackhead; a plug of keratin and sebum within a hair follicle that is blackened at the surface

_____ 18. The partial or complete absence of hair from areas of the body where it normally grows; baldness

_____ 19. Abnormal growth of hair on a person's face and body

_____ 20. A slough produced by a thermal burn, by a corrosive application, or by gangrene

_____ 21. A fungal infection of the fingernails or toenails

TRUE OR FALSE

Write T or F next to each statement.

_____ 1. The skin is one of the most abused organs of the body system.

_____ 2. The skin is one of the smallest organs in the body.

_____ 3. The lunula is the small white portion at the tip of the nail.

_____ 4. Growths on the surface of the skin are common and not all are cancerous.

_____ 5. UV exposure may be used as treatment for psoriasis.

_____ 6. Psoriasis is an uncommon and infectious inflammatory skin disorder.

_____ 7. Burns range in severity from first degree to fourth degree with fourth degree as the most severe.

_____ 8. Warts are not contagious.

_____ 9. Nails on both hands and feet endure daily abuse and can become damaged.

_____ 10. Onychomycosis infection normally starts at the base of one or more toenails.

SYSTEM IDENTIFIER

Label the following parts of the skin.

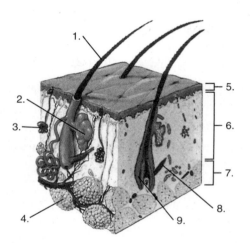

1. _____

2. _____

3. _____

4. _____

5. _____

6. _____

7. _____

8. _____

9. _____

Complete each question by circling the best answer.

1. The function of the skin is to protect the body against heat, cold, light, dehydration, and:
   A. Sunburn
   B. Injuries
   C. Infection
   D. Broken bones

2. The two glands that are within the layers of the skin are the sebaceous and _____ glands:
   A. Thyroid
   B. Sebum
   C. Sweat
   D. Lymph

3. Acne is a common condition caused by the inflammation of sebaceous glands that produce:
   A. Pustules
   B. Comedones
   C. Scars
   D. All of the above

4. _____ are used to treat the symptoms of urticaria.
   A. Decongestants
   B. Antihistamines
   C. Sunscreens
   D. Ibuprofen

5. Abnormal growth of new tissue on the skin that results in a malignancy is known as:
   A. Skin cancer
   B. A skin tag
   C. A wart
   D. A nodule

6. Psoriasis patients who have developed arthritic symptoms are often prescribed:
   A. Methotrexate
   B. NSAIDS
   C. Sulfasalazine
   D. All of the above

7. Treatment for herpes zoster includes:
   A. Neomycin
   B. Valacyclovir
   C. Clotrimazole
   D. Betamethasone

8. Treatment for plantar warts includes:
   A. Benzoyl peroxide
   B. Permethrin
   C. Salicylic acid
   D. Fluocinolone

9. Impetigo can be treated with:
   A. Mupirocin
   B. Fluorouracil
   C. Coal tar
   D. Hydrocortisone

10. The iPLEDGE program is aimed at preventing pregnancy during the use of _____ products.
    A. Tetracycline
    B. Tretinoin
    C. Diphenhydramine
    D. Isotretinoin

FILL IN THE BLANKS

Answer each question by completing the statement in the space provided.

1. The nerves allow the skin to detect _____, _____ and _____.

2. Hair and nails are composed of a protein called _____.

3. The most effective non–drug treatment for acne is to keep the skin clean and free from _____ by using cleansing agents that will _____ sebum production and exfoliate dead skin cells.

4. Hives are commonly caused by _____ reactions to food, the environment, or drugs, and can occur anywhere on the body.

5. Applying a _____, _____ compress helps to alleviate the itching that accompanies hives.

6. Topical _____ can also be used to alleviate symptoms of pruritus.

7. _____ are widely used to treat pruritus associated with eczema.

8. _____ may be used to cause mild sunburn of the skin and subsequent peeling in patients with more serious psoriasis disease.

9. Prolonged use of _____ is not recommended because of possible overgrowth of resistant bacteria.

10. Prescription treatments for lice include _____ and _____, which are reserved for resistant cases.

MATCHING

Match the trade and generic drug names.

_____ 1. Bactroban

_____ 2. Lamisil

_____ 3. Nizoral

_____ 4. Temovate

_____ 5. Retin-A

A. Clobetasol propionate
B. Terbinafine
C. Tretionoin
D. Mupirocin
E. Ketoconazole

Match the drugs with their indications.

_____ 1. Silvadene

_____ 2. Elidel

_____ 3. Desenex

_____ 4. Claravis

_____ 5. Remicade

A. Antifungal
B. Psoriasis
C. Burn wound infections
D. Acne
E. Eczema

442

SHORT ANSWER

Reply to each question based on what you have learned in the chapter.

1. List three common skin conditions that can be self-managed with OTC products.

   _____

   _____

2. List two topical agents that can be used to help treat mild acne and how they work.

   _____

   _____

3. List two medications used for the treatment of shingles.

   _____

   _____

4. List two prescription treatments for resistant cases of lice.

   _____

   _____

RESEARCH ACTIVITIES

Follow the instructions given in each exercise and provide a response.

1. Access the website *https://www.ipledgeprogram.com/PrescriberInformation.aspx.*

   A. What are the Isotretinoin prescribing requirements for females and males?

   B. What are the requirements for pharmacists when dispensing Isotretinoin?

   C. As a pharmacy technician, how can you help the pharmacist meet the necessary requirements to dispense Isotretinoin?

2. Access the website *http://www.cdc.gov/std/hpv/stdfact-hpv.htm.*

   A. What potential health problems are caused by HPV?

B. How can HPV be prevented?

C. What vaccinations are available for HPV? What is the vaccination schedule?

D. In your state, can this vaccination be administered by the pharmacist? If so, how can you help the pharmacist educate and administer the vaccination?

REFLECT CRITICALLY

CRITICAL THINKING

Reply to each question based on what you have learned in the chapter.

1. Jamie is a pharmacy technician in a local retail store. A patient is complaining that her skin condition is worsening while using the prescribed antibacterial agent. Jamie directs the patient to the pharmacist for counseling. What will the pharmacist most likely tell the patient?

2. A patient is prescribed a corticosteroid ointment for psoriasis. Describe some of the possible side effects, especially if used long term.

3. Cathy goes to the doctor shortly after giving birth and returning home from the hospital. She is complaining of vaginal itching. On further questioning, she reveals that her newborn has "white spots" in her mouth. What do you suspect may be the problem, and what might be prescribed?

4. Gus is a pharmacy technician in a specialty hospital. A patient is brought in with multiple severe burns. What special precautions would Gus need to observe when preparing medication for this patient?

LAB SCENARIOS

Therapeutic Agents for the Dermatologic System

Objective: To review with the pharmacy technician terms associated with the dermatologic system and review the brand and generic names, indications, contraindications, adverse effects, dosage forms, routes of administration, and daily dosage of medications used to treat disorders of the dermatologic system.

DID YOU KNOW?

- Acne is the most common disorder, affecting 40 to 50 million Americans.
- In 2004, over $2.2 billion were spent on acne treatment.
- Approximately 7.5 million Americans have psoriasis.
- In 2004, $1.2 billion were spent on the treatment of psoriasis.

Lab Activity #25.1: Define the following terms associated with the dermatologic system.

Equipment Needed:

- Medical dictionary
- Pencil/pen

Time needed to complete this activity: 30 minutes

1. Acne _____

2. Acne vulgaris _____

3. Allergy _____

4. Blister _____

5. Candidiasis _____

6. Comedone _____

7. Cysts _____

8. Decubitus ulcer _____

9. Dermatitis _____

10. Eczema _____

11. Fungus _____

12. Mycoses _____

13. Onychomycosis _____

14. Papule _____

15. Petechiae _____

16. Psoriasis _____

17. Pustule _____

18. Ringworm _____

19. Scabies _____

20. Tinea capitis _____

21. Tinea manus _____

22. Tinea pedis _____

23. Tinea unguium _____

24. Urticaria _____

25. Wheal _____

Lab Activity #25.2: Using a drug reference book, identify the generic name, drug classification, indications, contraindications, adverse effects, dosage forms, routes of administration, and daily dosage of medications used to treat conditions affecting the dermatologic system.

Equipment needed:

■ *Drug Facts & Comparisons* or *Physicians' Desk Reference*
■ Pencil/pen

Time needed to complete this activity: 60 minutes

Brand (Trade) Name	Generic Name	Drug Classification	Indication	List Two Contraindications	List Five Adverse Effects	Dosage Forms Available	Routes of Administration	Recommended Daily Dosage		Drug Interactions	Pregnancy Category	Patient Information
								Adult	Pedi			
Accutane												
Aclovate												
Azelex												
Bactroban												
Benzac												
BenzaClin												
Clindagel												
Clobex												
Differin												
Diflucan												
Dovonex												
Dynacin												
Gris-Peg												
Kenalog												
Lamisil												
Lidoderm												
Loprox												
MetroCream												
MetroGel												
Minocin												
Nizoral												
Renagel												
Renova												
Retin-A												
Silvadene												
Spectazole												
Sporanox												
Sumycin												
Tazorac												
Topicort												
Ultravate												
Vibramycin												
Westcort												

447

Using Therapeutic Agents for the Dermatologic System

Objective: To review with the pharmacy technician prescription orders, dosage calculations, and extemporaneous compounding.

Lab Activity #25.3: Answer the questions based on the prescription orders for each question.

Equipment needed:

- *Drug Facts and Comparisons* or *Physician's Desk Reference*
- Pencil/pen
- Calculator

Time needed to complete this activity: 15 minutes

The following are approved DAW codes:
- DAW 0: no product selection indicated
- DAW 1: substitution not allowed by provider
- DAW 2: substitution allowed: patient requested product dispensed
- DAW 3: substitution allowed: pharmacist selected product dispensed
- DAW 4: substitution allowed: generic drug not in stock
- DAW 5: substitution allowed: brand drug dispensed as generic
- DAW 6: override
- DAW 7: substitution not allowed: brand drug mandated by law
- DAW 8: substitution allowed: generic drug not available in marketplace
- DAW 9: other

---

1. Rx 1:
   Duac Gel 45 g
   app top to face qd hs
   Ref x3

   A. How much will be dispensed (use metric quantities)? _____

   B. How many days will the medication last? _____

   C. How many refills are permitted on the prescription? _____

   D. What DAW code will be used? _____

   E. Write directions as they would appear on the medication label.

   _____

   _____

   F. What auxiliary label(s) should be affixed to the medication label?

   _____

   _____

   _____

2. Rx 2:
   Monodox 100 mg 1 month supply
   i cap q12h
   Ref x 5

   A. How much will be dispensed? _____

   B. How many days will the medication last? _____

   C. How many refills are permitted on the prescription? _____

   D. What DAW code will be used? _____

   E. Write directions as they would appear on the medication label.

   _____

   _____

   F. What auxiliary label(s) should be affixed to the medication label?

   _____

   _____

   _____

3. Rx 3:
   Benzamycin 46 g
   app bid p washing face
   Ref x 6

   A. How much will be dispensed (use metric quantities)?_____

   B. How many days will the medication last? _____

   C. How many refills are permitted on the prescription? _____

   D. What DAW code will be used?

   E. Write directions as they would appear on the medication label.

   _____

   _____

   F. How should this medication be reconstituted? Where should it be stored after reconstitution?

   _____

   _____

   _____

   G. What auxiliary label(s) should be affixed to the medication label?

   _____

   _____

Chapter **25** **Therapeutic Agents for the Dermatologic System**

4. Rx 4:
   Bactroban ung 22 g
   app affected area tid x3d
   Ref

   A. How much will be dispensed (use metric quantities)? _____

   B. How many days will the medication last? _____

   C. How many refills are permitted on the prescription? _____

   D. What DAW code will be used? _____

   E. Write directions as they would appear on the medication label.

   _____

   _____

   F. What auxiliary label(s) should be affixed to the medication label?

   _____

   _____

   _____

5. Rx 5:
   Temovate Cr 45 g
   app affected area bid utd
   Ref

   A. How much will be dispensed (use metric quantities)? _____

   B. How many days will the medication last? _____

   C. How many refills are permitted on the prescription? _____

   D. What DAW code will be used? _____

   E. Write directions as they would appear on the medication label.

   _____

   _____

   F. What auxiliary label(s) should be affixed to the medication label?

   _____

   _____

   _____

6. Rx 6:
   Kenalog spray 100 g
   app affected area tid to qid utd
   Ref

   A. How much will be dispensed (use metric quantities)? _____

   B. How many days will the medication last? _____

   C. How many refills are permitted on the prescription? _____

D. What DAW code will be used? _____

E. Write directions as they would appear on the medication label.

_____

_____

F. What auxiliary label(s) should be affixed to the medication label?

_____

_____

_____

7. Rx 7:
   Lamisil 250 mg #30
   i tab daily
   Ref x3

   A. How much will be dispensed? _____

   B. How many days will the medication last? _____

   C. How many refills are permitted on the prescription? _____

   D. What DAW code will be used? _____

   E. Write directions as they would appear on the medication label.

   _____

   _____

   F. What auxiliary label(s) should be affixed to the medication label?

   _____

   _____

8. Rx 8:
   Lotrisone Lotion 1 oz
   app affected area bid, qam and qpm x1 week
   Ref

   A. How much will be dispensed (use metric quantities)? _____

   B. How many days will the medication last? _____

   C. How many refills are permitted on the prescription? _____

   D. What DAW code will be used? _____

   E. Write directions as they would appear on the medication label.

   _____

   _____

F. What auxiliary label(s) should be affixed to the medication label?

_____

_____

_____

9. Rx 9:
   Enbrel (1 carton)
   50 mg weekly
   Ref x3

   A. How much will be dispensed (use metric quantities)? _____

   B. How many days will the medication last? _____

   C. How many refills are permitted on the prescription? _____

   D. What DAW code will be used? _____

   E. Write directions as they would appear on the medication label.

   _____

   _____

   F. Where should this medication be stored? _____

   G. What auxiliary label(s) should be affixed to the medication label?

   _____

   _____

   _____

10. Rx 10:
    Differin Gel 0.3% 1.5 oz
    app qd hs utd
    Ref x3

    A. How much will be dispensed (use metric quantities)? _____

    B. How many days will the medication last? _____

    C. How many refills are permitted on the prescription? _____

    D. What DAW code will be used? _____

    E. Write directions as they would appear on the medication label.

    _____

    _____

    F. What auxiliary label(s) should be affixed to the medication label?

    _____

    _____

    _____

Lab Activity #25.4: Calculate the quantity of the ingredients needed to prepare the following topical medications.

Equipment needed:

- Calculator
- Pencil/pen
- Paper

Time needed to complete this activity: 30 minutes

1. You are to prepare 2 ounces of 1% hydrocortisone cream from 2.5% hydrocortisone cream and 0.25% hydrocortisone cream. How many grams of each ingredient will you need?

   2.5% hydrocortisone cream: _____

   0.25% hydrocortisone cream: _____

2. You are to prepare an ointment containing 20% coal tar from 1200 g of 5% coal tar ointment and concentrated coal tar. How many grams of coal tar should be added to the 1200 g of 5% coal tar ointment to prepare a 20% coal tar ointment?

   Coal tar: _____

3. You are to prepare 4 ounces of Deltasone Cream 0.025%. How many mg of Deltasone will you need?

   Deltasone: _____

4. You have 4 ounces of 0.1% betamethasone cream in stock. To prepare a 0.05% betamethasone cream you will have to dilute your stock. How many grams of diluent cream will you need to add to prepare 0.05% betamethasone cream?

   Diluent cream: _____

5. You are to prepare 8 ounces of a 4% zinc oxide ointment. How many grams of zinc oxide will you need?

   Zinc oxide: _____

Lab Activity #25.5: Compounding a paste.

Prepare 1 ounce of the following formula:
Zinc Oxide	7.5 g
Cornstarch	7.5 g
Glycerin	
White Petrolatum	15 g

Equipment needed:

- Calculator
- Pen
- Disinfecting agent/cleanser
- Sink with running hot and cold water
- Latex gloves
- Electronic balance or torsion balance with metric weights
- Weigh boats or weigh papers
- Ointment slab or parchment paper
- Spatula
- Mortar card
- Zinc oxide powder
- Cornstarch
- Glycerin
- White petrolatum
- Ziploc bag (if desired)

- 1-ounce jar or tube for dispensing
- Label
- Auxiliary labels

Procedure

1. Wash hands and dry thoroughly.
2. Gather all necessary supplies.
3. Double check recipe and calculations.
4. Put gloves on.
5. Weigh zinc oxide, cornstarch, and white petrolatum on electronic balance or torsion balance.
6. Mix the zinc oxide and cornstarch together on an ointment slab or parchment paper.
7. Levigate zinc oxide and cornstarch mixture with a few drops of glycerin to form a paste.
8. Levigate equal amounts of white petrolatum with zinc oxide/cornstarch paste using an "S" pattern with the spatula.
9. Levigate well.
10. Check product for uniformity and appearance.
11. Using a Ziploc bag, package the paste into an ointment jar or ointment tube ensuring pharmaceutical elegance.
12. Label product with all necessary information—including beyond-use date and auxiliary labels.
13. Document procedure and all necessary information on compounding log.
14. Clean equipment and put away.
15. Clean work area.

Packaging: Ointment jar or tube

Labeling: For external use only. Use only as directed.

BUD: 6 Months or the expiration date of any ingredient if sooner than 6 months

Storage: Room temperature

Time needed to complete this activity: 45 minutes

26 Therapeutic Agents for the Hematologic System

TERMS AND DEFINITIONS

Select the correct term from the following list and write the corresponding letter in the blank next to the statement.

A. Albumin
B. Bone Marrow
C. Erythropoiesis
D. Erythropoietin
E. Hemoglobin
F. Hydrostatic Pressure
G. Osmotic Pressure
H. Pallor
I. Plasma
J. Plasma Protein
K. Serum
L. von Willebrand's Disease

_____ 1. Most common inherited bleeding disorder associated with a deficiency in the clotting protein von Willebrand factor

_____ 2. Oxygen-carrying component of red blood cells

_____ 3. Any of the various dissolved proteins of blood plasma

_____ 4. Pressure exerted by the flow of water through a semipermeable membrane separating two solutions with different concentration of solutes

_____ 5. Major protein found in plasma

_____ 6. Clear, yellowish fluid portion of blood

_____ 7. Formation of erythrocytes

_____ 8. Pressure exerted by a fluid owing to the force of gravity

_____ 9. Tissue that fills the cavities within the long bones that is the source of red blood cells and many white blood cells

_____ 10. Deficiency in color, particularly of the face

_____ 11. Clear, yellowish fluid obtained by separating whole blood into its solid and liquid components after it has been allowed to clot; plasma minus clotting factors

_____ 12. Hormone secreted by the kidney that stimulates the production of red blood cells by stem cells in bone marrow

TRUE OR FALSE

Write T or F next to each statement.

_____ 1. The life span of a platelet is approximately 14 days.

_____ 2. Blood can be divided into two main groups, leukocytes and thrombocytes.

_____ 3. WBCs are cells of the immune system that help defend the body against infection.

_____ 4. Leukocytes are the most prevalent blood cells within the blood.

_____ 5. The main function of RBCs is to carry oxygen to the tissues and organs of the body.

_____ 6. Anemia is caused by a reduction in the total number of WBCs in the body or by a problem with the quality or quantity of hemoglobin present.

_____ 7. Iron deficiency anemia is the most common form of anemia worldwide.

_____ 8. Gastrointestinal bleeding can lead to iron deficiency anemia.

_____ 9. Hypoxia is a form of polycythemia that occurs in people who have a difficult time oxygenating their blood.

_____ 10. The principal treatment goal for thrombocytopenia is to prevent bleeding.

Components of Whole Blood

Identify each component in this system and enter the term next to the corresponding number.

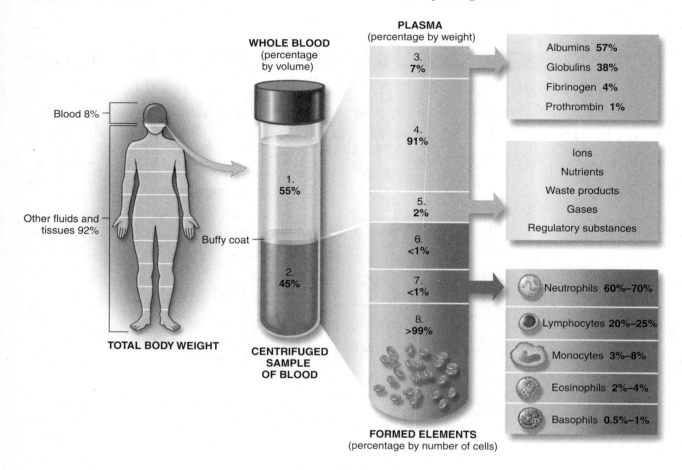

1. _____

2. _____

3. _____

4. _____

5. _____

6. _____

7. _____

8. _____

MULTIPLE CHOICE

Complete each question by circling the best answer.

1. Which of following medications can cause iron deficiency anemia because of GI bleeding?
   A. Droxia
   B. Naprosyn
   C. Hydrea
   D. DexFerrum

2. Mild anemia may be treated with dietary changes including an increase in:
   A. Spinach
   B. Broccoli
   C. Liver
   D. All of the above

3. Which of the following vitamins helps with the absorption of oral iron supplements?
   A. Vitamin A
   B. Vitamin B
   C. Vitamin C
   D. Vitamin D

4. _____ is indicated for iron deficiency anemia in people undergoing chronic dialysis and receiving epoetin alfa therapy.
   A. Ferrlecit
   B. Feosol
   C. Agrylin
   D. Droxia

5. Drug therapy for polycythemia vera involves treatments aimed at minimizing the risk of thrombosis with a myelo-suppressive agent such as:
   A. Vincristine
   B. Bleomycin
   C. Hydroxyurea
   D. Fluorouracil

6. Patients not responding to steroids, immunoglobulins, or splenectomy for thrombocytopenia treatment can take _____.
   A. Rituxan
   B. Gleevec
   C. Fludara
   D. Promacta

7. _____ can be used to treat idiopathic thrombocytopenic purpura (ITP).
   A. Neupogen
   B. Promacta
   C. Leukine
   D. Rheumatrex

8. The primary drugs used in the treatment of neutropenia are recombinant growth factors known as _____.
   A. Antimetabolites
   B. Antibiotics
   C. Colony-stimulating factors
   D. Miotic inhibitors

9. _____ are often used to treat leukemia.
   A. Antimetabolites
   B. Glucocorticoids
   C. Immunoglobulins
   D. Colony-stimulating factors

10. Treatment for von Willebrand's disease includes:
    A. Factor VIII concentrates
    B. DDAVP
    C. Estrogen therapy
    D. All of the above

FILL IN THE BLANKS

Answer each question by completing the statement in the space provided.

1. _____ _____ is a chronic condition where the body overproduces RBCs.

2. Overproduction of RBCs is believed to be caused by an increased sensitivity of stem cells in the bone marrow to the effects of _____.

3. Some of the most common causes of thrombocytopenia are _____, _____ _____ _____, and _____.

4. Transfusions to increase platelet levels may be necessary in individuals with low_____ _____.

5. Non–drug treatment for patients with chronic neutropenia includes avoidance of _____.

6. CSFs can be used _____ for chemotherapy-induced neutropenia as well as therapeutically for people with preexisting neutropenia.

7. Miotic inhibitors, which are used to prevent mitosis at the metaphase stage, are a group of _____ derived from plants.

8. The two major types of alkylating agents are the _____ _____ and _____.

9. Two broad categories of _____ include Hodgkin's disease and non-Hodgkin's.

10. _____ is the most common drug associated with adverse drug events leading to emergency department visits and hospitalization.

MATCHING

Matching I
Match the following trade and generic drug names.

_____ 1. Feosol

_____ 2. Hydrea

_____ 3. Agrylin

_____ 4. Ferrlecit

_____ 5. Promacta

_____ 6. Neupogen

_____ 7. Leukine

_____ 8. DDAVP

_____ 9. Epogen

_____ 10. Cytoxan

A. Anagrelide
B. Filgrastim
C. Epoetin alfa
D. Hydroxyurea
E. Eltrombopag
F. Ferrous sulfate
G. Sargramostim
H. Cyclophosphamide
I. Ferric gluconate
J. Desmopressin

Matching II

Match the following drugs with their classification.

_____ 1. Niferex

_____ 2. Neulasta

_____ 3. Epogen

_____ 4. Gleevec

_____ 5. Paraplatin

_____ 6. Purinethol

_____ 7. Rituxan

_____ 8. Hydrea

_____ 9. Cerubidine

_____ 10. Eldisine

A. Tyrosine kinase inhibitor
B. Antimetabolite
C. Purine nucleoside analogue
D. Oral iron salt
E. RBC stimulating agent
F. Alkylating agent
G. Mitotic inhibitor/vinca alkaloid
H. WBC stimulating agent
I. Monoclonal antibody
J. Anthracycline

SHORT ANSWER

Reply to each question based on what you have learned in the chapter.

1. List the classes of drugs used to treat leukemia.

_____

_____

_____

2. List two agents that cross the blood-brain barrier surrounding the central nervous system, which gives them the ability to treat cancers within the brain.

_____

_____

3. List five factors for the development of lymphoma.

_____

_____

_____

4. List two drugs people using warfarin should avoid taking because of the risk of bleeding.

_____

_____

Follow the instructions given in each exercise and provide a response.

1. Access the website *http://www.hematology.org/Patients/Blood-Disorders/5220.aspx.*

   A. What are eight common blood disorders that affect people?

   B. To what type of physician would you be referred for the diagnosis of a blood disorder?

   C. What clinical trials are currently available for blood disorders?

2. Access the website *http://www.cancer.gov/cancertopics/types/cancersbodylocation/hematologic.*

   A. List the many different types of blood cancers that are known.

   B. What types of treatment are available for blood cancers?

REFLECT CRITICALLY

CRITICAL THINKING

Reply to each question based on what you have learned in the chapter.

1. Why is dental care important for those with neutropenia?

2. Many scientists claim that the cure for cancer lies in the plants of the world's greatest forests. These forests are disappearing as a result of the growth in the world's population and the use of land for mining or agriculture. Should governments get involved in plant-targeted cancer research? Why or why not? What can be done to foster research in this area?

LAB SCENARIOS

Therapeutic Agents for the Hematologic System

Objective: To review with the pharmacy technician terms associated with the components of the hematologic system and review the brand and generic names, indications, contraindications, adverse effects, dosage forms, routes of administration, and recommended daily dosage of medications used to treat disorders of the hematologic system.

DID YOU KNOW?

- One person is diagnosed with a blood cancer every four minutes.
- 9% of new cancer cases will be caused by leukemia, lymphoma, and myeloma.
- Approximately 1,129,813 people are living with or are in remission from, leukemia, Hodgkin lymphoma, non-Hodgkin lymphoma or myeloma.
- 14% of children (<2 years) and 9% of women suffer from iron deficiency.
- 1n 2010, 209,000 emergency room visits were made with anemia as the primary diagnosis.
- In 2010, 4,852 deaths occurred from anemias.

Lab Activity #26.1: Define the following terms associated with the hematologic system.

Equipment needed:

- Medical dictionary
- Pencil/pen

Time needed to complete this activity: 30 minutes

1. Absolute neutrophil count _____

2. Acute lymphoblastic leukemia (ALL) _____

3. Acute myeloblastic leukemia (AML) _____

4. Anemia _____

5. Aplastic Anemia _____

6. Chronic lymphocytic leukemia (CLL) _____

7. Chronic myeloid leukemia (CML) _____

8. Colony stimulating factor (CSF) _____

9. Cryoprecipitate _____

10. Erythrocyte _____

11. Folate deficiency anemia _____

12. Granulocytopenia _____

13. Hemochromatosis _____

14. Hemolytic anemia _____

15. Hemophilia _____

16. Hypoxia _____

17. Idiopathic _____

18. Iron deficiency anemia _____

19. Leukemia _____

461

20. Leukocyte _____

21. Leukopenia _____

22. Lymphoid organ _____

23. Lymphoma _____

24. Myelodysplastic syndrome _____

25. Myeloma _____

26. Neutropenia _____

27. Osmosis _____

28. Pernicious anemia _____

29. Phlebotomy _____

30. Polycythemia _____

31. Sickle cell anemia _____

32. Sideroblastic anemia _____

33. Splenectomy _____

34. Thalassemia _____

35. Thrombocyte _____

36. Thrombocytopenia _____

37. White blood cells _____

Lab Activity #26.2: Using a drug reference book, identify the generic name, drug classification, indications, contraindications, adverse effects, dosage forms, routes of administration, and recommended daily dosage of medications used to treat conditions affecting the hematologic system.

Equipment needed:

- *Drug Facts & Comparisons* or *Physicians' Desk Reference*
- Pencil/pen

Time needed to complete this activity: 60 minutes

Brand (Trade) Name	Generic Name	Drug Classification	Indication	List Two Contraindications	List Five Adverse Effects	Dosage Forms Available	Routes of Administration	Recommended Daily Dosage Adult	Recommended Daily Dosage Pedi	Drug Interactions	Pregnancy Category	Patient Information
Aranesp												
Campath												
Cerubidine												
Cytosar												
Cytoxan												
DexFerrum												
Eldisine												
Epogen												
Feosol												
Ferate												
Ferrlecit												
Ferretts												
Fludara												
Gleevec												
Hydrea												
Leukeran												
Leukine												
Leustatin												
Neulasta												
Neupogen												
Niferex												
Nipent												
Paraplatin												
Purinethol												
Rheumatrex												
Rituxan												
Sprycel												
Tasigna												
Toposar												
Vincasar												
Venofer												
Vesanoid												

Chapter **26** **Therapeutic Agents for the Hematologic System**

Lab Activity #26.3: Using a drug reference book, identify the generic name, storage requirements, and expiration date (at room temperature) for hematologic agents.

Equipment needed:

■ *Handbook on Injectable Drugs*
■ Pencil/pen

Time needed to complete this activity: 30 minutes

Brand Name	Generic Name	Storage Requirements	Expiration Date
Aranesp			
Campath			
Cerubidine			
Cytosar			
Cytoxan			
DexFerrum			
Eldisine			
Epogen			
Ferrlecit			
Fludara			
Leukine			
Leustatin			
Neulasta			
Neupogen			
Nipent			
Paraplatin			
Rituxan			
Toposar			
Venofer			
Vincasar			

27 Over-the-Counter (OTC) Medications

TERMS AND DEFINITIONS

Select the correct term from the following list and write the corresponding letter in the blank next to the statement.

A. Analgesic
B. Antiinflammatory
C. Nutraceutical
D. Antitussive
E. Acetylsalicylic Acid
F. Bulk-Forming
G. Expectorant
H. Pruritus
I. Antipyretic
J. Sunscreen

_____ 1. A food or naturally occurring supplement thought to have a beneficial effect on human health

_____ 2. A drug that reduces fever

_____ 3. Medication relieves pain by reducing the perception of pain.

_____ 4. Aspirin

_____ 5. A drug that thins respiratory secretions, allowing the patient to cough up mucus from the lungs

_____ 6. A substance that protects the skin from ultraviolet (UV) light, thus protecting from sunburn; the skin protection factor (SPF) rates effectiveness

_____ 7. A drug that reduces swelling, redness, and pain and promotes healing

_____ 8. Fiber that can be used for helping both constipation and diarrhea

_____ 9. Itching of the skin

_____ 10. A drug that can reduce the coughing reflex

TRUE OR FALSE

Write T or F next to each statement.

_____ 1. The ability to buy drugs over the counter can lead to substantial savings for customers.

_____ 2. Most OTC drug labels recommend dosages for children younger than 2 years.

_____ 3. It is not important to ask patients if they are taking OTC medications when picking up their prescriptions.

_____ 4. Consumers need to be educated to follow the instructions on OTC products, including the appropriate duration of treatment with OTC medicines.

_____ 5. A potential and common side effect of ibuprofen is an increase in blood pressure.

_____ 6. Long-term PPI use has been linked to increased calcium absorption.

_____ 7. There are more OTC drugs available in different dosage forms, strengths, and combinations compared to legend drugs.

_____ 8. Standards of safety and effectiveness are lower for OTC drugs than for legend drugs.

_____ 9. Acne is a very serious skin conditions and should not be treated at home.

_____ 10. Strep throat can be treated with OTC medications.

MULTIPLE CHOICE

Complete each question by circling the best answer.

1. The number of OTC drugs available to consumers has increased since the:
   A. 1960s
   B. 1970s
   C. 1980s
   D. 1990s

2. When deciding to switch a prescription medication to OTC, the FDA must consider:
   A. If there is enough information proving the medication can be safely taken without a health care provider's prescription and oversight of treatment
   B. If the product's labeling can be read, understood, and followed by the consumer without the guidance of a health care provider
   C. Both A and B
   D. None of the above

3. The same standards of safety and effectiveness that are placed on _____ also are used to approve OTC drugs.
   A. Legend drugs
   B. Dietary supplements
   C. Behind-the-counter drugs
   D. Nutraceutical products

4. Considerations the FDA must take before approving an OTC product include all of the following *except*:
   A. Labeling can be read, understood, and followed without the guidance of a health care provider
   B. OTC product is proven to be half as effective as the corresponding legend drug
   C. OTC product is safe and effective
   D. OTC product can be safely taken without a prescription

5. An OTC monograph includes:
   A. Acceptable ingredients
   B. Formulations
   C. Labeling
   D. All of the above

6. Which condition cannot be treated with OTC drugs?
   A. High blood pressure
   B. Fever
   C. Cough
   D. Diarrhea

7. Children and teenagers should not take aspirin for chickenpox or flu, because it has been associated with:
   A. Toxic shock syndrome
   B. Reye's syndrome
   C. Sudden infant death syndrome
   D. Acquired immunodeficiency syndrome

8. Taking too much _____ on a daily basis can lead to liver toxicity.
   A. Benadryl (diphenhydramine)
   B. Mucinex (guaifenesin)
   C. Motrin (ibuprofen)
   D. Tylenol (acetaminophen)

9. NSAID stands for:
   A. Nonsafety caps for AIDS patients
   B. Not safe as an IUD service
   C. Nonsteroidal antiinflammatory drug
   D. Nonsteroidal antiinflammatory disease

466

10. A common side effect of first-generation antihistamines is:
    A. Drowsiness
    B. Diarrhea
    C. Agitation
    D. Constipation

FILL IN THE BLANKS

Answer each question by completing the statement in the space provided.

1. Unless a prescription is written for an OTC item, the pharmacist is not required to _____ patients on these products.

2. Parents should consult with their pediatrician before giving children younger than _____ years of age any OTC medication.

3. To meet the criteria for designation as an OTC product, drug companies must perform comprehensive studies on the drug's _____ to determine whether consumers can easily and safely take the medication in question.

4. Many drugs that are sold OTC are also marketed as _____ drugs.

5. A potential and common side effect of NSAIDs is an increase in _____ _____.

6. Patients may not realize that many of the products they take contain _____, placing them at risk for liver toxicity if they take too much on a daily basis.

7. _____ is an endogenous hormone secreted by the pineal gland that plays a role in regulating circadian rhythms.

8. OTC sleep aids are generally intended to be used for no more than _____ _____.

9. Antacids are generally reserved for _____ _____ relief of heartburn, whereas PPIs and H2 receptor antagonists can be used for _____ _____ with a prescription.

10. Any products containing _____ must be kept behind the pharmacy counter and information about individuals purchasing these products must be logged and maintained.

SHORT ANSWER

Write a short response to each question in the space provided.

1. List three reasons why consumers use OTC products.

    A. _____

    B. _____

    C. _____

2. Give three examples of anti-inflammatory products.

    A. _____

    B. _____

    C. _____

3. Which decongestant does not cause drowsiness? _____

4. Give two examples of sleep aide products

    A. _____

    B. _____

5. Give two classes of drugs used to reduce or relieve gastric acid secretions.

    A. _____

    B. _____

6. Give two examples of special population groups that are at particular risk for receiving an inappropriate medication, the wrong dose, or the wrong drug product.

    A. _____

    B. _____

7. How do sunscreens and sunblocks work?

    A. Sunscreens

    _____

    _____

    B. Sunblocks

    _____

    _____

8. What is the most common OTC product recommended to help dry out pimples? _____

9. Give two examples of OTC products that are kept behind the pharmacy counter.

    A. _____

    B. _____

10. Approximately how many OTC products are marketed today? _____

MATCHING

Matching I

Match the OTC drugs with their indications.

_____ 1. Benadryl

_____ 2. Tylenol

_____ 3. Zantac

_____ 4. Chloraseptic

_____ 5. Unisom

A. Insomnia
B. Allergies
C. Sore throat
D. Pain
E. GERD

Matching II

Match the trade and generic drug names.

_____ 1. Pepcid

_____ 2. Mucinex

_____ 3. Colace

_____ 4. Aleve

_____ 5. Lamisil

A. Docusate sodium
B. Terbinafine
C. Famotidine
D. Naproxen
E. Guaifenesin

RESEARCH ACTIVITIES

Follow the instructions given in each exercise and provide a response.

1. Access the website *www.fda.gov*. In the *Quick Info Links* section, locate *Drugs@FDA* under the *Approvals and Clearances* link; type in OTC.

   A. What legend drugs have been converted to OTC status? List the active ingredient, strength, dosage form, and route for each of the products.

   B. On what date, or the tentative approval date, did the legend drug status change to OTC status for each of the products listed?

2. Access the website *http://www.fda.gov/Safety/MedWatch/default.htm*. What OTC products, if any, are listed in the MedWatch Safety Alerts in the last month? What is the safety concern with those products?

REFLECT CRITICALLY

CRITICAL THINKING

Reply to each question based on what you have learned in the chapter.

1. In a chain store or mass merchandiser outlet, where is the pharmacy located? Why?

2. You have a sore throat, and none of the OTC lozenges are helping. You have been told to gargle with saltwater. How will this help your sore throat?

3. Sometimes people buy an OTC medication because someone they know tried it and it worked for that person. Why should you not base your decision to buy OTC medications on that reasoning?

4. The FDA recently allowed Allegra to become an OTC product. What other drugs do you think should become OTC medications, provided they are safe and effective for patients?

5. What special considerations should be made for those suffering from high blood pressure? Which OTC products would not be recommended for those with this medical condition?

RELATE TO PRACTICE

LAB SCENARIOS

Over-the-Counter (OTC) Medications

Objective: To introduce the pharmacy technician to various over-the-counter medications and their indication(s), warning(s), dosage form(s), and route(s) of administration.

DID YOU KNOW?

- 81% of adults use OTC products as their first response to minor ailments.
- 70% of parents have given their child an OTC product in the middle of the night to help treat a sudden medical symptom.
- 10% of physician office visits could be avoided by treating common ailments with OTC products.
- OTC product availability has created $102 billion in annual health care savings.
- OTC product sales account for 8% of pharmaceutical sales volume.

Lab Activity #27.1: Visit a local pharmacy and familiarize yourself with the OTC section of the store. Complete the following table of OTC products.

Equipment needed:

- Retail pharmacy
- *Drug Facts and Comparison* or *Physician's Desk Reference*
- Pencil/pen

Time needed to complete the exercise: 60 minutes

Brand (Trade) Name	Active Ingredient(s)	Medication Strength	Indication	Warning(s)	Dosage Form(s) Available	Route(s) of Administration	Section Location	Pregnancy Category	Drug Interactions	Available as a Prescription?	What Alternative OTC Products Are Available?
A-200											
Abreva											
Advil											
Afrin											
Alavert											
Aleve											
Allegra											
Anbesol											
Ayr											
Bayer Aspirin											
BC Headache Powder											
Benadryl											
Benefiber											
Betadine											
Bufferin											
Caltrate 600											
Citrucel Powder											
Claritin Reditabs											
Clearasil											
Debrox Drops											
Delsym Extended-Release 12-Hour Cough Suppressant											

Continued

471

Brand (Trade) Name	Active Ingredient(s)	Medication Strength	Indication	Warning(s)	Dosage Form(s) Available	Route(s) of Administration	Section Location	Pregnancy Category	Drug Interactions	Available as a Prescription?	What Alternative OTC Products Are Available?
Dimetapp											
Dimetapp-DM											
Domeboro											
Dulcolax											
Ecotrin											
Excedrin Extra Strength											
Ex-Lax											
Feosol											
FiberCon											
Gas-X											
Gaviscon											
Gly-Oxide											
Gyne-Lotrimin											
Imodium A-D											
Lactaid											
Lamisil											
Lotrimin											
Maalox											
Metamucil											
Mineral Ice											
Monistat 7											
Motrin IB											
Mylanta											
Neosporin											

Brand (Trade) Name	Active Ingredient(s)	Medication Strength	Indication	Warning(s)	Dosage Form(s) Available	Route(s) of Administration	Section Location	Pregnancy Category	Drug Interactions	Available as a Prescription?	What Alternative OTC Products Are Available?
NicoDerm											
Nicorette											
Nizoral A-D											
Nytol											
OsCal											
Pepcid A-C											
Pepto-Bismol											
Phazyme											
Polysporin											
Preparation H											
Prevacid											
Prilosec											
Robitussin											
Rogaine											
Sudafed PE											
Tagamet HB											
TheraFlu											
Tinactin											
Triaminic											
Tums											
Tylenol											
Vicks 44											
Vicks Dayquil											
Vicks Nyquil											

473

Lab Activity #27.2: Using information learned and resources available, determine OTC therapeutic options the pharmacist may choose for each case. (Remember, only the pharmacist is legally allowed to council a customer.)

Equipment needed:

- Retail pharmacy
- *Drug Facts and Comparison*, or *Pocket Guide for Nonprescription Product Therapeutics*
- Pencil/pen

Time needed to complete the exercise: 30 minutes

1. A mother approaches the pharmacy counter stating she would like OTC product recommendations for her 8-year-old child's runny nose. Upon further questioning, she states the nasal discharge is clear and her child's nose itches. She also states that her child sneezes often, sometimes feels tired, and does not have a fever.

    A. What may be wrong with this patient? Why?

    _____

    _____

    B. What OTC products would help for this patient? List the brand name(s) and generic name(s).

    _____

    _____

    _____

    C. Choose one of the products listed. What is the appropriate dose for this patient?

    _____

    _____

    D. What potential side effects may occur from taking this OTC product?

    _____

    _____

    _____

    E. Are there any other warnings or precautions that should be considered when taking this OTC product?

    _____

    _____

    _____

2. A woman approaches the pharmacy counter stating her eyes feel irritated. Upon further questioning, she states that she often feels the need to rub her eyes and that it sometimes feels like there is sandpaper in them. She states that she does not have a history of allergies. You also notice that her eyes do look a little red. She would like to know if an OTC product would help her eyes feel better.

    A. What may be wrong with this patient? Why?

    _____

B. What OTC products would help for this patient? List the brand name(s) and generic name(s).

_____

_____

_____

C. Choose one of the products listed. What is the appropriate dose for this patient?

_____

_____

D. What potential side effects may occur from taking this OTC product?

_____

_____

_____

E. Are there any other warnings or precautions that should be considered when taking this OTC product?

_____

_____

_____

3. A man approaches the pharmacy counter stating he would like an OTC product recommendation for his feet. Upon further questioning, he states that his feet are itchy and sometimes burn. He also states that the symptoms began after he started attending the gym on a daily basis.

A. What may be wrong with this patient? Why?

_____

B. What OTC products would help for this patient? List the brand name(s) and generic name(s).

_____

_____

_____

C. Choose one of the products listed. What is the appropriate dose for this patient?

_____

_____

D. What potential side effects may occur from taking this OTC product?

_____

_____

_____

E. Are there any other warnings or precautions that should be considered when taking this OTC product?

_____

_____

_____

4. A man approaches the pharmacy counter stating his stomach often feels upset after he eats, especially after eating tomatoes and acidic foods. Upon further questioning, he also states that it is sometimes worse if he lies down after eating. He also informs the pharmacy that he does not have a history of a heart condition.

A. What may be wrong with this patient? Why?

_____

B. What OTC products would help for this patient? List the brand name(s) and generic name(s).

_____

_____

_____

C. Choose one of the products listed. What is the appropriate dose for this patient?

_____

_____

D. What potential side effects may occur from taking this OTC product?

_____

_____

_____

E. Are there any other warnings or precautions that should be considered when taking this OTC product?

_____

_____

_____

28 Complementary and Alternative Medicine (CAM)

TERMS AND DEFINITIONS

Select the correct term from the following list and write the corresponding letter in the blank next to the statement.

A. Alternative Medicine
B. Ayurveda
C. Biofeedback
D. Chiropractic Medicine
E. Complementary Medicine
F. Diagnosis
G. Herb
H. Homeopathy
I. Prophylaxis
J. Synthetic Medicine
K. Traditional Chinese Medicine

_____ 1. To prevent disease

_____ 2. A holistic medical system that originated in India

_____ 3. A system of therapy based on the belief that dilutions of medicinal substances that cause a specific symptom can be used to treat an illness that yields the same symptoms

_____ 4. A physician's assessment of the cause of a condition

_____ 5. A range of medical therapies that falls beyond the scope of Western medicine that may be used in a complementary fashion with traditional medicine practices

_____ 6. CAM whole medical system including a range of traditional medicine practices originating in China

_____ 7. Manual manipulation of the joints and muscles

_____ 9. Medication made in a laboratory from synthetic processes

_____ 10. The use of electronic monitoring of an automatic bodily function to train someone to acquire voluntary control of that function

_____ 11. Any plant that is valued for its aromatic, medicinal, flavorful, or other properties

TRUE OR FALSE

Write T or F next to each statement.

_____ 1. Traditional medicine has been in existence for thousands of years, whereas alternative approaches have been practiced for only a few hundred years.

_____ 2. Traditional medicine is the standard for the Western world today.

_____ 3. Probiotics are used as complimentary alternative medicine.

_____ 4. Herbs are considered a form of traditional medication.

_____ 5. Herbal medicines account for some of the first attempts to improve human health.

_____ 6. Many people do not report herbal use to their health care providers.

_____ 7. Biofeedback should be practiced only with a biofeedback instructor present.

_____ 8. The use of daily multivitamins and other such supplementation is generally not considered CAM.

_____ 9. Herbs are natural and therefore are not harmful.

_____ 10. Herbs that are brewed for teas usually are less potent than those prepared in capsule form.

477

MULTIPLE CHOICE

Complete each question by circling the best answer.

1. Traditional medicine includes all of the following *except*:
   A. Physician visits
   B. Prescription drugs
   C. Laboratory tests
   D. Visits to a chiropractor

2. Complementary alternative medicine includes all of the following *except*:
   A. Herbs
   B. X-rays
   C. Acupuncture
   D. Yoga

3. Eastern medicine includes treatments originating from all of the following *except*:
   A. Eastern Asia
   B. India
   C. Eastern United States
   D. Far East countries

4. A reason people may turn to alternative medicines is:
   A. Rising cost of health care
   B. Increasing age of the population
   C. Rising cost of traditional medications
   D. All of the above

5. Which of the following is *not* considered a nondrug treatment?
   A. Massage
   B. Herbs
   C. Meditation
   D. Biofeedback

6. Herbs used in Chinese medicine can:
   A. Cure the body of illness
   B. Prevent future problems
   C. A and B
   D. None of the above

7. Biofeedback has proved effective for all of the following *except*:
   A. Love life
   B. Heart rate
   C. Hypertension
   D. Gastrointestinal activity

8. Chiropractic treatment can include all of the following *except*:
   A. Adjustments of the joints
   B. Heat therapy
   C. Massage
   D. Chemotherapy

9. Homeopathy was first used in the United States in the:
   A. 1700s
   B. 1800s
   C. 1900s
   D. 2000s

10. Homeopathy is also sometimes referred to as:
    A. The placebo effect
    B. Law of opposites
    C. Law of similars
    D. Manipulation therapy

FILL IN THE BLANKS

Answer each question by completing the statement in the space provided.

1. The FDA does not regulate herbs as drugs because they are considered to be _____ _____.

2. _____ believed that consideration of attitude, environmental factors, and natural remedies were all integral components of medical treatment.

3. The use of needles at specific points throughout the body to release energy channels, and bring the body into harmony once again is known as _____.

4. The heart of Chinese medicine is the _____ and _____, which represent _____ and _____ entities.

5. Chiropractic therapy is a(n) _____ approach to treating pain from _____ of the bones and joints.

6. Massage is used for a variety of health-related purposes such as to relieve _____, rehabilitate _____, induce _____, decrease _____, and to reduce _____.

7. Ayurveda is based on the person knowing and understanding the _____ _____.

8. Biofeedback is a way of connecting the _____ to the body.

9. A homeopathic drug must meet standards for strength, quality, purity, and other parameters established in the _____ _____.

MATCHING

Match the following herbs with their treatment targets.

_____ 1. Black cohosh

_____ 2. Chamomile

_____ 3. Cranberry

_____ 4. Milk thistle

_____ 5. Echinacea

_____ 6. Garlic

_____ 7. Ginkgo biloba

_____ 8. Ginseng

_____ 9. Saw palmetto

_____ 10. Soy

_____ 11. St. John's wort

A. Benign prostatic hyperplasia (BPH)
B. Overall wellness
C. Common cold, vaginal candidiasis
D. Depression
E. GI disturbances, skin conditions
F. Vascular dementia, memory
G. Diabetes, nephropathy, hyperlipidemia, menopausal symptoms, osteoporosis
H. Liver health
I. Support hormonal changes
J. Support heart health
K. Urinary tract infections

SHORT ANSWER

Write a short response to each question in the space provided.

1. What are the three main goals of NCCAM?

   A. _____

   B. _____

   C. _____

2. List three prescription medications that can be affected by taking garlic and explain the potential interactions.

   A. _____

   B. _____

   C. _____

3. List three prescription medications that can be affected by taking gingko biloba and explain the potential interactions.

   A. _____

   B. _____

   C. _____

4. List three prescription medications that can be affected by taking ginseng and explain the potential interactions.

   A. _____

   B. _____

   C. _____

5. List three prescription medications that can be affected by taking St. John's wort and explain the potential interactions.

   A. _____

   B. _____

   C. _____

RESEARCH ACTIVITIES

Follow the instructions given in each exercise and provide a response.

1. Access the website *www.rxlist.com*. Under the supplements tab, list the featured supplement.

   Featured supplement: _____

   A. Was this supplement discussed in the chapter?

   B. By what other names is this supplement known?

C. How does the supplement work?

D. What are the safety concerns for this supplement?

E. What are the dosing considerations for this supplement?

2. Access the website *http://nccam.nih.gov/health.*

   A. What resources are available for health care providers?

   B. What resources are available for consumers?

REFLECT CRITICALLY

CRITICAL THINKING

Reply to each question based on what you have learned in the chapter.

1. Alternative medicine has been on the rise the past few years. Many people are not aware that the FDA does not regulate many of the "natural" products being marketed. As a consumer, how can you be sure that these "natural" products really contain the ingredients reported on the labels? As a pharmacy technician, how can you help make consumers aware of "natural" products?

2. Besides the various therapies and herbal products discussed in the chapter, what other forms of alternative medicine are available?

3. Spiritual healing brings another dimension to alternative medicine. Why is it so different from the other forms discussed in the chapter?

4. You are trying to convince your classmates that trying alternative medicine is better than seeing a physician every time you feel ill. How would you make your case for this form of therapy?

RELATE TO PRACTICE

LAB SCENARIOS

Complementary Alternative Medicine

Objective: To introduce the pharmacy technician to complementary alternative medicine and its usage in the prevention and treatment of illness.

DID YOU KNOW?

Complementary and alternative medicine (CAM) is defined as a "medical products and practices that are not part of standard care." Conventional medicine is medicine practiced by holders of M.D. and O.D. degrees and by all allied health professionals. Complementary and alternative medicine is gaining in popularity in the United States. As a member of the allied health team, pharmacy technicians need to be familiar with complementary and alternative medicine because of the changing demographics of our society.

Lab Activity #28.1: Using the National Center for Complementary and Alternative Medicine website (*www.nccam.nih. gov*) or resources available, complete the following table of herbal products.

Equipment needed:

- Computer with Internet access
- Paper
- *PDR for Herbal Medicines*
- Pencil/pen

Time needed to complete this activity: 60 minutes

Herbal Product	Common Name(s)	Latin Name	Indication	Therapeutic Category	Approved Use	Unapproved Use	Dosage Forms Available	List Two Side Effects	Drug Interactions
Alfalfa									
Aloe vera									
Astragalus									
Basil									
Belladonna									
Bilberry									
Bitter orange									
Black cohosh									
Brewer's yeast									

Herbal Product	Common Name(s)	Latin Name	Indication	Therapeutic Category	Approved Use	Unapproved Use	Dosage Forms Available	List Two Side Effects	Drug Interactions
Cat's claw									
Cayenne									
Chamomile									
Chaste tree									
Cinnamon									
Cranberry									
Dandelion									
Echinacea									
Ephedra									
Eucalyptus									
European elder									
Evening primrose									
Fenugreek									
Feverfew									
Flaxseed									
Garlic									
Ginger									
Ginkgo									
Ginseng									
Green tea									
Hawthorn									
Hoodia									
Horse chestnut									
Ipecac									
Kava									
Kelp									
Lavender									
Licorice root									
Melatonin									
Milk thistle									
Mistletoe									
Noni									
Oats									
Peppermint Oil									
Psyllium									

Continued

483

Herbal Product	Common Name(s)	Latin Name	Indication	Therapeutic Category	Approved Use	Unapproved Use	Dosage Forms Available	List Two Side Effects	Drug Interactions
Quinine									
Red clover									
Rosemary									
Sage									
Saw palmetto									
Senna									
Soybean									
St. John's wort									
Thunder god vine									
Turmeric									
Valerian									
Yew									
Yohimbe									

Lab Activity #28.2: Using the National Center for Complementary and Alternative Medicine website (*www.nccam.nih.gov*), answer the following questions on complementary and alternative treatments.

Equipment needed:

- Computer with Internet access
- Paper
- Pencil/pen

Time needed to complete this activity: 60 minutes

1. Acupuncture

   A. Where did acupuncture originate?

   _____

   B. Approximately how many people in the United States receive acupuncture each year?

   _____

   C. Who regulates the needles used in acupuncture?

   _____

   D. Does an acupuncture practitioner require a license to practice in the United States?

   _____

   E. Would you consider acupuncture as a therapy? Why or why not?

   _____

   _____

   _____

2. Aromatherapy

    A. What are two examples of essential oils that may be used in aromatherapy?

    _____

    _____

    B. What is one theory of how aromatherapy works in the treatment of symptoms and side effects of cancer therapy?

    _____

    _____

    _____

    C. What are two routes of administration for essential oils?

    _____

    D. What is one side effect that may be experienced by an individual undergoing aromatherapy?

    _____

    E. Would you consider aromatherapy as a therapy? Why or why not?

    _____

    _____

    _____

3. Ayurvedic medicine

    A. Where did Ayurvedic medication originate?

    _____

    B. What does the term *Ayurveda* mean?

    _____

    C. What are the three key concepts of Ayurvedic medicine?

    _____

    _____

    _____

    D. How many Americans use Ayurvedic medicine each year?

    _____

    E. What is a dosha?

    _____

    _____

    F. What do the three dosha represent?

    _____

    _____

    _____

485

G. What are four treatment practices used in Ayurvedic medicine?

_____

_____

H. What are two concerns regarding Ayurvedic medications?

_____

_____

I. Would you use Ayurvedic medicine? Why or why not?

_____

_____

_____

4. Chiropractic

A. On what area of the body does chiropractic practice focus?

_____

_____

B. What does the term chiropractic mean?

_____

C. What percentage of American adults have used chiropractic alignments within the past year?

_____

D. What requirements must an individual possess to practice as a chiropractor?

_____

_____

_____

E. Who regulates the chiropractic practice?

_____

_____

F. Would you use a chiropractor to treat a condition? Why or why not?

_____

_____

_____

5. Massage therapy

A. What is massage therapy?

_____

_____

B. How many Americans receive a massage each year?

_____

C. What conditions may be treated by using massage therapy?

_____

_____

D. What licenses or certifications may a massage therapist possess?

_____

_____

_____

_____

E. Would you use massage therapy to treat a condition? Why or why not?

_____

_____

_____

6. Meditation

A. Why might a patient use meditation as a form of treatment?

_____

_____

B. What are the four meditation techniques?

_____

_____

_____

_____

C. What are the four elements of meditation?

_____

_____

_____

_____

D. How many Americans have meditated within the past year?

_____

E. Where does Mindfulness originate?

_____

F. Where does Transcendental Meditation originate?

_____

G. What is hypothesized as the mechanism of action for meditation?

_____

_____

_____

H. Do you meditate? If yes, how has it helped you?

_____

_____

_____

7. Naturopathy

A. Where did naturopathy originate?

_____

B. How many Americans participate in naturopathy?

_____

C. What are the six principles of naturopathy?

_____

_____

_____

_____

_____

D. What type of education does a naturopathic physician require?

_____

E. How many states have licensing requirements for naturopathic physicians?

_____

F. What methods of treatment does a naturopathic physician use?

_____

_____

_____

G. Would you use a naturopathic physician? Why or why not?

_____

_____

_____

_____

8. Reiki

    A. Where did Reiki originate?

    _____

    B. What is the belief behind Reiki?

    _____

    _____

    C. How many Americans use Reiki?

    _____

    D. Is training required for Reiki?

    _____

    E. Would you use Reiki? Why or why not?

    _____

    _____

    _____

    _____

9. Tai Chi

    A. Where did Tai Chi originate?

    _____

    B. What does Tai Chi mean?

    _____

    C. What Chinese concepts does Tai Chi use?

    _____

    _____

    D. How many Americans use Tai Chi?

    _____

    E. Why do individuals practice Tai Chi?

    _____

    _____

    _____

    _____

    F. Would you use Tai Chi as a form of treatment? Why or why not?

    _____

    _____

    _____

    _____

10. Yoga

    A. Where did yoga originate?

    _____

    B. What techniques are used in yoga?

    _____

    _____

    C. What percentage of adults in the United States practice yoga?

    _____

    D. What is Iyengar yoga?

    _____

    _____

    E. What is Ashtanga yoga?

    _____

    _____

    F. What is Vini yoga?

    _____

    _____

    G. What is Kundalini yoga?

    _____

    _____

    H. What is Bikram yoga?

    _____

    _____

    I. Would you use yoga as a form of therapy? Why or why not?

    _____

    _____

    _____